PHARMACOLOGY RECALL, 2E

RECALL SERIES EDITOR

LORNE H. BLACKBOURNE, MD
Trauma, Burn, and Critical Care Surgeon
San Antonio, Texas

PHARMACOLOGY RECALL
2nd Edition

EDITOR
ANAND RAMACHANDRAN, MD
Comprehensive Ophthalmologist
Columbus, Ohio

Wolters Kluwer | Lippincott Williams & Wilkins
Health

Philadelphia · Baltimore · New York · London
Buenos Aires · Hong Kong · Sydney · Tokyo

Acquisitions Editor: Donna M. Balado
Managing Editor: Cheryl W. Stringfellow
Marketing Manager: Emilie Linkins
Production Editor: Paula C. Williams
Designer: Terrry Mallon
Compositor: Nesbitt Graphics, Inc.
Printer: R.R. Donnelley

Copyright © 2007 Lippincott Williams & Wilkins

351 West Camden Street
Baltimore, MD 21201

530 Walnut Street
Philadelphia, PA 19106

Printed in China

First Edition, 2000

Library of Congress Cataloging-in-Publication Data

Pharmacology recall / editor, Anand Ramachandran.—2nd ed.

   p. ; cm.—(Recall)

 Includes index.

 ISBN 0-7817-5562-X (alk. paper)

1. Pharmacology—Outlines, syllabi, etc. I. Ramachandran, Anand. II. Series: Recall series.

 [DNLM: 1. Pharmacology—Examination Questions. 2. Drug Therapy—Examination Questions. QV 18.2 P5355 2006]

 RM301.14.P473 2006

 615'.1076—dc22

2006035064

The publishers have made every effort to trace the copyright holders for borrowed material. If they have inadvertently overlooked any, they will be pleased to make the necessary arrangements at the first opportunity.

To purchase additional copies of this book, call our customer service department at **(800) 638-3030** or fax orders to **(301) 223-2320**. International customers should call **(301) 223-2300**.

Visit Lippincott Williams & Wilkins on the Internet: http://www.LWW.com.
Lippincott Williams & Wilkins customer service representatives are available from 8:30 am to 6:00 pm, EST.

10 11 12 13
4 5 6 7 8 9 10

RRS1006

Dedication

For my parents and my wife, Sandhya, whose love and support make anything possible.

Anand Ramachandran

Preface

Pharmacology Recall was written with the busy health science student and house officer in mind. The fundamental principle behind the design of *Pharmacology Recall* is that in order to learn printed material, two essential events must occur: (1) the text must be read and (2) the information must be memorized and added to a framework of knowledge already acquired. *Pharmacology Recall* offers its readers a distinct advantage in that it *minimizes the time spent reading and identifying important material* and *maximizes the time available for actual learning.* As with the other titles in the Lippincott Williams & Wilkins *Recall* series, *Pharmacology Recall* accomplishes this with a concise two-column question-and-answer format to facilitate quick learning.

By using the bookmark provided to cover the answers on the right-hand side of the page, revealing them only after attempting to answer the questions, you can easily identify weak points. With the second reading, you can focus only on those questions answered incorrectly the first time and not waste time rereading information you have already learned. This, in essence, is the *Recall* advantage.

As an additional aid, *Pharmacology Recall* includes a **Pharmacology Power Review** (Chapter 53). This chapter provides a unique birds-eye view of the subject and can be used to review large amounts of high-yield information quickly, before medical school and USMLE examinations. Also, mnemonics appear throughout the book to facilitate memorization; the mnemonic icon is illustrated at the end of this preface. Common board questions are indicated by a pencil symbol (✎). Illustrations are provided to clarify important concepts.

Pharmacology Recall is the end result of professors, residents, and students working cooperatively to produce a complete yet concise text. We anticipate that you will find it an extremely useful tool while learning the discipline of pharmacology.

Comments and suggestions are always encouraged. If your ideas are used, they will be acknowledged in future revisions. Please send them to me via the publisher, Lippincott Williams & Wilkins, at the web site LWW.com/medstudent.

Anand Ramachandran, MD

Disclaimer
This book is intended to be a study guide for the acquisition of basic pharmacologic facts and should not be used to guide patient care.

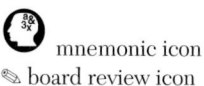 mnemonic icon
✎ board review icon

Preface

CONTRIBUTORS

Sumathi Balaraman, MD
Michael Bess, MD
Angela Chandler, MD
Mark Dellinger, MD
Erin Donahen, MD
John Hagopian, MD
Sara Hirschfeld, MD
Johanna Jensen, MD
Steve Lee, MD
Markus Leong, MD
Jimmy Lyions (Medical Student)
Joseph Mack, MD
Jaishree Manohar (Medical Student)
Csaba Mihaly, MD
Uma Murthi, RPH

Tann Nichols (Medical Student, 3rd year)
Mitesh K. Patel, MD
Nikesh K. Patel, MD
Arun Raghupathy, MD
Vimala Ramachandran, MD
Doug Reader, MD
John A. Scherschel (Medical Student, 3rd year)
Maralyn Seavolt, MD
Samir Shah, MD
Mark Szewczyk, RPH
Randy Vanvooris, MD
John Vaughn, MD
Michael Weinstock, MD

FACULTY REVIEWERS FROM THE FIRST EDITION

Miriam Chan, PharmD
Riverside Methodist Hospitals
Columbus, Ohio

Richard Fertel, PhD
Professor of Pharmacology
Ohio State University Medical School
Columbus, Ohio

Daniel A. Koechel, PhD
Professor of Pharmacology
Medical College of Ohio
Toledo, Ohio

Benedict R. Lucchesi, PhD, MD
Professor of Pharmacology
University of Michigan Medical School
Ann Arbor, Michigan

Kathy Morman, PharmD
Riverside Methodist Hospital
Columbus, Ohio

Ronald Mellgren, PhD
Professor of Pharmacology
Medical College of Ohio
Toledo, Ohio

Keith Schendler, PhD
Professor of Pharmacology
Medical College of Ohio
Toledo, Ohio

Angela Swerlein, PharmD
Riverside Methodist Hospitals
Columbus, Ohio

Acknowledgments

I would like to extend thanks to the staff at Lippincott Williams & Wilkins for their enthusiastic assistance. I am also grateful to the many students who have provided feedback via email or through websites. Their comments have been invaluable in perfecting the text.

Contents

Section I:
PRINCIPLES OF PHARMACOLOGY

Section II:
AUTONOMIC NERVOUS SYSTEM

Section III:
CENTRAL NERVOUS SYSTEM

Section IV:
CARDIOVASCULAR SYSTEM

Section V:
RESPIRATORY SYSTEM

Section VI:
ENDOCRINE SYSTEM

Section VII:
MUSCULOSKELETAL SYSTEM

Section VIII:
GASTROINTESTINAL SYSTEM

Section IX:
IMMUNE SYSTEM

Section X:
ANTIMICROBIAL DRUGS

Section XI:
TOXICOLOGY

APPENDICES

Section I

Principles of
Pharmacology

1

Introduction to Pharmacology

What is pharmacology?

The study of the interaction between chemicals and living systems

What is a drug?

A drug is broadly defined as any chemical agent that affects biological systems.

Name and define the four major subdivisions of pharmacology.

1. **Pharmacokinetics**—describes "what the body does to the drug." This includes topics such as the absorption, distribution, metabolism, and excretion of drugs.
2. **Pharmacodynamics**—describes "what the drug does to the body." Specifically, it deals with the biochemical and physiological effects of drugs and their mechanisms of action.
3. **Pharmacotherapeutics**—describes the use of drugs for the prevention, diagnosis, and treatment of disease.
4. **Toxicology**—describes the undesirable effects of therapeutic agents, poisons, and pollutants on biological systems.

For each of the following endings, name the classification of drug and give an example:

    -azine

phenothiazine-like antipsychotics (e.g., **chlorpromazine**)

    -ane

volatile general anesthetics (e.g., **halothane**)

    -azepam

antianxiety drugs (e.g., **diazepam**)

-bital	barbiturate sedative hypnotic drugs (e.g., **phenobarbital**)
-caine	local anesthetics (e.g., **cocaine**)
-cillin	penicillins (e.g., **nafcillin**)
-cycline	tetracycline-type antibiotics (e.g., **doxycycline**)
-olol	β-blockers (e.g., **propranolol**)
-opril	ACE inhibitors (e.g., **captopril**)
-statin	HMG-CoA reductase inhibitors (e.g., **lovastatin**)
-zosin	postsynaptic α-receptor blockers (e.g., **terazosin**)

Should trade names be memorized for the boards?

✎ In the past the boards have not tested trade names. It is best to first learn the generic name. Trade names have been provided only for future reference.

Do I need to know every characteristic of every drug?

No. However, it is absolutely critical that you at least remember the classification, mechanism of action, therapeutic use, and life-threatening or unique adverse effects of all the major drugs.

How is a drug developed?

The creation of a safe and effective drug involves numerous steps. Once a drug is synthesized, it must undergo animal testing. After animal testing and prior to human testing, the manufacturer must submit an Investigational New Drug Exemption (IND) application.

Describe the four phases of human clinical testing.

Phase I: The proposed drug's pharmacokinetics is studied in a relatively small number of *normal* human volunteers. Acute effects of the drug, from negligible to mildly toxic, are monitored over a wide range of doses.

Phase II: The drug is evaluated in moderate number of patients with the target disease. Also, a placebo drug is included in a single- or double-blinded design. The goal is to see whether the drug works in the affected patients at a nontoxic level.

Phase III: Similar to phase II except on a much larger scale. The drug is now used in centers across the country in a manner very similar to its final intended use. A control drug is also used in this phase. Once this stage is completed, a New Drug Application (NDA) is submitted to the FDA for approval.

Phase IV: This stage occurs after the drug hits the market. Toxicities are monitored and long-term effects determined (Figure 1–1).

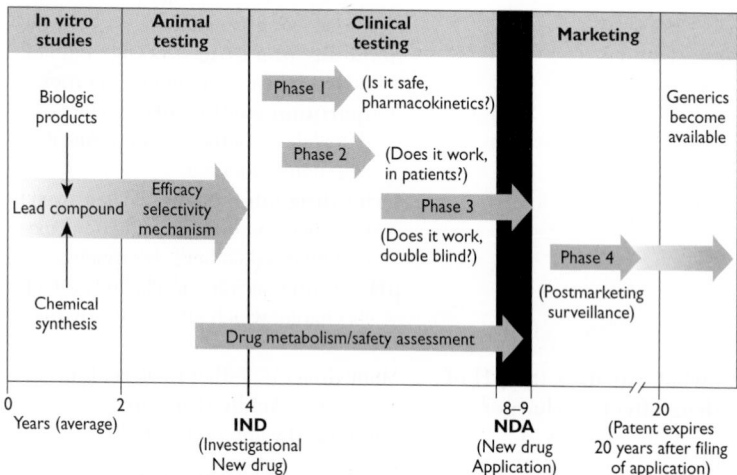

Figure I–I. The development and testing process required to bring a drug to market in the United States. Some of the requirements may be different for drugs used in life-threatening diseases. (Adapted with permission from Katzung BG. *Basic & Clinical Pharmacology,* 9th ed. New York: McGraw-Hill, 2004, p. 65.)

2   Pharmacokinetics

Define pharmacokinetics.

Pharmacokinetics comprises **actions of the body on drugs**, including the principles of drug **absorption, distribution**, **biotransformation (metabolism)**, and **excretion**.

ABSORPTION

Define absorption.

Absorption is the rate at and extent to which a drug moves from its site of administration.

What does the rate and efficacy of absorption depend on?

Route of administration—The intravenous route is most effective.

Blood flow—Highly vascularized organs such as the small intestine have the greatest absorbing ability.

Surface area available—Absorption of a drug is directly proportional to the surface area available.

Solubility of a drug—A drug's ratio of hydrophilic to lipophilic properties **(partition coefficient)** will determine whether it can permeate cell membranes.

Drug–drug interactions—When given in combination, drugs can either enhance or inhibit each other's absorption.

pH—A drug's acidity or alkalinity affects its charge, which affects absorption.

In what way does the pH of a drug affect its charge?

Many drugs are either weak acids or weak bases. **Acidic drugs are uncharged** when protonated:

$$HA \rightleftarrows H^+ + A^-$$

Basic drugs are charged when protonated:

$$BH^+ \rightleftarrows B + H^+$$

How does charge affect a drug's ability to permeate a cell membrane?

Generally, a drug will pass through cell membranes more easily if it is uncharged. Therefore the amount of drug absorbed depends on its ratio of charged to uncharged species, which is determined by the ambient pH and the pK_a (negative log of dissociation constant) of the drug. (Figure 2–1).

Define bioavailability.

The fraction of administered drug that gains access to its site of action or a biological fluid that allows access to the site of action.

What is the bioavailability of an intravenously injected drug?

100%—because all of the drug enters the systemic circulation.

What is the bioavailability of any drug that is not intravascularly injected?

Less than 100%—because some of the drug will not be absorbed, or it may become inactivated.

What factors affect bioavailability?

1. First-pass metabolism.

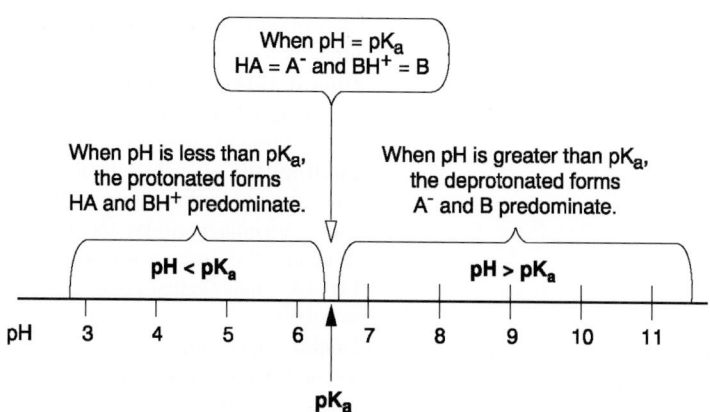

Figure 2–1. The distribution of a drug between its ionized and un-ionized forms depends on the ambient pH and pK_a of the drug. For illustrative purposes, the drug has been assigned a pK_a of 6.5. (Redrawn with permission from Howland RD, Mycek MJ [Harvey RA, Champe PC, eds.]. *Lippincott's Illustrated Reviews: Pharmacology,* 3rd ed. Baltimore: Lippincott Williams & Wilkins, 2006, p. 6.)

2. All of the factors that affect absorption (i.e., pH, blood flow, drug solubility, drug-drug interactions, route of administration).

What is first-pass metabolism?

Biotransformation that occurs before the drug reaches its site of action. It most commonly occurs in the liver. (For example, orally administered **nitroglycerin** is said to have a high first-pass metabolism because 90% of it is inactivated by the liver. **Morphine** is another important drug that has a high first-pass metabolism.)

What are the major routes of drug administration?

Alimentary
Parenteral
Inhalation
Topical
Transdermal
Subcutaneous

Name the four types of alimentary routes of administration and state the advantage of each.

1. **Oral**—commonest route. *Advantages* include convenience/patient compliance and the utilization of the small intestine, which is specialized for absorption because of its large surface area.
2. **Buccal** (between gum and cheeks). *Advantage:* Allows direct absorption into the venous circulation.
3. **Sublingual** (under the tongue)— Nitroglycerin is often given by this route. *Advantage:* Allows the drug to drain into the superior vena cava, thus bypassing hepatic first-pass metabolism.
4. **Rectal** (suppository)—Useful when the oral route is unavailable due to vomiting or loss of consciousness. *Advantage:* Approximately 50% of drug absorbed from the rectum will bypass the liver.

Name the four parenteral routes of administration and state the advantage of each.

1. **Intravenous**—direct injection into the vascular system. *Advantage:* Most rapid and potent mode of administration, because 100% of drug enters the circulation.
2. **Intramuscular**—*Advantages:* Usually more rapid and complete absorption than with oral administration. Minimizes hazards of intravascular injection.
3. **Subcutaneous**—*Advantages:* Same as intramuscular.
4. **Intrathecal**—*Advantage:* In cases of acute CNS infections or spinal anesthesia, drugs can be more effective if injected directly into the spinal subarachnoid space.

What category of drugs is commonly administered by inhalation?

Pulmonary agents

How are inhaled drugs administered?

By machine aerosolization or vaporization

When is topical administration used?

Usually for treatment of localized disease (e.g., psoriasis, acne, eye infections)

When is transdermal administration used?

For sustained release of a drug—for example, **nicotine** patches

DISTRIBUTION

What is distribution?

The process by which a drug leaves the bloodstream and enters the interstitium or the cells of the tissues

By what three biochemical mechanisms are drugs absorbed into cells?

1. **Passive diffusion**—governed by a concentration gradient across a membrane, which makes a drug move from an area of high concentration to one of low concentration. It is the **most common** mode of drug transport.

2. **Transport by special carrier proteins**—a form of passive diffusion that is facilitated by a carrier protein.
3. **Active transport**—transport against a concentration gradient. The energy for this mechanism comes from dephosphorylation of adenosine triphosphate.

What does distribution depend on?

Blood flow

Capillary permeability—The structure of capillaries varies depending on the organ. For example, in the brain, the junction between cells is very tight. In the liver and spleen, the junction between endothelial cells is wide, which allows large molecules to pass through.

Binding to plasma proteins such as albumin—This will limit access to cellular compartments.

Drug structure—Small lipophilic molecules will be able to distribute across cell membranes more easily than will large polar molecules.

BIOTRANSFORMATION

Why does the body biotransform drugs?

The lipophilic properties of drugs that allow them to pass through cell membranes hinder their elimination. Therefore drugs are modified to become more polar, so that elimination can occur more quickly. In some cases, however, drugs are *activated* from their prodrug state through biotransformation.

What are the two general sets of modifications that occur in biotransformation?

They are known as phase I and phase II reactions.

What happens in a phase I reaction?

Lipophilic molecules are converted into more polar molecules by the introduction (or unmasking) of a polar functional group.

What types of phase I reactions occur?

Oxidation, reduction (dehydrogenation), and hydrolysis

What happens in phase II conjugation reactions?

Formation of a covalent linkage between functional groups on the parent drug and another substrate

Specifically, what substrates are added in phase II conjugation reactions?

Glucuronate—Quantitatively, addition of this substrate constitutes the most important conjugation reaction.
Acetic acid
Glutathione
Sulfate

In what organ do phase I and phase II reactions occur?

Primarily in the liver

Where do these reactions occur on a cellular level?

Phase I reactions occur predominantly in the cytochrome P-450 system.
Phase II reactions occur in the cytosol.

Do phase II reactions always follow phase I reactions?

No. In a few cases a drug will undergo a phase II reaction first. In general, however, phase I precedes phase II; once a drug completes phase II, it is usually inactive.

What factors affect drug biotransformation?

Genetic differences—The capacity to metabolize a drug through a given pathway varies in each individual. (For example, some individuals are slow acetylators and therefore cannot rapidly inactivate drugs such as **isoniazid**, **procainamide**, and **hydralazine**.)
Induction of the cytochrome P-450 system—may increase biotransformation
Inhibition of the cytochrome P-450 system—if two drugs or compounds are competing for the active site of the same enzyme, then one of the drugs will have a decreased rate of transformation.

Disease—especially of the liver.

Age and gender—neonates, for example, are deficient in conjugating enzymes.

Are the rates for drug biotransformation predictable?

Yes. In general, drugs will be inactivated or biotransformed according to one of two general chemistry principles: first-order and zero-order kinetics.

What is first-order kinetics?

A process whereby a constant **percentage** of substrate is metabolized per unit of time. (For example, if 10% of a certain drug [concentration, 100 mg/dL] is eliminated every 2 hr, the concentration will be 90 mg/dL 2 hr later; in 4 hr, it will be 81 mg/dL; and so on.) The higher the concentration of drug, the greater the absolute amount of drug biotransformed or excreted per unit of time.

What is zero-order kinetics?

The process by which a constant **amount** of drug is metabolized per unit of time regardless of the drug concentration. (For example, if a drug concentration is 100 mg/dL and the body can remove 5 mg/dL every hour, then 1 hr later the concentration will be 95 mg/dL; 2 hr later, it will be 90 mg/dL; and so on.) **Ethanol**, **phenytoin**, and **aspirin** are all important drugs that are metabolized according to zero-order kinetics.

EXCRETION

What is excretion?

The process by which a drug or metabolite is removed from the body.

What is the difference between excretion and secretion?

Excretion is the removal of a drug from the body.

Secretion occurs when the drug is actively transported from one compartment into another. (For example, drugs are *secreted* into the renal tubule from the medullary capillaries.)

What are the major routes of excretion?

Renal—urine is one of the most common routes of elimination for hydrophilic compounds. Acidification of the urine can enhance excretion of weak bases, while alkalinization promotes excretion of weak acids.

Fecal

Respiration—primarily for anesthetic gases and vapors.

Breast milk

Skin

3   Pharmacodynamics

What is pharmacodynamics?

Pharmacodynamics describes the actions of a drug on the body and includes the principles of receptor interactions, mechanisms of therapeutic and toxic action, and dose-response relationships.

How is pharmacodynamics related to pharmacokinetics?

The pharmacokinetic processes of absorption, distribution, biotransformation, and excretion determine how quickly and to what extent a drug will appear at a target site. The concepts of pharmacodynamics explain the pharmacological effects of drugs and their mechanism of action (Figure 3-1).

RECEPTOR INTERACTIONS

What is a receptor?

A receptor is a macromolecule typically made of proteins that interacts with either an endogenous ligand or a drug to mediate a pharmacological or physiological effect.

What are the two main functions of receptors?

1. Ligand binding
2. Activation of an effector system (message propagation)

What is an effector?

Effectors transduce drug-receptor interactions into cellular effects. There are four types of well-known effector mechanisms:
1. **Transmembrane**—Some ligands, such as **insulin**, bind to receptors that have both an extracellular and intracellular component. Binding of the extracellular component stimulates the intracellular component, which is

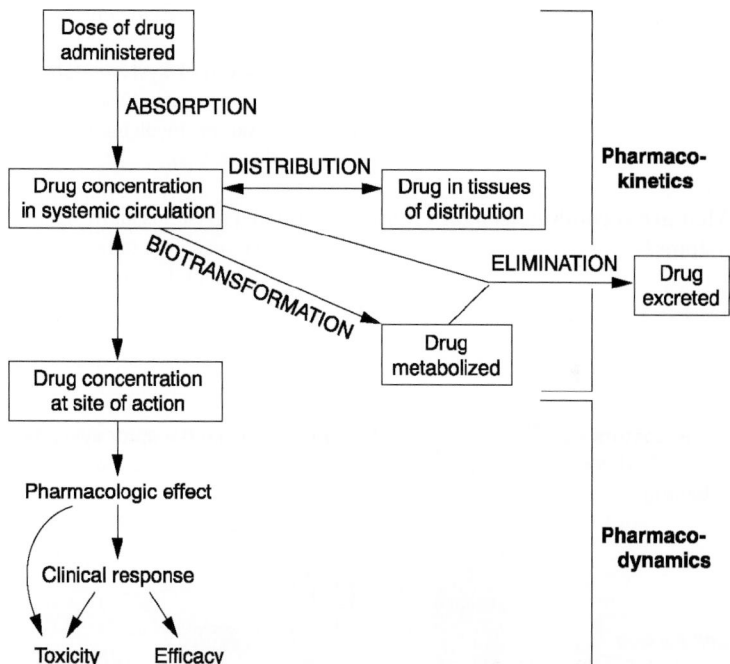

Figure 3–1. The relationship between dose and effect can be separated into pharmacokinetic (dose-concentration) and pharmacodynamic (concentration-effect) components. Concentration provides the link between pharmacokinetics and pharmacodynamics and is the focus of the "target concentration" approach to rational dosing. The three primary processes of pharmacokinetics are absorption, distribution, and elimination. (Redrawn with permission from Katzung BG. *Basic and Clinical Pharmacology,* 7th ed. Stamford, CT: Appleton & Lange, 1998, p. 35.)

coupled to an enzyme—for example, tyrosine kinase.
2. **Ligand-gated ion channels**—Drugs bind to these receptors, which then alter the conductance of ions through the cell membrane channels. Examples of ligand-gated ion channel drugs are **benzodiazepines** and **acetylcholine**.
3. **Intracellular**—Thyroid and steroid hormones bind to nuclear receptors to form complexes that interact with

DNA, causing changes in gene expression.

4. **Second-messenger system**—Drugs bind to receptors that activate second-messenger systems involving G proteins (Figure 3-2).

What are second-messenger systems?

Second-messenger systems allow signals from cell surface receptors to be converted and amplified into a cellular response.

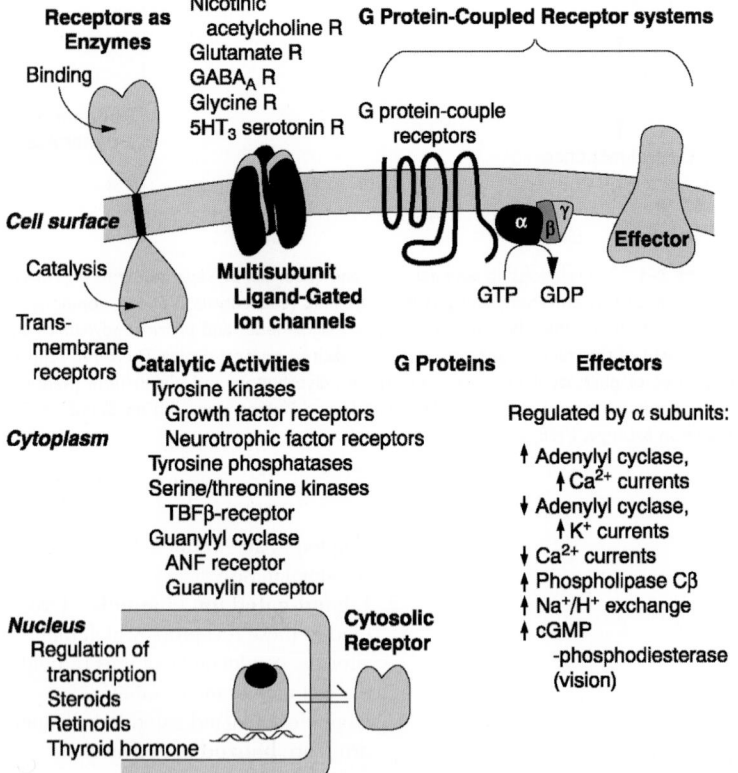

Figure 3–2. Classification of physiological receptors and their relationships to signaling pathways. (Redrawn with permission from Hardman JG, Limbird LE [eds.]. *Goodman and Gilman's The Pharmacological Basis of Therapeutics,* 9th ed. New York: McGraw-Hill, 1996, p. 32.)

What are the three best-known second-messenger systems, and which enzyme produces each?	1. Cyclic adenosine monophosphate (cAMP)—produced by adenylate cyclase
	2. Cyclic guanosine monophosphate (cGMP)—produced by guanylate cyclase
	3. Inositol triphosphate (IP_3)—produced by phospholipase C

MECHANISMS OF THERAPEUTIC AND TOXIC ACTION

What is an agonist?	A drug that binds to and activates receptors
What is a full agonist?	A drug that, when bound to a receptor, produces 100% of the maximum possible biological response
What are partial agonists?	Drugs that produce less than 100% of the maximum possible biological response no matter how high their concentration
What are antagonists?	Drugs that bind to receptors or other drugs and *inhibit* a biological response
What does a competitive antagonist do?	It binds *reversibly* to the same active site of an enzyme as an agonist.
How can a competitive antagonist be overcome?	By increasing the concentration of the drug (agonist). The maximum efficacy of the drug will not change in the presence of a competitive antagonist.
What does a noncompetitive antagonist do?	It binds irreversibly to a different site on the enzyme than the antagonist. Noncompetitive agonists *cannot* be overcome by increasing concentrations of the drug.
How will the maximum efficacy of a drug be affected by such noncompetitive antagonists?	Maximum efficacy will be *reduced* in the presence of a noncompetitive antagonist (Figure 3-3).

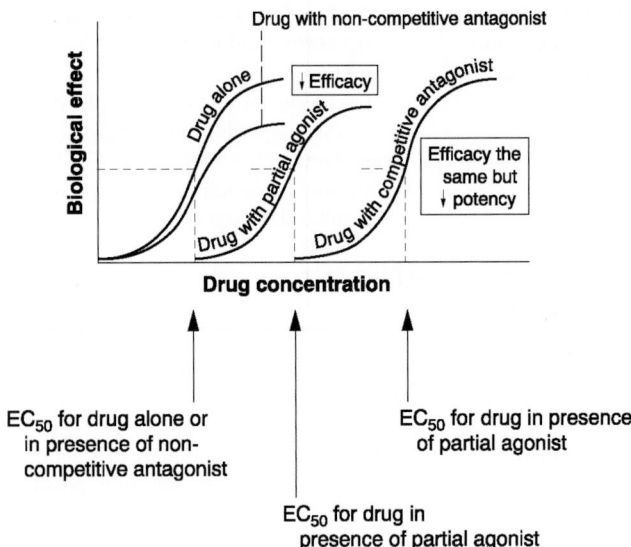

Figure 3–3. Effects of drug antagonists and partial agonist. EC_{50} = drug dose that shows 50% of maximal response. (Redrawn with permission from Mycek MJ, Harvey RA, Champe PC [Harvey RA, Champe PC, eds.]. *Lippincott's Illustrated Reviews: Pharmacology,* 2nd ed. Philadelphia, Lippincott-Raven Publishers, 1997, p. 22.)

DOSE-RESPONSE RELATIONSHIPS

What is the difference between efficacy and potency?	Efficacy is the ability to produce a biological effect. Potency is related to the amount of drug necessary to cause a biological effect.
Give an example of efficacy.	If two drugs, A and B, are both claimed to reduce a patient's heart rate by 25%, they both have the same efficacy.
Give an example of potency.	Only 1 mg of drug A needs to be given to achieve a reduction in heart rate, whereas 10 mg of drug B is needed. Therefore it can be inferred that drug A is more potent.

What is K_d?

The concentration of drug yielding 50% occupancy of its corresponding receptor (dissociation constant)

What is EC_{50}?

The drug concentration that produces 50% of the maximum possible response in a graded dose-response curve (see Figure 3-3).

4

Drug Dosing and Prescription Writing

DRUG DOSING

What three factors are involved in determining an appropriate drug dose for a patient?

1. Type of infection or disease
2. Patient variables (e.g., weight, liver or kidney disease)
3. *Plasma concentration* needed to achieve efficacy

What are the two major water compartments in the body?

Intracellular and extracellular. The extracellular compartment is further subdivided into the plasma (vascular) compartment and the interstitium (Figure 4-1).

What is volume of distribution (V_d)?

The ratio of the amount of drug in the body to the plasma concentration

How is V_d calculated?

V_d = total drug in the body ÷ plasma concentration of the drug. Realize that this number is calculated; it does not have a physical equivalent. That is why it is known as the *apparent* volume of distribution. For example, some drugs, such as **quinacrine**, can have a V_d of 50,000 L. The actual volume of the human body, however, is much less.

What is the significance of a large V_d?

Based on the equation presented above, a large V_d signifies that most of the drug is being sequestered in some tissue or compartment. Therefore the drug is not being eliminated and its half-life is extended.

What is the significance of a small V_d?

If a drug has a small V_d, a large amount of the drug is bound to plasma proteins

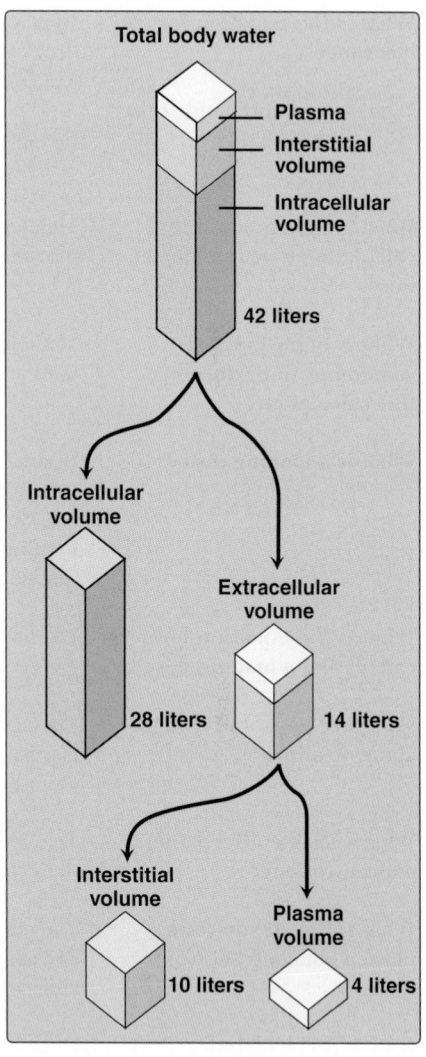

Figure 4–1. Relative size of various distribution volumes within a 70-kg individual. (Reproduced with permission from Howland RD, Mycek MJ [Harvey RA, Champe PC, eds.]. *Lippincott's Illustrated Reviews: Pharmacology,* 3rd ed. Baltimore, Lippincott Williams & Wilkins, 2006, p. 9.)

(i.e., albumin) and only a small fraction of the drug has diffused outside of the vascular compartment.

What is clearance?

Clearance is defined as the volume of plasma cleared of drug per unit of time.

What is the equation for clearance?

(Rate of elimination of drug)/(plasma drug concentration)

What is a maintenance dose?

A dose of a drug given to achieve a therapeutic plasma concentration over an extended period of time

What is the equation for calculating a maintenance dose?

Maintenance dose = clearance × desired plasma concentration = bioavailability

What is important to remember in performing this calculation?

You must be absolutely certain that the units are correct.

What is a loading dose?

In some clinical situations, the desired plasma concentration of a drug must be achieved rapidly. In these cases a single **loading dose** is injected, followed by a routine maintenance dose.

What is the equation for calculating a loading dose?

Loading dose = V_d × desired plasma concentration / bioavailability

What are peak and trough concentrations?

These are maximum and minimum plasma concentrations, respectively, observed during dosing intervals.

What variable affects these concentrations?

They will fluctuate around the steady-state plasma concentration (C_{ss}).

What is the steady-state plasma concentration?

The point at which the rate of drug availability is equal to the rate of drug elimination

How is it calculated?

Dosage = plasma level × clearance

How does frequency of dosing affect the steady-state concentration?

It will not change.

What factors will dosing frequency affect?

Using smaller doses more frequently will help minimize swings in drug concentration (i.e., maximum and minimum plasma concentrations) (Figure 4-2).

What is a half-life?

The half-life is the amount of time required for the drug concentration in the body to change by one-half. It is derived from volume of distribution and clearance.

How is a drug's half-life calculated?

$T_{1/2} = 0.693 \times V_d/CL$

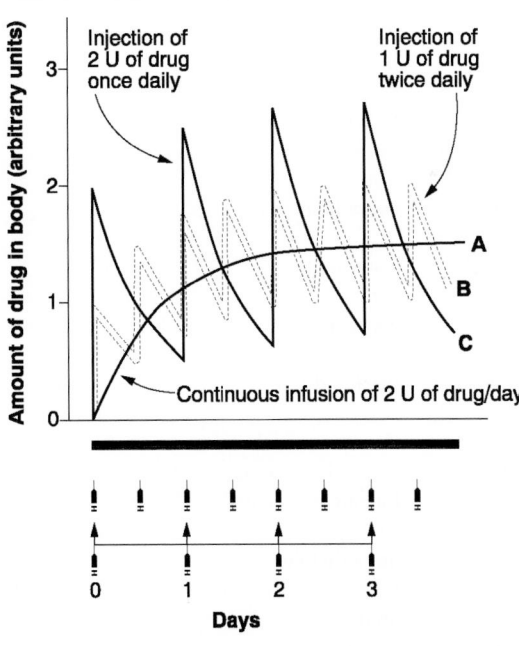

$!$ = Rapid injection of drug

Figure 4–2. Variations in predicted plasma concentration of a drug given by infusion (*A*), twice-daily injection (*B*), or once-daily injection (*C*). The model assumes rapid mixing in a single body compartment and a $t_{1/2}$ of 12 hr. (Reproduced with permission from Howland RD, Mycek MJ [Harvey RA, Champe PC, eds.]. *Lippincott's Illustrated Reviews: Pharmacology*, 3rd ed. Baltimore, Lippincott Williams & Wilkins, 2006, p. 21.)

How many half-lives are required to reach steady-state concentration?

Approximately 4 1/2 half-lives. At $3.3t_{1/2}$ the drug will reach 90% of its effective steady state.

What is an excretion rate?

The rate at which a drug is eliminated from the body, which is measured by clearance × plasma concentration

What is a therapeutic index?

The ratio of a drug's toxic dose to its therapeutic dose. A safe drug will have a high therapeutic index. See **Appendix A** for sample problems illustrating these concepts.

PRESCRIPTION WRITING

Is prescription writing tested on the boards?

No. It is presented only for your background knowledge.

Define the following abbreviations:

q

every hour

qhs

every night

qd

every day

bid

twice a day

tid

three times a day

qid

four times a day

stat

immediately

po

orally

gtt

drops

prn

as needed

qs

quantity sufficient (i.e., the pharmacist will dispense the appropriate number of pills.)

How is a standard pre-scription written?

See Figure 4-3.

The first line contains the drug name and dose:

Lasix 40 mg

The second line contains the directions for use:

Sig: ┬ tab po bid

This line states, "take one tablet by mouth twice a day."

The third line contains the number of tablets to be dispensed:

#14 (When writing for a controlled substance such as **oxycodone** (Percocet), this number should also be written in longhand [*fourteen*].)

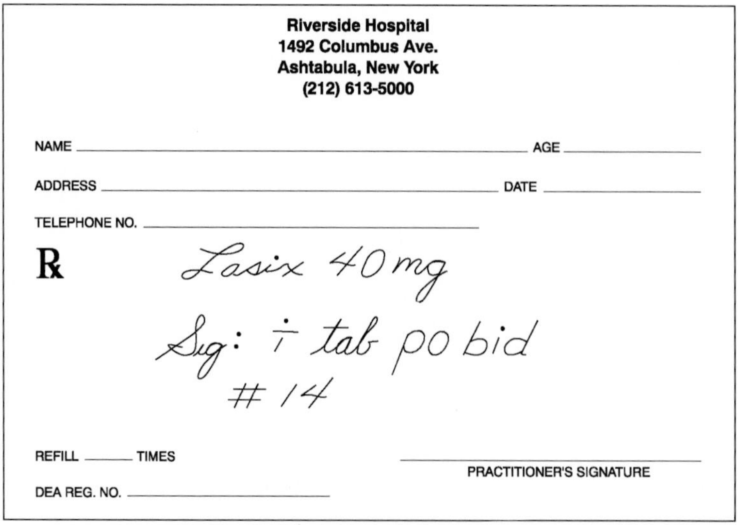

Riverside Hospital
1492 Columbus Ave.
Ashtabula, New York
(212) 613-5000

NAME _____ AGE _____

ADDRESS _____ DATE _____

TELEPHONE NO. _____

R   *Lasix 40 mg*

      Sig: ┬ tab po bid
        # 14

REFILL _____ TIMES

                    _____
                    PRACTITIONER'S SIGNATURE

DEA REG. NO. _____

Figure 4–3. A sample prescription.

Section II

Autonomic Nervous System

5

Introduction to Autonomic Nervous System Pharmacology

Name the two branches of the human nervous system.

1. Central nervous system
2. Peripheral nervous system

What are the two subdivisions of the peripheral nervous system?

1. Somatic nervous system, which innervates skeletal muscle
2. Autonomic nervous system (ANS)

What is the autonomic nervous system?

A collection of nuclei, cell bodies, nerves, ganglia, and plexuses that provides afferent and efferent innervation to smooth muscle and visceral organs

Why is this system important?

The ANS regulates functions that are not under conscious control, such as blood pressure, heart rate, and intestinal motility. (✎ Also, ANS drugs have traditionally been a favorite topic of USMLE examiners.)

What are the two major subdivisions of the ANS?

1. Sympathetic nervous system
2. Parasympathetic nervous system

What are the anatomic differences between these two systems?

The **sympathetic nervous system** originates in the thoracolumbar portion of the spinal cord. The *preganglionic neurons* are short and usually synapse somewhere in the paravertebral ganglia (sympathetic chain). The *postganglionic neurons* are long and terminate at the visceral organs.

The **parasympathetic nervous system** originates from cranial nerve nuclei III, VII, IX, and X as well as the third and fourth sacral spinal roots (craniosacral

Table 5–1. Autonomic Nervous System: Sympathetic vs. Parasympathetic Responses

Effector Organs[a]	Sympathetic		Parasympathetic	
	Receptor	Response	Receptor	Response
Eye				
Radial muscle (iris)	α_1	Contraction (mydriasis)	—	—
Circular muscle (iris)	—	—	M_3	Contraction (miosis)
Ciliary muscle	β_2	Relaxation	M_3	Contraction (accommodation)
Heart				
SA node	β_1	$\uparrow$ HR	M_2	$\downarrow$ HR
AV node	β_1	$\uparrow$ conduction velocity and automaticity	M_2	$\downarrow$ conduction velocity
Contractility	β_1	$\uparrow$ force of contraction (atria & ventricles)	M_2	$\downarrow$ contractility (atria)
Lung				
Bronchial muscle	β_2	Relaxation (bronchodilation)	M_3	Contraction (bronchoconstriction)
Blood vessels				
Most (except skeletal muscle)	α_1	Constriction	—	—
Skeletal muscle	β_2	Relaxation	—	—
GI (stomach and intestine)				
Sphincter	α_1	Constriction (retention)	M_3	Relaxation (defecation)
Motility and tone	α, β_2	$\downarrow$	M_3	$\uparrow$ motility and tone

GU				
Urinary sphincter	α_1	Constriction	M_3	Relaxation
Bladder wall	β_2	Relaxation (retention)	M_3	Contraction
Uterus, pregnant	α_1; β_2	Contraction; relaxation	—	—
Uterus, nonpregnant	β_2	Relaxation	—	—
Penis, seminal vesicles	α_1	Ejaculation	M	Erection
Secretory glands				
Sweat	α_1	Localized secretion	M	Generalized secretion
Intestinal	α_2	Inhibition	M_3	↑ secretion
Bronchial	—	—	M	↑ secretion
Lacrimal	α	↑ secretion (moderate)	M	Profuse secretion
Metabolism				
Adrenal medulla	N_N	Secretion of catecholamines	—	
Kidney	β_1	↑ renin release	—	
Skeletal muscle	β_2	Glycogenolysis, ↑ contractility	—	
Pancreas (beta cells)	α_2	↓ insulin release	—	
Fat cells	β_3	Lipolysis	—	

[a]The parasympathetic system controls most organs except blood vessels, which are regulated by the sympathetic nervous system.
N_N = nicotinic receptors; M = muscarinic receptors
(Adapted from Gallia G, Hann CL, Hewson WH. *The Pharmacology Companion*. Ann Arbor, MI: Alert & Oriented Publishing Company, 1997.)

origins). The preganglionic neurons take a long path and synapse onto short postganglionic neurons in or near the target organ.

What are the functions of the sympathetic nervous system?

The sympathetic nervous system is normally active even at rest; however, it assumes a dominant role when the body becomes stressed in some way. For example, if you sense danger, your heart rate increases, blood pressure rises, eyes dilate, blood sugar rises, bronchioles expand, and blood flow shifts from the skin to skeletal muscles (Table 5-1). The sympathetic nervous system prepares you for **"flight or fight"** situations.

With what major receptors is the sympathetic nervous system associated?

Adrenergic receptors—alpha-1 (α_1), alpha-2 (α_2), beta-1 (β_1), beta-2 (β_2), and dopamine receptors

What are the actions of the parasympathetic system?

The parasympathetic nervous system is predominant under tranquil conditions. It slows heart rate, lowers blood pressure, increases intestinal activity, constricts the pupils, and empties the urinary bladder (Table 5-1). The parasympathetic nervous system is also known as the **rest and digest** system.

What receptors does the parasympathetic system act on?

Cholinergic receptors—muscarinic and nicotinic

How are the parasympathetic and sympathetic systems related?

These two systems oppose each other's actions. Remember that both systems are working at all times; however, which system predominates over an organ will depend on the situation. The heart, for example, is predominantly controlled by the parasympathetic system except under stress, when it is controlled by the sympathetic system.

What are the two principal neurotransmitters in the ANS?

1. Acetylcholine—cholinergic transmission
2. Norepinephrine—adrenergic transmission (Figure 5-1)

Which ion is required for the release of these neurotransmitters from their storage vesicles?

The calcium ion (Ca^{2+}) is required for the release of *most* neurotransmitters from their storage vesicles.

How do autonomic drugs function?

ANS drugs achieve their effects by acting as either agonists or antagonists at cholinergic and adrenergic receptors. The following four chapters discuss each of these drug classes in greater detail.

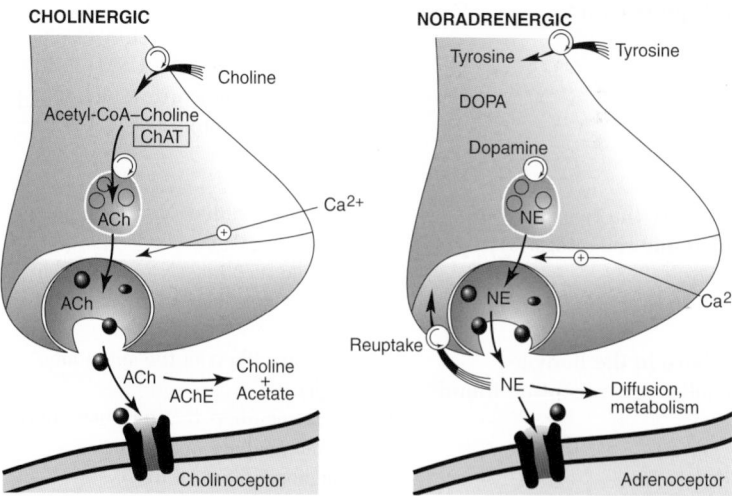

Figure 5–1. Circles with rotating arrows represent transporters; ChAT, choline acetyltransferase; ACh, acetylcholine; AChE, acetylcholinesterase; NE, norepinephrine. (From Bhushan V, Le T. *First Aid for the USMLE Step 1*. New York: McGraw-Hill, 2005, p. 296. Adapted with permission from Katzung BG, Trevor AJ. *Examination & Board Review: Pharmacology*, 5th ed. Stamford, CT: Appleton & Lange, 1998, p. 42.)

6   Cholinergic Agonists

What are cholinergic agonists?

Cholinergic agonists are drugs that mimic or potentiate the actions of **acetylcholine**.

What are the two major families of cholinergic receptors?

1. **Muscarinic**—This receptor family earned its name because it was first identified using muscarine, an alkaloid found in certain poisonous mushrooms.
2. **Nicotinic**

What pharmacologic subtypes of muscarinic receptors exist?

There are several different subtypes of muscarinic receptors, namely, M_1 to M_5. They are found in ganglia, smooth muscle, myocardium, secretory glands, and the CNS. (✎ For the USMLE, it is not necessary to memorize which subtype of muscarinic receptors a drug will act on.)

Identify the two types of nicotinic receptors.

1. Neuronal nicotinic (N_N), located in autonomic ganglia
2. Muscular nicotinic (N_M), located in the neuromuscular junction

Where in the body are cholinergic receptors found?

Preganglionic fibers of the autonomic ganglia

Preganglionic fibers that terminate in the adrenal medulla

Postganglionic fibers of the parasympathetic system

Voluntary muscles of the somatic system

CNS

Sweat glands innervated by the postganglionic sympathetic nervous system

See Figure 6-1.

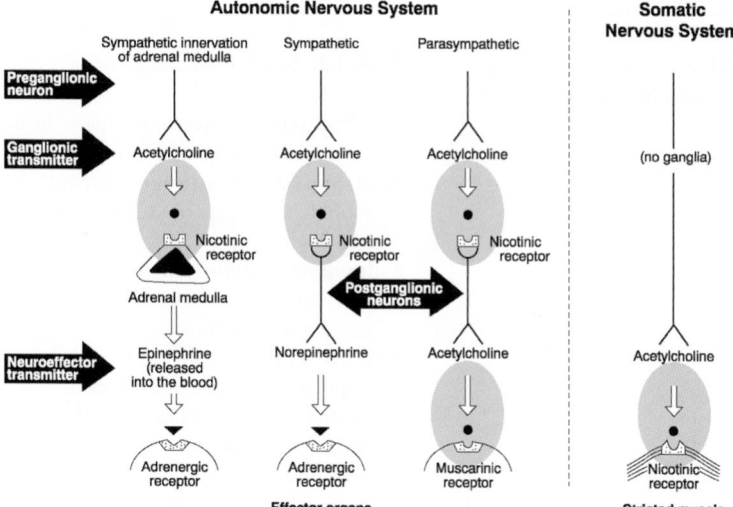

Figure 6–1. Sites of action of cholinergic agonists in the autonomic and somatic nervous systems. (Redrawn with permission from Howland RD, Mycek MJ [Harvey RA, Champe PC, eds.]. *Lippincott's Illustrated Reviews: Pharmacology*, 3rd ed. Baltimore: Lippincott Williams & Wilkins, 2006, p. 44.)

What types of cholinergic agonists are available for clinical use?

Cholinergic agonists can be divided into two major groups:

1. **Direct-acting agonists** chemically bind with and activate muscarinic and nicotinic receptors in the body.
2. **Indirect-acting agonists** inhibit the enzyme acetylcholinesterase and therefore increase the concentration of **acetylcholine** within the synapse.

DIRECT-ACTING AGONISTS

Give six examples of direct-acting agonists.

1. **Acetylcholine**—prototype
2. **Bethanechol**
3. **Carbachol**
4. **Pilocarpine**
5. **Methacholine**
6. **Nicotine** (discussed in *Chapter 17—CNS Stimulants*)

ACETYLCHOLINE

What are the physiological actions of acetylcholine?

Acetylcholine affects almost every system within the body:

Cardiovascular system—decreases heart rate, contractility, and blood pressure.

Gastrointestinal system— increases motility of the gastrointestinal tract and bladder.

Pulmonary system— increases secretions of the bronchioles and constricts bronchi.

The eye—causes constriction of the pupillary sphincter muscle and contraction of the ciliary muscle, which causes miosis and accommodation.

Peripheral nervous system—causes contraction of skeletal muscle.

Central nervous system—serves as a neurotransmitter.

Endocrine system—causes release of epinephrine from the adrenal medulla (via nicotinic receptor) and it stimulates sweat gland secretions.

What receptors does acetylcholine activate?

Both muscarinic and nicotinic

What are the clinical indications?

Acetylcholine is sometimes used to achieve miosis during ophthalmic surgery. In general, it is rarely used because it has widespread effects and is so rapidly hydrolyzed by acetylcholinesterase.

What are the adverse reactions?

The adverse effects result from excessive generalized cholinergic stimulation. They include:

Diarrhea and **d**ecreased blood pressure
Urination
Miosis
Bronchoconstriction and **b**radycardia
Excitation of skeletal muscle

Lacrimation
Salivation and sweating
DUMBELS
NOTE: These adverse effects
are typical of *all* direct and
indirect cholinergic agonists,
not just **acetylcholine**.

BETHANECHOL (Urecholine)

**What type of chemical
compound is bethanechol?**

A carbamic acid ester

**What receptors does it work
on?**

Bethanechol works primarily on
muscarinic receptors, but it also has some
mild nicotinic properties.

**What are its therapeutic
uses?**

Bethanechol increases intestinal
motility, especially after surgery. Because
this drug also stimulates the detrusor
muscle of the bladder, it is also
used to treat urinary retention.
BBB—**B**ethanechol stimulates
the **B**ladder and **B**owel.

**What are the adverse effects
of bethanechol
administration?**

The adverse effects are those that result
from generalized cholinergic stimulation
(see above).

CARBACHOL (Carbastat)

**What type of compound is
carbachol?**

A carbamic acid ester similar to
bethanechol

What is its clinical use?

This drug is rarely used clinically today,
but it was once used for glaucoma and to
stimulate miosis during ophthalmic
surgery.

**What receptors does
carbachol work on?**

Both muscarinic and nicotinic receptors

What are its adverse effects?

Those that result from excessive
generalized cholinergic stimulation

PILOCARPINE (Pilocar)

What type of compound is pilocarpine?	An alkaloid
What are pilocarpine's physiological actions?	Causes miosis and contraction of the ciliary muscle (accommodation) Decreases heart rate Causes bronchial smooth muscle contraction Increases secretions from salivary, lacrimal, and sweat glands
Is it cleaved by acetylcholinesterase?	No, the drug is unaffected by this enzyme.
State the clinical use.	Pilocarpine is extremely good for stimulating miosis and opening the trabecular meshwork around the canal of Schlemm. Therefore pilocarpine can be used for the treatment of glaucoma.
How is it administered?	Usually given topically
What receptors does this drug work on?	Primarily muscarinic receptors
What are the adverse effects?	Unlike the other direct-acting agonists previously discussed, **pilocarpine** is able to enter the brain and cause CNS disturbances such as hallucinations and convulsions, along with generalized cholinergic stimulation.

METHACHOLINE (Mecholyl)

What is methacholine used for?	Diagnosis of asthma and bronchial hyperreactivity
What receptors does it stimulate?	Muscarinic receptors
What are the adverse effects?	Generalized cholinergic stimulation

INDIRECT-ACTING AGONISTS

Give six examples of indirect-acting cholinergic agonists.	1. **Isoflurophate** 2. **Echothiophate** 3. **Parathion** 4. **Edrophonium** 5. **Physostigmine** 6. **Neostigmine**
How do they work?	By inhibiting the enzyme acetylcholinesterase, which is responsible for the hydrolysis of acetylcholine. Neuronal response to acetylcholine is therefore enhanced.
Which receptors do they act on?	Because they increase the synaptic concentration of acetylcholine, indirect-acting agonists stimulate both nicotinic and muscarinic receptors.
Which indirect-acting cholinergic agonists have the ability to *irreversibly* inhibit acetylcholinesterase?	Only the organophosphates (**isoflurophate**, **echothiophate**, and **parathion**) irreversibly inhibit acetylcholinesterase.
Why are physostigmine, neostigmine, edrophonium, and pyridostigmine considered to be reversible?	Because they do not bind covalently to acetylcholinesterase

ORGANOPHOSPHATES (ISOFLUROPHATE, ECHOTHIOPHATE, PARATHION)

Describe the mechanism of action.	Organophosphates bind covalently to acetylcholinesterase and can permanently inactivate the enzyme. The effects of organophosphates can last as long as a week, which is approximately the time needed to synthesize a new molecule of acetylcholinesterase.
Is it at all possible to reverse the effects of organophosphates?	In most cases, no. However, if **pralidoxime** (a cholinesterase reactivator) is given before the organophosphate binds to

acetylcholinesterase and loses one if its alkyl groups (a process called aging), it may be possible for pralidoxime to remove the organophosphate from acetylcholinesterase (Figure 6-2).

What were these drugs used for in the past?

Organophosphates were used in wars as nerve gases. They produce an immense stimulation at cholinoreceptors throughout the body, causing respiratory muscle paralysis and convulsions.

What are these drugs used for today?

Isoflurophate and **echothiophate** are used occasionally for accommodative esotropia.

What drug is used to treat organophosphate poisoning?

Atropine is used, along with gastric lavage and charcoal.

What are the toxicities of the organophosphates?

Excessive cholinergic stimulation

PHYSOSTIGMINE (Eserine)

When is physostigmine administered?

For glaucoma (rarely)
For overdoses of **atropine**, phenothiazines, and tricyclic antidepressants
For intestinal and bowel atony
For accommodative esotropia (rarely)

Can physostigmine enter the CNS?

Yes, because it is a tertiary amine.

What are the adverse effects?

Convulsions
Muscle paralysis secondary to overstimulation
Cataracts
Generalized excessive cholinergic stimulation

NEOSTIGMINE (PROSTIGMIN)

Does this drug enter the CNS?

No, because it is a polar quaternary carbamate.

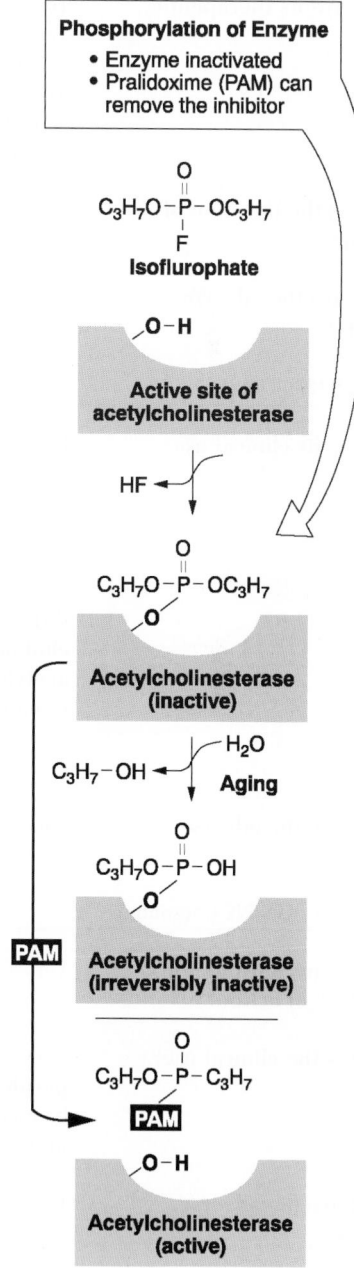

Figure 6–2. Covalent modification of acetylcholinesterase by isoflurophate. (Redrawn with permission from Howland RD, Mycek MJ [Harvey RA, Champe PC, eds.]. *Lippincott's Illustrated Reviews: Pharmacology,* 3rd ed. Baltimore: Lippincott Williams & Wilkins, 2006, p. 52.)

What are its therapeutic uses?	Treatment of myasthenia gravis
	Treatment of urinary retention and paralytic ileus
	Antidote for nondepolarizing neuromuscular blockade, as with **tubocurarine** (See *Chapter 7.*)

What is the duration of action?

Usually 2 to 4 hr

What are the adverse effects?

Excessive cholinergic stimulation

EDROPHONIUM (Enlon)

What is its clinical use?

Edrophonium is similar to **neostigmine** except that it is used in the **diagnosis of myasthenia gravis.** It is not useful for maintenance therapy because of its short duration of action (approximately 5 to 15 min). Edrophonium is also used **to differentiate myasthenia gravis from cholinergic crisis (excessive acetylcholine).** Both conditions can result in muscle weakness; however, administration of edrophonium helps myasthenia but worsens cholinergic crisis.

What are the adverse effects?

Excessive cholinergic stimulation

PYRIDOSTIGMINE (Mestinon)

What is pyridostigmine's duration of action?

Very long—usually 3 to 6 hr

What is the clinical use?

Because of its long duration of action, **pyridostigmine**, like **neostigmine**, can be used for long-term treatment of myasthenia gravis.

What are the adverse effects?

Excessive cholinergic stimulation

7

Cholinergic Antagonists

What are cholinergic antagonists?

Drugs that bind to cholinergic receptors (muscarinic and/or nicotinic) but do not trigger the usual intracellular response

Name three subclasses of cholinergic antagonists.

1. **Muscarinic blockers**
2. **Neuromuscular blocking agents**—inhibit the efferent impulses to skeletal muscle via the nicotinic muscle receptor (N_M)
3. **Ganglionic blockers**—inhibit the nicotinic neuronal receptor (N_N) of both parasympathetic and sympathetic ganglia

MUSCARINIC ANTAGONISTS

Give six examples of muscarinic blockers.

1. **Atropine** (prototype)
2. **Scopolamine**
3. **Homatropine**
4. **Cyclopentolate**
5. **Tropicamide**
6. **Pirenzepine**

Are there other drugs that exhibit antimuscarinic properties?

Yes—these include the anti-Parkinson's drugs (e.g., **benztropine**), the antidepressants (e.g., **chlorpromazine** [Thorazine]), antihistamines (e.g., **diphenhydramine**), and antiasthmatics (e.g., **ipratropium**), which are discussed further in later chapters.

ATROPINE

To what family of compounds does atropine belong?

Atropine comes from the plant *Atropa belladonna* and is known as a belladonna alkaloid.

What is the significance of the plant's name?

Belladonna in Latin means **pretty lady.** During the Roman era, the plant was used to dilate women's pupils, which was considered to be attractive.

What is atropine's mechanism of action?

It causes **reversible, nonselective** blockade of muscarinic receptors.

What agent can be used to counteract the effects of atropine?

High concentrations of **acetylcholine** or an equivalent muscarinic agonist

Does this drug cross the blood-brain barrier?

No. Atropine does not readily cross the blood-brain barrier.

What are the pharmacologic actions of atropine?

CNS—At toxic doses, it can cause restlessness, hallucinations, and delusions.

Cardiovascular system—At low doses, **atropine** reduces heart rate through central stimulation of the vagus nucleus. At high doses, **atropine** blocks muscarinic receptors of the heart and thus induces tachycardia.

Gastrointestinal system—reduces salivary gland secretion and GI motility

Pulmonary system—reduces bronchial secretions and stimulates bronchodilation

Urinary system—blocks muscarinic receptors in the bladder wall, which results in bladder wall relaxation

Eye—causes paralysis of the sphincter muscle of the iris and ciliary muscle of the lens, resulting in mydriasis and cycloplegia (My*d*riasis = *d*ilation.)

Sweat glands—suppresses sweating, especially in children

You will more readily remember the actions of **atropine** if you recognize that blocked cholinergic receptors result in an unopposed sympathetic response.

List the therapeutic uses of atropine.

Treatment of bradycardia
Mydriasis and cycloplegia—beneficial when an accurate refraction is required. Also used in amblyopia therapy for young children
Gastrointestinal spasms
Cystitis—decreases urgency
Organophosphate poisoning

When is the use of atropine to effect mydriasis and cycloplegia contraindicated?

Do not dilate the eyes of a patient who has narrow-angle glaucoma, because this may result in an acute crisis due to closure of the canal of Schlemm.

What is atropine's duration of action?

Approximately 4 hr except when it is placed in the eye, where it usually lasts about 7 to 10 days

How is atropine absorbed and excreted?

It is well absorbed from the gastrointestinal system and conjunctival membrane. It is excreted through both hepatic metabolism and renal filtration.

What are the toxic effects of this drug?

Toxic Effect:	*Mnemonic:*
Dry mouth	"Dry as a bone"
Inhibition of sweating (most toxic effect in young children and infants)	"Hot as a hare"
Tachycardia and cutaneous vasodilation	"Red as a beet"
Blurring of vision	"Blind as a bat"
Hallucinations and delirium	"Mad as a hatter"

SCOPOLAMINE

What is the classification of scopolamine?

Like **atropine**, this drug is a belladonna alkaloid.

What is its mechanism of action?

Nonselective competitive blockade of muscarinic receptors

How is scopolamine used therapeutically?
Prevention of motion sickness—"lotion for motion"

How does this drug differ from atropine?
It has a longer duration of action and more potent CNS effects.

What is scopolamine's route of administration?
It is often given transdermally.

Are there any adverse effects?
Yes—similar to those of **atropine**: "Dry as a bone, red as a beet, hot as a hare, blind as a bat, mad as a hatter."

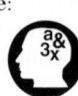

HOMATROPINE, CYCLOPENTOLATE (Cyclogyl), AND TROPICAMIDE (Mydriacyl)

What are these drugs used for?
In ophthalmology, they are given topically for mydriasis and cycloplegia.

What are the adverse effects?
Similar to those of **atropine** but much milder because systemic absorption is very low

PIRENZEPINE

What is it?
A selective M_1 muscarinic inhibitor

How is this drug used?
For treating gastric ulcers

What are the adverse effects?
Similar to those of **atropine**

NEUROMUSCULAR BLOCKING AGENTS

Name the two major subdivisions of neuromuscular agents.
1. Nondepolarizing blocking agents
2. Depolarizing blocking agents

NONDEPOLARIZING BLOCKING AGENTS

Name four nondepolarizing agents.
1. **Tubocurarine**—prototype
2. **Pancuronium**—longer duration of action than **tubocurarine**

3. **Atracurium**—suitable for short surgical procedures
4. **Vecuronium**

What is their mechanism of action?

These drugs competitively block cholinergic transmission at the nicotinic neuromuscular receptors (N_M) by preventing the binding of **acetylcholine** to its receptor. (See Figure 6-1.)

What is the therapeutic use of these agents?

They are used as adjuvant drugs for anesthesia—they promote muscle relaxation.

Are all muscles equally affected?

No. The muscles of the eye and face are affected first, whereas the respiratory muscles are affected last.

What is the route of administration?

All neuromuscular junction blockers must be given IV because oral absorption is poor.

What are the adverse effects?

Bronchoconstriction and hypotension, caused by histamine release

What can be used to counteract the effects of these drugs?

Because neuromuscular junction blockers are competitive inhibitors, their actions can be reversed with edrophonium or neostigmine.

DEPOLARIZING NEUROMUSCULAR BLOCKING AGENTS

Name the only depolarizing neuromuscular blocking agent used in the United States.

Succinylcholine

What is this drug's mechanism of action?

Phase 1—*Succinylcholine* binds to the nicotinic receptor, opens the Na^+ channels, and causes membrane depolarization, which initially results in transient fasciculations. Flaccid paralysis will follow in a few minutes, because **succinylcholine** is resistant to acetylcholinesterase and will cause prolonged depolarization of the membrane.

Phase II—Eventually the membrane will at least partially repolarize. However, the receptor is now desensitized to **acetylcholine**, thus preventing the formation of further action potentials.(Figure 7-1.)

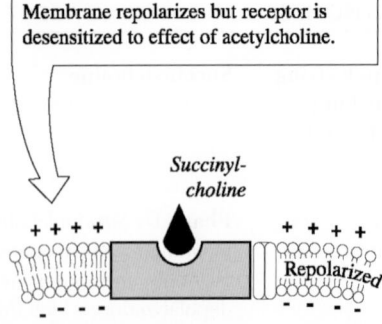

Figure 7–1. Mechanism of action of depolarizing neuromuscular agents. (Redrawn with permission from Howland RD, Mycek MJ [Harvey RA, Champe PC, eds.]. *Lippincott's Illustrated Reviews: Pharmacology,* 3rd ed. Baltimore: Lippincott Williams & Wilkins, 2006, p. 63.)

What is the duration of action?

3 to 6 min if given as a single dose

What substance metabolizes succinylcholine?

Plasma cholinesterase

How is succinylcholine used clinically?

As an adjuvant to general anesthesia
To facilitate rapid intubation

What are the adverse effects?

Bronchoconstriction caused by histamine release
Hypotension
Arrhythmias
Apnea due to respiratory paralysis
Malignant hyperthermia when used with **halothane**

How is malignant hyperthermia treated?

By rapid cooling and the administration of **dantrolene**. **Dantrolene** blocks the release of Ca^{2+} from the sarcoplasmic reticulum, which reduces skeletal muscle contraction and subsequently heat production.

Do neuromuscular blocking agents block autonomic ganglia as well?

In general, no. The skeletal muscle end plate and autonomic ganglia use different subtypes of nicotinic receptors.
Tubocurarine can, however, produce a small amount of ganglionic blockade.

GANGLIONIC BLOCKERS

Name four ganglionic blockers.

1. **Nicotine**
2. **Hexamethonium**
3. **Mecamylamine**
4. **Trimethaphan**

What exactly do these drugs do?

Ganglionic inhibitors compete with acetylcholine to bind with nicotinic receptors of both parasympathetic and sympathetic ganglia.

What is the mechanism of action?

Ganglionic blockers can be divided into two groups:

1. Drugs such as **nicotine**, which initially stimulate the ganglia and then block them because of a persistent depolarization
2. Drugs such as **hexamethonium**, **mecamylamine**, and **trimethaphan**, which block ganglia without any prior stimulation

Describe the physiological effects.

The physiological effects of ganglionic blockers can be predicted if you remember which division of the autonomic nervous system exercises dominant control of the organ in question:

Heart—Tachycardia results because the parasympathetic system is normally dominant on the heart.

Arterioles and veins—vasodilation, increased peripheral blood (sympathetic normally dominant)

Eye—cycloplegia, mydriasis (parasympathetic normally dominant)

GI system—reduced motility; diminished gastric and pancreatic secretions (parasympathetic normally dominant)

Urinary system—urinary retention (parasympathetic normally dominant)

Glands—reduced sweating, lacrimation, salivation (parasympathetic normally dominant)

What is their therapeutic use?

Because they lack selectivity, the ganglionic blockers have been largely phased out of clinical use. In the past, these drugs were used in hypertensive emergencies.

What are the adverse effects?

The toxicities of ganglionic blockers are identical to their physiological effects, described above.

8   Adrenergic Agonists

What are adrenergic agonists?

Drugs or endogenous catecholamines that activate α and/or β receptors. These drugs are also knows as **sympathomimetics**.

How can these substances be classified?

According to mechanism of action (direct vs. indirect) as well as receptor-site specificity (α_1, α_2, β_1, β_2, dopamine)

Name the important α-selective direct-acting agonists.

Phenylephrine
Methoxamine
Clonidine
Methyldopa

Identify the major β-selective direct-acting agonists.

Dobutamine
Isoproterenol
Albuterol
Metaproterenol
Terbutaline

List the major α- and β-selective direct-acting agonists.

Epinephrine
Norepinephrine
Dopamine

Which of the direct-acting agonists are considered endogenous catecholamines?

Epinephrine, norepinephrine, and **dopamine. Isoproterenol** and **dobutamine** are synthesized catecholamines.

Why is that significant?

Endogenous catecholamines are rapidly hydrolyzed by COMT (catechol-*O*-methyltransferase). Thus these agents have a short half-life and are ineffective when given orally due to the action of intestinal enzymes. It is also important to remember that these drugs are polar and do not easily penetrate the blood-brain barrier.

Name two indirect-acting adrenergic agonists.

Tyramine and **amphetamine**

Name two mixed (direct and indirect) agonists.

Ephedrine and **metaraminol**

DIRECT-ACTING α-SELECTIVE RECEPTOR AGONISTS

Where are α_1 and α_2 receptors located?

The α_1 receptors are located on the postsynaptic membrane.
The α_2 receptors are predominantly located on the presynaptic membrane. Postsynaptic α_2 receptors are limited to the CNS and blood vessels.

What physiological responses occur when α-selective receptors are stimulated?

Stimulation of α_1 receptors leads to the release of intracellular calcium from the endoplasmic reticulum via inositol triphosphate (IP_3). This leads to vascular constriction, decreased intestinal tone and motility, contraction of the bladder's internal sphincter, ejaculation, contraction of the pregnant uterus, and mydriasis. (See Table 5-1 in *Chapter 5— Introduction to Autonomic Nervous System Pharmacology.*) (Figure 8-1).

Name the direct-acting agonists that are selective for α_1- and α_2-adrenergic receptors.

α_1 receptors—phenylephrine and methoxamine
α_2 receptors—chlonidine and methyldopa (discussed in *Chapter 20—Antihypertensive Drugs*)

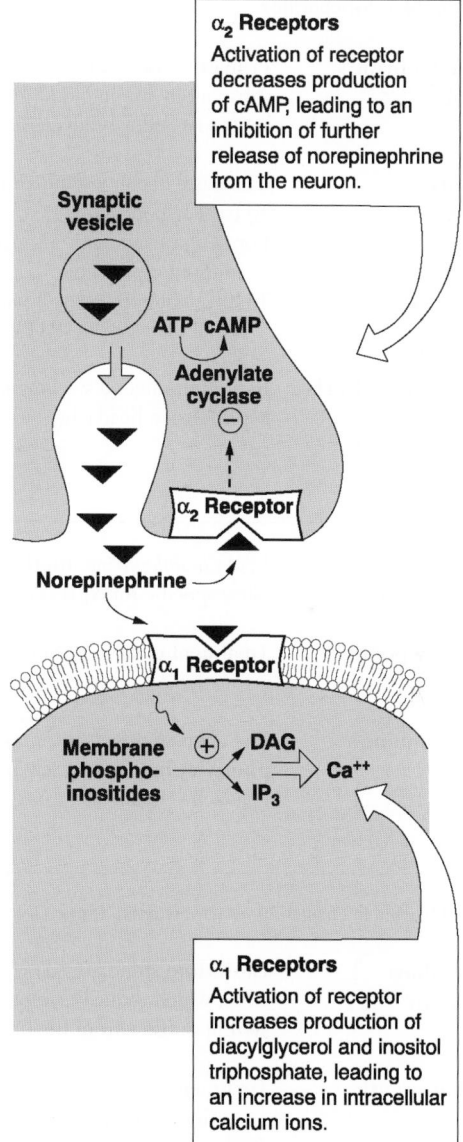

α₂ Receptors

Activation of receptor decreases production of cAMP, leading to an inhibition of further release of norepinephrine from the neuron.

Synaptic vesicle

ATP cAMP

Adenylate cyclase
⊖

α₂ Receptor

Norepinephrine

α₁ Receptor

Membrane phospho-inositides
⊕ **DAG**
IP₃ Ca⁺⁺

α₁ Receptors

Activation of receptor increases production of diacylglycerol and inositol triphosphate, leading to an increase in intracellular calcium ions.

Figure 8–1. Second messengers mediate the effects of α receptors. DAG = diacylglyc-erol; IP = inositol triphosphate. (Redrawn with permission from Howland RD, Mycek MJ [Harvey RA, Champe PC, eds.]. *Lippincott's Illustrated Reviews: Pharmacology,* 3rd ed. Baltimore: Lippincott Williams & Wilkins, 2006, p. 69.)

PHENYLEPHRINE (Neo-Synephrine)

What are phenylephrine's physiological actions?	Primarily vasoconstriction. The subsequent rise in blood pressure also leads to a reflex bradycardia.
Describe this drug's therapeutic uses.	As a nasal decongestant (primary use) To treat hypotension For ocular examinations: mydriasis without cycloplegia To terminate episodes of paroxysmal atrial tachycardia (PAT)
What are the adverse effects associated with phenyl-ephrine administration?	Rebound mucosal swelling and hypertensive headache

METHOXAMINE

What receptors does methoxamine work on?	Like *phenylephrine*, **methoxamine** is fairly specific for α_1 receptors.
Describe the therapeutic uses.	Treatment of hypotension and PAT
What are methoxamine's adverse effects?	The adverse effects are similar to those of **phenylephrine**—namely hypertensive headache. It can also cause vomiting.

CLONIDINE

Clonidine is also discussed in *Chapter 20—Antihypertensive Drugs.*

What receptors does clonidine work on?	**Clonidine** stimulates α_2 receptors in the CNS, which reduces sympathetic nervous system outflow from the brain.
Describe its therapeutic uses.	Treatment of hypertension—especially in patients with renal disease, since it does not decrease kidney perfusion Withdrawal from benzodiazepines and opiates Treatment of diarrhea in diabetic patients who have autonomic neuropathies

What toxicities may patients experience while using clonidine?

Sedation
Dry mouth
Sexual dysfunction
Orthostatic hypotension

DIRECT-ACTING β-SELECTIVE AGONISTS

Where are the β receptors located?

The β_1 receptors are primarily located on the postsynaptic membrane of organs such as the heart. The β_2 receptors are found on both the pre- and postsynaptic membranes.

What are the physiological responses once β receptors are stimulated?

Stimulation of β_1 receptors activates adenylate cyclase, which opens calcium channels, leading to cardiac stimulation with both increased inotropic and chronotropic effects. β_1 stimulation also leads to increased lipolysis. **β_2 receptors** work via adenylate cyclase stimulation as well. In this case, however, bronchial smooth muscle as well as the vasculature of skeletal muscle are dilated. The uterus, ciliary, and detrusor muscles are relaxed and glucagon release is increased. **Both β_1 and β_2 receptors** produce decreased intestinal tone and motility (just as the α-adrenergic receptors do). See also Table 5-1 in *Chapter 5—Introduction to Autonomic Nervous System Pharmacology.*

DOBUTAMINE

What is it?

A dopamine analogue

What receptors does dobutamine act on?

Primarily β_1, but it does have some action on β_2 receptors as well.

What are the physiological effects of dobutamine?

Increased heart rate and contractility (β_1) and some smooth muscle relaxation (β_2). This combination allows the heart to pump forcefully while not having to overcome the increased peripheral

	vascular resistance seen with other pressors.
What is dobutamine's therapeutic use?	Treatment of unstable CHF and shock
What is the route of administration?	IV
What are this drug's adverse effects?	Arrhythmias Headache Hypertension Palpitations Angina Nausea

ISOPROTERENOL

Which receptors mediate the effects of isoproterenol?	**Isoproterenol** has direct actions on β_1 and β_2 receptors equally.
What are its physiological actions?	Increases cardiovascular inotropic and chronotropic response (β_1) Lowers peripheral vascular resistance (β_2) and subsequently diastolic blood pressure Relaxes smooth muscles (β_2)
In what clinical situations is it appropriate to use isoproterenol?	Stimulation of heart rate in patients suffering from heart block and bradycardia In the past, used for treatment of asthma
What is the route of administration?	IV
What are the toxicities of isoproterenol?	Arrhythmias Palpitations Tachycardia Headache

ALBUTEROL, METAPROTERENOL, SALMETEROL, AND TERBUTALINE

What are the pharmacologic actions of these β_2 direct-acting agonists?	Smooth muscle relaxation, especially around bronchioles Can stimulate β_1 receptors at higher doses
What is the route of administration?	Albuterol and metaproterenol are usually inhaled. **Terbutaline** can be given orally or subcutaneously.
List the therapeutic uses.	Treatment of bronchospasm/asthma Treatment of chronic obstructive pulmonary disease Treatment of bronchitis Terbutaline and ritodrine can be used to relax the uterus during premature labor.
What are the potential adverse effects of the β_2-selective drugs?	Arrhythmias Tremor Tachycardia Headache Nausea and vomiting

DIRECT-ACTING α AND β AGONISTS

EPINEPHRINE

Which receptors does epinephrine act on?	It stimulates α_1, α_2, β_1, and β_2 receptors. At low doses, epinephrine stimulates β receptors; at high doses, it stimulates α receptors.
What are the physiological responses to epinephrine?	Cardiovascular—increased heart rate and contractility as well as vasoconstriction of arterioles in the skin, viscera, and mucous membranes Respiratory—bronchodilation through activation of β_2 receptors Metabolic—increased glycogenolysis, release of glucagon, and a decreased release of insulin result in hyperglycemia. Epinephrine also increases the concentration of free fatty acids in blood.

What are the therapeutic uses?

Given for bronchospasm secondary to acute asthma or anaphylactic shock.

Used in anaphylaxis and cardiac arrest to increase cardiac electrical activity.

Used in conjunction with local anesthetics to prolong the duration of anesthesia.

Used to achieve hemostasis.

What are epinephrine's adverse effects?

Cardiac arrhythmias

Hypertension

Palpitations

Dizziness, anxiety, headache, tremor

Myocardial infarction due to increased cardiac work

Pulmonary edema

To what does the term "epinephrine reversal" refer?

When **epinephrine** is administered alone, it will cause an increase in systemic systolic blood pressure because of its α activity. When given in conjunction with an α blocker such as **phenoxybenzamine**, **epinephrine** will cause a decrease in systolic blood pressure because of its β_2 activity. This effect is known as **epinephrine reversal**.

NOREPINEPHRINE (Levophed)

What receptors does norepinephrine stimulate?

α_1, α_2, and β_1 receptors.

Norepinephrine has a stronger affinity for α receptors than for β receptors. It does not stimulate β_2 receptors.

What are its physiological effects?

Powerful vasoconstriction of skeletal muscle and renal vasculature, increased myocardial contractility

Reflex bradycardia via a rise in vagal activity

What is its therapeutic use?

It is one of the last-line agents in the treatment of shock.

What are norepinephrine's adverse effects?

Tissue hypoxia secondary to potent vasoconstriction

Decreased perfusion to the kidneys
Tissue necrosis due to extravasation
  during intravenous administration
Arrhythmias

DOPAMINE

Where is this agonist found?	It is synthesized in the CNS, sympathetic ganglia, and adrenal medulla. It is the metabolic precursor to norepinephrine.
What receptors does dopamine act on?	On α_1, β_1, and β_2 receptors. It also stimulates its own **dopamine** (D_1 and D_2) receptors located in the peripheral mesenteric and renal vascular beds. **Dopamine** receptors are stimulated at low dose, β receptors at moderate dose, and α_1 receptors at higher doses. **Dopamine** does not cross the blood-brain barrier.
What are dopamine's therapeutic uses?	Treatment of shock—it raises blood pressure by stimulating the β_1 receptors of the heart. Used in acute renal failure to increase renal blood flow. Treatment of acute congestive heart failure.
How is it administered?	IV
What are dopamine's adverse effects?	Decreased renal perfusion at higher doses Arrhythmias Tachycardia Hypertension Tissue necrosis can occur if dopamine extravasates during infusion.

INDIRECT-ACTING AGONISTS

TYRAMINE

What is tyramine?	Tyramine is a by-product of **tyrosine** metabolism; **tyrosine** is a precursor to

dopamine, **epinephrine**, and **norepinephrine**.

What is the mechanism of action of tyramine?

Tyramine is taken up by sympathetic neurons, which causes a release of catecholamines.

Is there a therapeutic use for tyramine?

No. It is a normal by-product of tyrosine metabolism, which is usually eliminated by MAO.

What are tyramine's adverse effects?

It can cause a **hypertensive emergency** in patients who take MAO-inhibiting drugs, since MAO is responsible for the metabolism of tyramine. It is important to **warn patients who are taking MAO inhibitors** not to eat foods with high tyramine concentrations, such as red wine, beer, chocolate, and cheese.

AMPHETAMINE

What are its pharmacological actions?

It releases stores of **norepinephrine** and **dopamine** from presynaptic terminals. It can readily enter the CNS.
Amphetamine can also raise blood pressure through vasoconstriction.

When is it appropriate to administer amphetamine?

Amphetamine's clinical uses are limited by the psychological and physical dependence it can induce. It is, however, used to treat attention deficit hyperactivity disorder (ADHD) and narcolepsy. It can also be used for appetite suppression.

What are the adverse effects?

Psychological and physical dependence
Psychosis
Confusion
Insomnia
Headache
Restlessness
Palpitations
Tachycardia
Impotence
See *Chapter 17—CNS Stimulants*, for further discussion of amphetamines.

MIXED (DIRECT AND INDIRECT) AGONISTS

EPHEDRINE

How does ephedrine work?	It stimulates the release of **norepinephrine** from nerve terminals. It also acts as a direct adrenergic agonist on α and β receptors.
What are ephedrine's therapeutic uses?	**Ephedrine** is used in the treatment of nasal congestion, bronchospasm, and hypotension.
What are the adverse effects?	Arrhythmias Palpitations Insomnia Hypertension

METARAMINOL

Describe this drug's actions.	**Metaraminol** acts indirectly by releasing **norepinephrine** from presynaptic terminals. It can also directly stimulate α receptors.
What are its therapeutic uses?	Treatment of hypotension and termination of PAT episodes
What are the adverse effects?	Similar to those of **norepinephrine**

9

Adrenergic Antagonists

What are adrenergic antagonists?	They are drugs that bind to adrenergic receptors but do not initiate the usual intracellular response.
Name the two major subdivisions of this drug class.	1. α blockers 2. β blockers
Is there another class of adrenergic antagonists?	Yes—the indirect adrenergic antagonists

α BLOCKERS

Name seven α blockers.	1. **Prazosin** (Minipress)—α_1-adrenergic selective, reversible 2. **Doxazosin** (Cardura)—α_1-adrenergic selective, reversible 3. **Terazosin** (Hytrin)—α_1-adrenergic selective, reversible 4. **Phenoxybenzamine** (Dibenzyline)— nonselective, **irreversible.** Remember, **phenoxybenzamine** is the only α-adrenergic receptor mentioned that is nonreversible. (✎ board question) 5. **Tamsulosin** (Flomax)—α_1-adrenergic selective, reversible 6. **Yohimbine** (Yocon)—α_2-adrenergic selective, reversible 7. **Phentolamine** (Regitine)— nonselective, reversible

PRAZOSIN, TERAZOSIN, AND DOXAZOSIN

What is their mechanism of action?

They competitively and selectively block α_1-adrenergic receptors.

Describe the physiological sequelae of α_1 blockade.

Blockade of α_1-adrenergic receptors on vascular smooth muscle **inhibits** constriction of arterioles and veins. This results in decreased peripheral vascular resistance and a lower blood pressure.

Blockade of α_1-adrenergic receptors in bladder smooth muscle results in relaxation and decreased resistance to urine flow.

What are the clinical uses?

Treatment of hypertension

Prevention of urinary retention in patients who have benign prostatic hypertrophy

Are there adverse effects?

Prazosin and structural analogues can cause:

Gastrointestinal hypermotility

Orthostatic hypertension, **especially after the initial dose**

Sexual dysfunction, dry mouth, and dizziness

PHENOXYBENZAMINE

How does this drug work?

Phenoxybenzamine is unique in that it works by noncompetitively blocking the α_1 postsynaptic receptor and α_2 presynaptic receptors.

Describe the physiological actions of phenoxybenzamine.

It blocks peripheral vasoconstriction.
It induces a reflex tachycardia.

How is phenoxybenzamine administered?

Orally

What is the duration of action?

Because it binds covalently to the receptor, this drug has a very long duration of action (approximately 14 to 48 hr).

Describe the therapeutic use.	Treatment of patients with ***pheochromocytoma-induced hypertension*. Phenoxybenzamine** is useful because of its long duration of action.
	Treatment of patients with benign prostatic hypertrophy. **Phenoxybenzamine** reduces the size of the prostate.
	Spinal cord injuries may lead to autonomic hyperreflexia, which results in high blood pressure. **Phenoxybenzamine** blunts this response.
	Treatment of patients with Raynaud's disease
What are the toxicities associated with the use of phenoxybenzamine?	Orthostatic hypotension
	Reflex tachycardia—If severe, it may induce anginal pain; therefore, phenoxybenzamine is contraindicated in patients with coronary disease.
	Inhibition of ejaculation due to lack of smooth muscle contraction in the vas deferens

YOHIMBINE

What is it?	A selective α_2-receptor antagonist
Describe the clinical use.	Erectile dysfunction

TAMSULOSIN

How does it work?	**Tamsulosin** specifically inhibits the alpha$_{1A}$ adrenoreceptor. Approximately 70% of the α_1 receptors in the prostate are α_{1A} .
What is its clinical use?	Benign prostatic hyperplasia
Can it be used with other α-blocking drugs?	No. This combination of drugs should be avoided.

What are its adverse effects?   Orthostatic hypotension, ejaculatory problems

PHENTOLAMINE

What is it?   An imidazole derivative

Describe the mechanism of action.   Reversibly blocks α_1 and α_2 receptors

How is this drug used clinically?   Because it has a half-life of only 4 hr, **phentolamine** is used for the short-term control of pheochromocytoma-induced hypertension.

What is the route of administration?   IV or IM—poorly absorbed orally

What are the adverse effects of phentolamine administration?   Orthostatic hypotension
Gastrointestinal stimulation, which may lead to peptic ulcers
Tachycardia, anginal pain, myocardial infarction, or effects due to reflex sympathetic response

β BLOCKERS

How are β blockers subclassified?   All of the β blockers are competitive antagonists; however, they can be subgrouped according to three major properties:
1. Selectivity of receptor blockade
2. Possession of intrinsic sympathomimetic activity
3. Capacity to block α-adrenergic receptors

β_1-SELECTIVE BLOCKERS

Name four β_1-selective blockers.
1. **Atenolol** (Tenormin)
2. **Esmolol** (Brevibloc)
3. **Acebutolol** (Sectral)
4. **Metoprolol** (Lopressor)

Is their β_1 selectivity absolute?

No. At high doses these drugs will block β_2 receptors.

What is the main advantage of β_1 selectivity?

These drugs are sometimes called cardioselective because they lack the unwanted bronchoconstrictive and hypoglycemic effects of nonselective blockers.

What clinical conditions warrant the use of cardioselective β blockers?

Atenolol—hypertension, myocardial infarction

Esmolol—Because of its very short duration of action (10 min), it is used when immediate β blockade is needed, as for thyroid storm. It is administered only IV.

Acebutolol—hypertension

Metoprolol—hypertension, anginal pain, myocardial infarction

NONSELECTIVE β-ADRENERGIC ANTAGONISTS

What is the prototype nonselective β blocker?

Propranolol (Inderal)

Name the pharmacologic actions of nonselective β blockers.

Decreased cardiac output and blood pressure

Reduction of sinus rate and conduction through the atria

Peripheral vasoconstriction

Bronchoconstriction

Decreased glycogenolysis and glucagon secretion

Increased VLDL and decreased HDL

How is propranolol absorbed?

This drug is almost completely absorbed after oral administration, but only approximately 25% reaches the systemic circulation because of first-pass metabolism.

What is the site of propranolol's metabolism?

The liver

In what clinical situations are nonselective β blockers indicated?

Hypertension
Angina, tachycardia
Arrhythmia
Thyroid storm
Acute panic syndrome
Migraine headaches

Name two other nonselective β-adrenergic antagonists.

Timolol (Blocadren) and **nadolol** (Corgard).

What are the clinical uses of these two drugs?

Similar to those of propranolol. Timolol also comes in an ophthalmic solution, which is used to treat glaucoma. See Table 9–1 for a summary of other key drugs used to treat glaucoma.

Table 9–1. Drugs Used in Glaucoma

Group, Drugs	Mechanism

Cholinometics
  Pilocarpine, carbachol,
  physostigmine, echothiophate
  (rarely used)
	Ciliary muscle contraction, opening of trabecular meshwork; increased outflow

α Agonists, nonselective
  Epinephrine, dipivefrin
  (rarely used)
	Increased outflow, probably via the uveoscleral veins

α$_2$-selective agonists Apraclonidine, brimonidine	Decreased aqueous secretion

β Blockers
  Timolol, betaxolol, carteolol,
  levobunolol, metipranolol
	Decreased aqueous secretion from the ciliary epithelium

Diuretics Acetazolamide, dorzolamide	Decreased aqueous secretion due to lack of HCO_3^- ion
Prostaglandin analogues Latanoprost	Increased uveoscleral outflow

Adapted with permission from Katzung BG (ed.). *Basic & Clinical Pharmacology*, 8th ed. New York: McGraw-Hill, 2001.

What are the adverse effects of nonselective β blockers?

Bradycardia, which could lead to congestive heart failure

Bronchoconstriction—can result in an asthmatic attack

May hide warning signs of hypoglycemia such as tachycardia; therefore, it is critical to monitor diabetics who are receiving β blockers.

Fatigue

Decreased glycogenolysis and glucagon secretion

Depression

Sexual dysfunction

How does this compare with cardioselective β₁ blockers?

Remember that cardioselective β_1 blockers lack the bronchoconstrictive and hypoglycemic effects of nonselective β blockers. The other side effects are common to both.

β BLOCKERS WITH INTRINSIC SYMPATHOMIMETIC ACTIVITY

Name two drugs that are classified as β blockers but also have some β-agonistic properties.

Acebutolol (Sectral) and **Pindolol** (Visken)

Why are these drugs considered to be partial agonists?

They very mildly stimulate both β_1- and β_2-adrenergic receptors. However, their intrinsic effects are not as strong as those of a full agonist, such as isoproterenol.

What are these two drugs used for?

Treatment of hypertension in patients prone to bradycardia

Are there any advantages to using these agents?

Acebutolol and pindolol produce bronchoconstriction only at extremely high doses. They do not induce bradycardia to the degree that full antagonists do, and they cause very minimal disruption of lipid and carbohydrate metabolism.

β BLOCKERS WITH α-BLOCKING CAPACITY

Labetalol (Normodyne)

What is this drug's mechanism of action?	Nonselective β-blockade along with α_1-adrenergic selective blockade, which results in peripheral vasodilation rather than the vasoconstriction that occurs with the other β blockers
What is the clinical use?	Treatment of hypertension and atrial fibrillation
What are the adverse effects?	Orthostatic hypotension and dizziness

Carvedilol (Coreg)

What is it?	A nonselective β blocker that also has α_1-blocking properties
List the clinical uses.	Treatment of hypertension Treatment of chronic CHF—Although it may seem paradoxical to use β blockers in the treatment of CHF, since they can also worsen symptoms, they appear to benefit the patient by reducing sympathetic activity. They may also improve diastolic dysfunction by prolonging diastolic filling time.
What are the mechanisms of action?	Reduction of sympathetic activity Improvement of diastolic dysfunction by prolonging diastolic filling time
What are the contraindications to use?	β blockers are contraindicated in the treatment of acute CHF or heart block. They are used only when the patient is hemodynamically stable

β_2-SELECTIVE BLOCKERS

Butoxamine

What is it?	A selective β_2-adrenergic antagonist
Does this drug have any clinical use?	No—not currently

NEW β-BLOCKING DRUGS

Are there many other β blockers?	Yes. New β blockers are produced yearly.
How do these new drugs differ from the β blockers discussed here?	Primarily in their pharmacokinetics
How can physicians recognize these new drugs?	By the **-olol** ending in their names
What are the indications and adverse effects of the new β blockers?	Generally they will be similar to those of other β blockers.

INDIRECT ADRENERGIC ANTAGONISTS

Why are guanethidine and reserpine considered indirect adrenergic antagonists?	Although they do not directly block α- or β-adrenergic receptors, they block the release of norepinephrine from nerve endings. They antagonize the effects of the sympathetic system.

GUANETHIDINE (Ismelin)

What is this drug's mechanism of action?	It enters the peripheral adrenergic nerve by a reuptake mechanism for norepinephrine and **binds to storage vesicles**, the action of which subsequently blocks the release of stored norepinephrine.
Does guanethidine have a clinical use?	Rarely for the treatment of hypertension

What are the adverse effects?	Orthostatic hypotension and sexual dysfunction

RESERPINE (Serpalan)

What is it?	A rauwolfia alkaloid
What is reserpine's mechanism of action?	It blocks norepinephrine **transport** from cytoplasm into intracellular storage vesicles. Subsequently, the neuron is not able to release any catecholamines.
How is this drug used clinically?	For treating hypertension (very rarely used)
What are the adverse effects?	CNS depression and bradycardia

Section III

Central Nervous System

10

Introduction to Central Nervous System Pharmacology

Name the major CNS neurotransmitters.

Acetylcholine
Norepinephrine
Dopamine
Serotonin
Gamma-aminobutyric acid (GABA)
Glycine
Glutamate

What types of receptors are most commonly found in the CNS?

Ion-gated receptors (Na^+, K^+, Cl^-, Ca^{2+})
Ligand-gated receptors (Figure 10-1)

What are the primary functions of a neurotransmitter?

To bind a receptor and subsequently either excite or inhibit the postsynaptic neuron

What are EPSPs?

Excitatory postsynaptic potentials—initiated when an excitatory neurotransmitter activates Na^+ or Ca^{2+} channels

Give five examples of excitatory neurotransmitters.

1. Norepinephrine
2. Dopamine
3. Acetylcholine
4. Glutamate
5. Aspartate

What are IPSPs?

Inhibitory postsynaptic potentials—initiated when an inhibitory neurotransmitter opens Cl^-, channels and the cell membrane becomes hyperpolarized. IPSPs make it more difficult for the neuron to become activated.

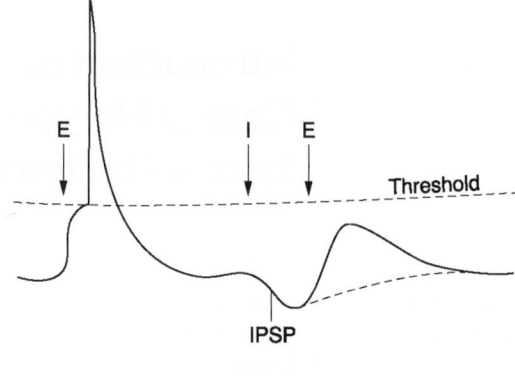

Figure 10–1. Interaction of excitatory and inhibitory synapses. On the left, a suprathreshold stimulus is given to an excitatory pathway (E). On the right, this same stimulus is given shortly after stimulating an inhibitory pathway (I), which prevents the excitatory potential from reaching threshold. (Redrawn with permission from Katzung BG. *Basic and Clinical Pharmacology,* 7th ed. Stamford, CT: Appleton & Lange, 1998, p. 345.)

Give two examples of inhibitory neurotransmitters.

1. Glycine
2. GABA

In general, how do drugs affecting the CNS work?

Most drugs will affect the production, storage, release, reuptake, or metabolism of a neurotransmitter. Other agents may directly affect the postsynaptic receptor.

What are the major differences between the autonomic nervous system and the central nervous system?

There are three major differences:
1. The number of neurotransmitters is greater in the CNS.
2. The number of synapses is greater in the CNS.
3. The CNS, unlike the autonomic nervous system, has a large array of inhibitory neurons that serve to modulate action.

11

Anxiolytics, Hypnotics, and Sedatives

Define anxiety.

An unpleasant emotional state consisting of apprehension, tension, and feelings of danger without a real or logical cause

What are some of the physical symptoms seen with anxiety?

Tachycardia
Tachypnea
Sweating
Trembling
Weakness

What are the major classes of drugs used to treat anxiety?

Benzodiazepines—the most frequently used drugs for anxiety
Azapirones— **buspirone**
Barbiturates—rarely used today because of severe side effects and a low therapeutic index. These drugs have generally been replaced by the benzodiazepines.

BENZODIAZEPINES

Give some examples of benzodiazepines and their approximate duration of action.

Short-Acting (2 to 8 hr):
Triazolam (Halcion)
Oxazepam (Serax)
Midazolam (Versed)
Clonazepam (Klonopin)
Intermediate-Acting (10 to 20 hr):
Temazepam (Restoril)
Lorazepam (Ativan)
Alprazolam (Xanax)

Long-Acting (1 to 3 days):
Chlordiazepoxide (Librium)
Diazepam (Valium)
Flurazepam (Dalmane)

What is GABA?

GABA (γ-aminobutyric acid) is the major inhibitory neurotransmitter of the CNS.

How do benzodiazepines work?

When benzodiazepines bind to specific receptors that are separate from but adjacent to the $GABA_A$ receptor, they potentiate the binding of GABA to its own receptor. The binding of GABA to its own receptor results in increased chloride ion conductance, cell membrane hyperpolarization, and decreased initiation of action potentials.
Remember that benzodiazepines do not bind to GABA receptors—they bind adjacent to them (Figure 11-1).

What are the therapeutic indications for benzodiazepines?

These drugs are used clinically as muscle relaxants and in the treatment of the following:
Anxiety disorders
Panic disorders—alprazolam is the drug of choice.
Status epilepticus—diazepam is the drug of choice.
Sleep disorders—flurazepam or temazepam.
Alcohol withdrawal—diazepam is most commonly used.

Are benzodiazepines effective for controlling pain as well as anxiety?

No. They have little analgesic effect.

What is their route of administration?

PO, IV, or IM

Where are benzodiazepines metabolized?

They are metabolized in the liver and excreted in the urine. Many of the benzodiazepines have active metabolites.

Receptor Empty (No Agonists)

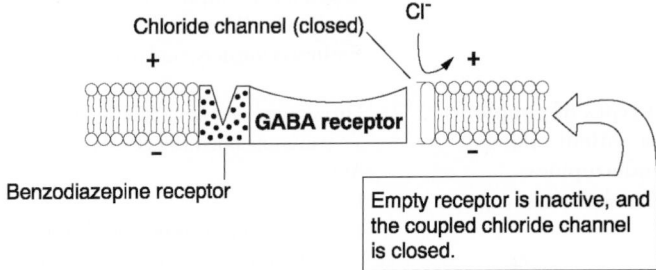

Receptor Binding GABA

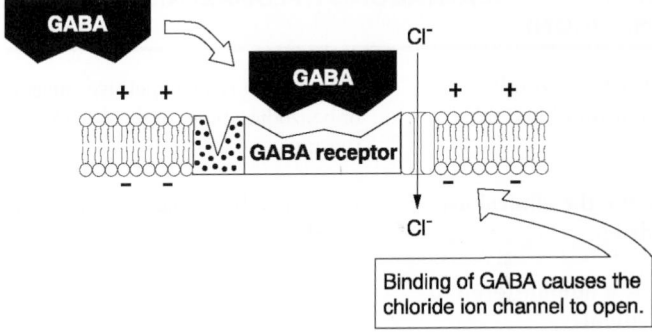

Receptor Binding GABA and Benzodiazepine

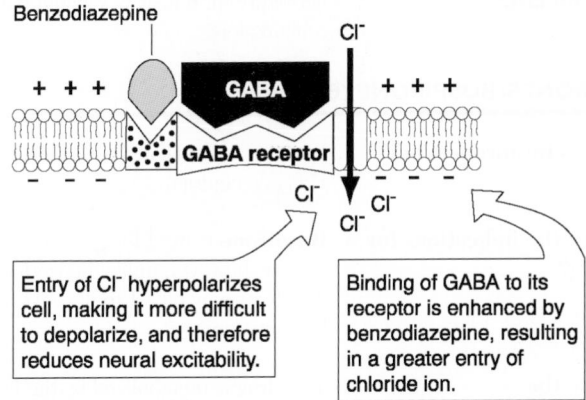

Figure 11–1. Schematic diagram of benzodiazepine-GABA-chloride ion channel complex. GABA = γ-aminobutyric acid. (Redrawn with permission from Mycek MJ, Harvey RA, Champe PC [Harvey RA, Champe PC, eds.]. *Lippincott's Illustrated Reviews: Pharmacology,* 2nd ed. Philadelphia: Lippincott-Raven Publishers, 1997, p. 91.)

Does dependence occur?

Yes. Prolonged use can result in dependence. Abrupt discontinuation can result in withdrawal symptoms, including confusion, anxiety, and agitation.

What types of symptoms may a patient taking benzodiazepines experience?

Drowsiness and confusion—the most common side effects

Ataxia

Dizziness

Respiratory depression and death if taken with other CNS depressants such as ethanol

BENZODIAZEPINE ANTAGONIST: FLUMAZENIL (ROMAZICON)

What is flumazenil's mechanism of action?

Flumazenil is a competitive antagonist of benzodiazepines at the $GABA_A$ receptor.

Describe the clinical use of this drug.

Reversal of benzodiazepine sedation or overdose

How is it administered to the patient?

IV use only

How long do the effects of flumazenil last?

Only 1 hr—Repeat doses may be necessary for a heavily sedated patient to remain alert.

AZAPIRONES: BUSPIRONE (BuSpar)

How does buspirone work?

It acts as a partial agonist at serotonin (5-HT_{1A}) receptors.

What are the indications for this drug?

Buspirone is used for generalized anxiety; however, unlike benzodiazepines, its effects may take 1 to 2 weeks to become apparent.

What are the pharmacokinetic properties of buspirone?

This drug is metabolized by the liver and excreted in the urine; its half-life is 2 to 11 hr.

How do the actions of buspirone differ from those of the benzodiazepines?

Buspirone lacks the muscle relaxant and anticonvulsant properties of the benzodiazepines.

What advantages does buspirone have over benzodiazepines?

Minimal sedation
Low abuse potential
No overdose fatalities reported
No withdrawal symptoms

What toxic effects are associated with buspirone?

Headache, nausea, dizziness

BARBITURATES

Give four examples of barbiturates and their duration of action.

1. **Phenobarbital** (Luminal) —long-acting/1–2 days.
2. **Pentobarbital** (Nembutal)—short-acting/2–8 hours.
3. **Amobarbital** (Amytal)—short-acting
4. **Thiopental** (Pentothal)—ultra–short-acting/10–20 minutes.

How do these drugs work?

Like benzodiazepines, barbiturates increase the duration of GABA action on Cl- entry into the cell, which results in membrane hyperpolarization and a decrease in neuron excitability. Barbiturates do not, however, bind to benzodiazepine receptors.

What are the therapeutic indications for barbiturate administration?

Induction of anesthesia—thiopental
Anticonvulsants—phenobarbital
Anxiety—rarely

Why are benzodiazepines favored over barbiturates for the treatment of anxiety?

Benzodiazepines have a much higher therapeutic index, cause less physiological dependence, and do not induce hepatic enzymes (Figure 11-2).

By what routes can barbiturates be administered?

IV, PO, or IM

What are the pharmacokinetic properties of barbiturates?

They are metabolized in the liver and excreted in the urine.

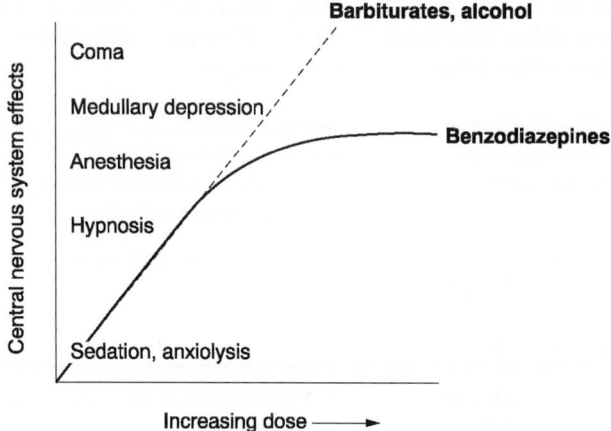

Figure 11–2. Comparison of dose-response relationships of benzodiazepines and barbiturates. (Redrawn with permission from Gallia G, Hann CL, Hewson WH. *The Pharmacology Companion.* Ann Arbor, Michigan: Alert & Oriented Publishing Company, 1997, p. 33, Fig. 3.1.)

What determines the duration of action of thiopental?	Redistribution to the other tissues
Does barbiturate dependency occur?	Yes. Abrupt cessation can lead to severe withdrawal symptoms (tremor, restlessness, nausea, seizures, and cardiac arrest).
For whom are barbiturates contraindicated?	For patients who have acute intermittent porphyria, because they increase porphyrin synthesis
What are the adverse effects of these drugs?	Drowsiness and decreased motor control Induction of the P-450 system, which can therefore decrease the effect of other drugs metabolized by these enzymes Addiction In high doses, respiratory depression and coma Allergic reactions, especially in patients with asthma

OTHER SEDATIVES

ZOLPIDEM (Ambien)

Describe this drug's clinical use.	Treatment of insomnia
What are its adverse effects?	Ataxia, nightmares, headache and confusion

CHLORAL HYDRATE

What are its clinical uses?	Hypnosis Sedation (in children)
Describe this drug's adverse effects.	Gastrointestinal distress Unpleasant taste

ALCOHOL

See *Chapter 18—Alcohol and Other Drugs of Abuse.*

12

Antipsychotics

What are antipsychotic drugs?

Antipsychotics, also known as neuroleptics, are drugs used primarily to treat psychotic states such as schizophrenia, delusional disorder, and other hallucinatory states.

What is their mechanism of action?

Antipsychotics block various receptors including cholinergic, adrenergic, serotoninergic, muscarinic, and histamine receptors. However, their antipsychotic actions are primarily thought to be due to blocking of **dopamine receptors** in the central nervous system, particularly the D_2 receptors in the mesocortical and mesolimbal systems of the brain.

Do antipsychotic agents differ in potency?

Yes—a drug's potency parallels its affinity for D_2 receptors. **Haloperidol** and **thiothixene** are high-potency drugs because they have high affinity for the D_2 receptors, whereas **chlorpromazine** and **thioridazine** are low-potency drugs because they have low affinity for D_2 receptors.

Do antipsychotics differ in efficacy?

No. The traditional antipsychotics are all considered to be equivalent in efficacy.

How are antipsychotics usually administered?

In most cases these drugs are given orally; they can be given intramuscularly if the patient is noncompliant.

Describe the absorption and metabolism of the traditional antipsychotics.

They are variably absorbed orally but they pass into the brain easily and have a large volume of distribution. Metabolism occurs by the cytochrome P-450 system in the liver.

What is the onset of action?   Antipsychotics may not become effective for several weeks to months. However, sedation and other side effects can occur rapidly.

Can these drugs cure illnesses such as schizophrenia?   No! Antipsychotics only reduce the symptoms of the illness; they cannot cure the illness.

How are the antipsychotics classified?   Classification is based on structural differences. The major classes include phenothiazines, butyrophenones, dibenzoxazepines, thioxanthines, and benzisoxazoles.

TRADITIONAL ANTIPSYCHOTICS

PHENOTHIAZINES

What are some examples of phenothiazines?
Chlorpromazine (Thorazine)—prototype
Fluphenazine (Prolixin)
Trifluoperazine (Stelazine)
Thioridazine (Mellaril)
Perphenazine (Trilafon)

What distinctive side effects does thioridazine cause?
Pigmentary retinopathy
May cause cardiac arrhythmias and conduction block

BUTYROPHENONES

Name two drugs in this class.
Haloperidol (Haldol)
Droperidol (Inapsine)

Other than psychotic states, for what can haloperidol be used?
Tourette's syndrome
Huntington's disease
Phencyclidine overdose—drug of choice

What type of side effect is especially pronounced with haloperidol?
Extrapyramidal side effects (✎ common board question)

DIBENZOXAZEPINES

Name a drug that belongs to this class.	*Loxapine* (Loxitane)

THIOXANTHENES

Name a drug that belongs to this class.	*Thiothixene* (Navane)

CLINICAL USES AND SIDE EFFECTS

What are the clinical applications of traditional antipsychotic agents?

Traditional neuroleptics have several therapeutic uses, but the most important to remember are:

Treatment of any agitated or psychotic state, such as bipolar disease or schizophrenia (These agents are especially effective for the positive symptoms of schizophrenia, such as delusions, thought disorders, and hallucinations.)

Antiemetic therapy—phenothiazines with the exception of **thioridazine**

Treatment of Tourette's syndrome— haloperidol

Treatment of intractable hiccups— chlorpromazine

Antipruritic therapy—promethazine (because of histamine blockade)

What is an easy way to remember the side effects of the traditional antipsychotics?

With a few exceptions, all of the traditional antipsychotics have similar toxicities—namely, sedation, extrapyramidal effects, anticholinergic effects, and α-adrenergic effects (hypotension).

Do all traditional antipsychotics produce the same degree of each type of side effect?

No. The severity of each adverse effect varies among the classes of antipsychotic drugs. For example, high-potency drugs such as **haloperidol** and **fluphenazine** produce the greatest extrapyramidal effects, and low-potency drugs such as thioridazine and chlorpromazine produce the greatest anticholinergic effects (Table 12–1).

Table 12–1. Side-Effect Profiles of Neuroleptic Drugs

Potency	Drug	Side Effects			
		Sedation	Extrapyramidal Effects	Anticholinergic Effects	α-Adrenergic Effects
HIGH	Haloperidol	1	4	1	1
	Fluphenazine	1	4	2	1
	Thiothixene	2	3	2	1
	Trifluoperazine	2	3	2	1
	Loxapine	2	2	2	2
	Chlorpromazine	4	2	3	4
LOW	Thioridazine	4	1	4	4

1 = low, 4 = high

Describe the toxicities of traditional antipsychotic agents.

CNS sedation—seen markedly with the phenothiazines

Endocrine alteration—galactorrhea, amenorrhea, and infertility, likely due to blockade of dopamine release from the pituitary

Anticholinergic effects—dry mouth, constipation, urinary retention, and blurry vision

Antiadrenergic effects—watch for light-headedness and orthostatic hypotension secondary to α-adrenergic blockade. Phenothiazines can cause sexual dysfunction (failure to ejaculate).

Extrapyramidal side effects—akathisia (motor restlessness), parkinsonian syndrome (bradykinic rigidity, tremor), acute dystonic reactions, neuroleptic malignant syndrome, and tardive dyskinesia (✎ common board question)

What is tardive dyskinesia?

Tardive dyskinesia is a symptom that may occur after prolonged therapy with neuroleptics (4 months to 1 year). It is characterized by rhythmic involuntary movements of the tongue, lips, or jaw. Patients may also demonstrate puckering of the mouth or even chewing movements.

Is tardive dyskinesia reversible?

There is no known treatment for established cases of tardive dyskinesia. The syndrome may remit partially or completely if neuroleptic treatment is withdrawn, although in many cases it is irreversible. Anticholinergic agents actually increase the severity of tardive dyskinesia.

What is an acute dystonic reaction?

Prolonged muscle spasms of tongue, neck, or face

How are acute dystonic reactions treated?	Patients are given **diphenhydramine** (Benadryl) or an injection of **benztropine**.
What is neuroleptic malignant syndrome?	Patients who receive neuroleptics for long-term treatment may experience rigidity, altered mental status, cardiac arrhythmias, hypertension, and life-threatening hyperpyrexia.
What is the therapy for neuroleptic malignant syndrome?	This disorder is treated with **dantrolene**, a skeletal muscle relaxant (✎ common board question).

ATYPICAL ANTIPSYCHOTIC DRUGS

Name six examples of atypical antipsychotic drugs.	1. *Clozapine* (Clozaril) 2. *Risperidone* (Risperdal) 3. *Olanzapine* (Zyprexa) 4. *Aripiprazole* (Abilify) 5. *Quetiapine* (Seroquel) 6. *Ziprasidone* (Geodon)
Why are these drugs considered "atypical"?	They are newer and in addition to blocking dopamine receptors, atypical antipsychotics also produce significant therapeutic effects through the blockade of serotonin ($5\text{-}HT_2$) receptors. They are also rarely associated with extrapyramidal side effects.
Are they more effective than traditional antipsychotics?	Most physicians consider them a better choice for therapy because of their decreased side effects.
Describe the actions of clozapine.	This agent is a dibenzodiazepine derivative. It differs from traditional antipsychotics in its potent blockade of serotonin ($5\text{-}HT_2$) receptors, along with the usual dopamine blockade.
What is it used for?	Clozapine has been effective in treating cases of schizophrenia that are refractory to other neuroleptic drugs. It is especially effective in treating the **negative symptoms** of schizophrenia (blunted emotion, withdrawal, reduced ability to form relationships).

What are the side effects?

Clozapine causes fewer extrapyramidal side effects than traditional neuroleptics. **Clozapine** does cause seizures and a very dangerous **agranulocytosis** in 1% to 2% of patients (✎ common board question). Weekly blood tests are required for patients receiving clozapine therapy. Although weight gain can occur with extended treatment of most antipsychotics, it is especially prominent with clozapine. This can lead to hypertension and other diseases.

Describe the actions of risperidone.

Risperidone (Risperdal) is a benzisoxazole drug that, like clozapine, has a very high affinity for 5-HT_2 receptors. It also has antidopaminergic (D_2) activity. However, **risperidone** exhibits no anticholinergic effects and diminished extrapyramidal effects. **Risperidone** is a first-line agent for the treatment of schizophrenia, since it is effective for both the positive and negative symptoms of the disease. The drug is also known to prolong QT intervals and therefore should be used with caution in patients who have abnormal QT intervals.

Describe the actions of olanzapine.

Like **risperidone** and **clozapine**, **olanzapine** blocks both dopamine and serotonin receptors. Effective in the treatment of both positive and negative symptoms of schizophrenia, depression, or obsessive-compulsive disorder (OCD), it can produce anticholinergic effects and orthostatic hypotension. Also causes significant weight gain.

Describe the actions of aripiprazole, quetiapine, and ziprasidone.

These three drugs are the newer atypical antipsychotics. They cause very little extrapyramidal side effects. Aripiprazole is unique in that it is the only drug that is a partial agonist at D_2 receptors.

13   Drugs Used to Treat Depression and Mania

ANTIDEPRESSANTS

What is depression?

An affective syndrome characterized by intense sadness, general loss of interest in the everyday aspects of life, insomnia, changes in appetite, and low self-esteem.

What does the biogenic amine theory of depression propose?

That depression is due to a deficiency of norepinephrine, serotonin, and dopamine in the synapses of the CNS.

List the major categories of antidepressants.

Tricyclics
Selective serotonin reuptake inhibitors (SSRIs)
Monamine oxidase inhibitors (MAOIs)
Heterocyclics (atypical antidepressants)

Which of these agents are now considered first-line treatment for depression?

SSRIs
Heterocyclics

TRICYCLICS

Give some examples of tricyclic antidepressants.

Tertiary Amine Tricyclics
Amitriptyline (Elavil)—prototype
Imipramine (Tofranil)—prototype
Doxepin (Sinequan)
Clomipramine (Anafranil)
Trimipramine (Surmontil)

Secondary Amine Tricyclics
Amoxapine (Asendin)
Maprotiline (Ludiomil)
Protriptyline (Vivactil)

Desipramine(Norpramin)
Nortriptyline (Pamelor, Aventyl)

What are the physiological differences between tertiary amine and secondary amine tricyclics?

The secondary amine tricyclics in general are less likely to cause sedation, hypotension, and anticholinergic effects. However, they are more likely to induce psychosis.

What is the mechanism of action of all the tricyclics?

These drugs are thought to increase levels of norepinephrine and serotonin in the synaptic cleft by blocking reuptake. They also block histamine, cholinergic, and α-adrenergic receptors, which accounts for a large proportion of their side effects. Tricyclics are also thought to cause a down-regulation of monoamine receptors; this may account for some of their therapeutic benefit.

Do these drugs elevate mood in normal individuals?

No. These drugs are not CNS stimulants.

What are the clinical indications for tricyclics?

Mood disorders (depression primarily)
Panic disorder
Generalized anxiety disorder
Posttraumatic stress disorder
Obsessive-compulsive disorder
    (**clomipramine**)
Pain disorders
Enuresis in children (**imipramine**)
    causes contraction of the internal
    sphincter of the bladder.

How are tricyclics administered?

They are well absorbed orally and penetrate into the CNS easily.

How are these drugs metabolized?

They undergo significant first-pass metabolism in the liver; they are conjugated with glucuronic acid and excreted through the kidneys.

Which of the tricyclics are most efficacious?

All are equally efficacious.

When should a physician expect to see a change in the patient's mood?

Although the uptake mechanism is inhibited almost immediately, antidepressant clinical effects may require 2 to 8 weeks to become apparent. This suggests that their mechanism of action is not completely understood.

What are the signs and symptoms of tricyclic toxicity?

Anticholinergic side effects—blurred vision; dilated pupils; hot, dry skin; constipation; confusion, especially in the elderly; urinary retention

Autonomic effects—orthostatic hypotension secondary to α-adrenergic blockade. This leads to reflex tachycardia.

ECG changes—widening of the QRS complex, arrhythmias

Lowering of the seizure threshold

Weight gain

Sedation due to histamine blockade

Watch for the "Three C's of TriCyclic Toxicity: **C**holinergic blockade, **C**ardiac arrhythmias, **C**onvulsions

Can tricyclics and MAOIs be given together for added benefit?

No! This combination can lead to severe convulsions and coma.

SELECTIVE SEROTONIN REUPTAKE INHIBITORS (SSRI)

Give some examples of SSRIs.

Fluoxetine (Prozac)—prototype
Sertraline (Zoloft)
Paroxetine (Paxil)
Fluvoxamine (Luvox)
Citalopram (Celexa)
Escitalopram (Lexapro)

What is their mechanism of action?

Inhibition of serotonin reuptake without significant effects on norepinephrine, muscarinic, histaminic, or α-adrenergic receptors.

Which one is the most effective?

Different patients may respond better to one drug over another, but no drug in this class has been shown to be superior in all patients.

When would these drugs be indicated?

Clinical depression is the primary reason for prescribing these drugs. They are also used to treat obsessive-compulsive disorder (fluvoxamine) and anxiety.

How are SSRIs administered?

Orally

How are they metabolized?

By the cytochrome P-450 system. Fluoxetine and paroxetine are potent P-450 inhibitors. Therefore plasma levels of other coadministered drugs that are metabolized through the cytochrome P-450 system may rise to dangerous levels.

Describe the side-effect profile of SSRIs.

In general SSRIs have fewer side effects (anticholinergic, antihistaminic, α-adrenergic blockade) than other classes of antidepressants.

What adverse symptoms may a patient taking SSRIs experience?

Nausea
Diarrhea
Nervousness
Sleep disturbances
Dizziness
Sexual dysfunction (impotence and decreased libido)

When are SSRIs contraindicated?

SSRIs are contraindicated in combination therapy with MAOIs because this combination may result in the **"serotonin syndrome,"** characterized by hyperthermia, muscle rigidity, myoclonus, and rapid changes in mental status.

MONOAMINE OXIDASE INHIBITORS (MAOIs)

What is monoamine oxidase?

MAO is a mitochondrial enzyme that is involved in the metabolism of catecholamine neurotransmitters.

Where are the highest concentrations of this enzyme?

In the liver, GI tract, and CNS

Name four MAOIs.

Tranylcypromine (Parnate)
Phenelzine (Nardil)
Isocarboxazid (Marplan)
Selegiline (Deprenyl)

Describe the mechanism of action of the MAOIs.

Two types of MAO exist: MAO-A and MAO-B.

Within the neurons, MAO-A is responsible for the inactivation of any serotonin or norepinephrine that may leak out of presynaptic storage vesicles. When MAO-A is blocked, these neurotransmitters accumulate in the vesicles and are released into the synapse.

MAO-B is responsible for the metabolism of dopamine and works in a similar manner. In general, the MAOIs except for selegiline—which is a specific inhibitor of MAO-B—are nonspecific inhibitors of MAO.

What are the MAOIs indicated for?

Treatment of atypical depression (with phobia or psychotic features). Other classes of antidepressants are more frequently used today because they have fewer toxic effects.

Describe the pharmacological properties of MAOIs.

They are well absorbed orally.

They are metabolized by acetylation in the liver (half-life, 2 to 3 hr).

They require 2 to 4 weeks of treatment to reach a steady-state plasma level.

What are the adverse effects of MAOIs?

Hypertensive crisis (headache, hypertension, arrhythmias, and possibly stroke) if the patient does not avoid eating foods high in tyramine which is normally inactivated by MAO. At increased levels, tyramine will release catecholamines from storage vesicles and therefore will act as a pressor agent. Hypertensive crisis can also occur when MAOIs are administered with **meperidine** (Demerol).

Orthostatic hypotension

Agitation, seizure
Dry mouth, blurred vision
Weight gain

**When are MAOIs
contraindicated?**

They should not be coadministered with
SSRIs or β agonists.

HETEROCYCLIC (ATYPICAL) ANTIDEPRESSANTS

**What is a heterocyclic
antidepressant?**

The drugs included in this class of
antidepressants are varied in organic
structure and mechanism of action. These
drugs are also known as *atypical
antidepressants* because they vary in
structure and sites of action. Heterocyclics
or atypicals are further divided into so-
called second- and third-generation drugs.
Tricyclics are considered to be the original
first-generation drugs.

**Give two examples of
second-generation
heterocyclic antidepressants.**

*Trazodone (Desyrel)
Bupropion (Wellbutrin)*

Trazodone

What is it?

An antidepressant similar in structure to
the benzodiazepine **alprazolam** (Xanax)
but more specific for the inhibition of
serotonin reuptake

**When is trazodone
indicated?**

To treat depression. It is particularly
effective for improving sleep.

**Where is this drug
metabolized?**

In the liver (excreted by the kidneys)

**Describe the adverse
effects.**

Sedation
Orthostatic hypotension
Nausea
Headache and dizziness
Agitation
Rarely priapism

Bupropion

**Describe this drug's
mechanism of action.**

This is not clearly known, but it is
thought to work through dopaminergic
and noradrenergic systems.

What are the indications for bupropion?	Clinical depression; also used for smoking cessation
What toxicities are associated with bupropion?	Headache, Nausea, dry mouth Tachycardia, Restlessness
What is the advantage of using bupropion?	There are no side effects related to sexual dysfunction, such as those that occur with SSRIs.
Which drugs are considered to be third-generation heterocyclics?	*Venlafaxine (Effexor)* *Nefazodone (Serzone)* *Mirtazapine (Remeron)*
How do these drugs work?	**Venlafaxine** and **nefazodone**: block the reuptake of both serotonin and norepinephrine. **Mirtazapine**: A potent inhibitor of presynaptic alpha$_2$ adrenoreceptors, which are involved in the feedback mechanism. This results in an increase of amine release from nerve endings. **Mirtazapine** also antagonizes serotonergic 5HT$_2$ and 5HT$_3$ receptors.
What are the side effects of these drugs?	**Venlfaxine:** nausea, anxiety, sustained increase in blood pressure, headache **Nefazodone:** dry mouth, nausea, sedation, liver impairment **Mirtazapine:** sedation, weight gain and increased serum cholesterol

ANTIMANIC AGENTS

What is mania?	Elevated mood with grandiose ideas, expansiveness, pressured speech, flight of ideas, decreased sleep, and increased activity
In what conditions is mania seen?	Affective disorders such as bipolar disorder
Give some examples of antimanic agents.	**Lithium**—drug of choice Anticonvulsants (**valproic acid** and **carbamazepine**)—See *Chapter 14— Anticonvulsants,* for further discussion of anticonvulsants.

LITHIUM

What is it?	A light alkali metal available in carbonate, slow-release, and controlled-release forms
How does lithium work?	The mechanism is unclear; it is thought to block the enzyme inositol-1-phosphatase, which affects neurotransmitters.
What is lithium's major indication?	It is primarily used in bipolar disorder—both manic and depressive episodes respond.
Describe some other uses.	This drug is also used as an adjuvant with antidepressants to treat major depression and with antipsychotics to treat schizophrenia.
What are the pharmacokinetic properties of lithium?	It is well absorbed orally and excreted in the urine.
When is lithium contraindicated?	Pregnancy—it is teratogenic.
What adverse effects should physicians watch for when administering lithium?	Acute intoxication—severe tremor, ataxia, seizures, confusion, and coma Nephrogenic diabetes insipidus Weight gain, vomiting, abdominal cramps, and diarrhea Disturbances in thyroid function (Monitor TSH for **lithium**-induced hypothyroidism.) Depression of T wave on ECG Leukocytosis
What substances affect lithium plasma levels?	Excessive intake of sodium lowers **lithium** levels Thiazide diuretics increase plasma levels of the drug.
How is lithium toxicity treated?	Overdoses are cleared by diuretics. As previously mentioned, *do not use thiazides* because they increase plasma levels of the drug. Use sodium bicarbonate or dialysis if necessary.

14   Anticonvulsants

What is a seizure?

An abnormal, synchronized electrical depolarization of neurons in the central nervous system

Name five major causes of seizures.

1. Idiopathic
2. CNS infections
3. Fever
4. Metabolic defects
5. Cerebral trauma

List the different types of seizures.

Partial (simple and complex)
Generalized tonic-clonic
Status epilepticus
Absence
Febrile
Myoclonic

What is a partial (focal) seizure?

A seizure in which abnormal discharges occur from a focal area within the brain. There are two types of partial seizures: simple and complex.

What are the characteristics of a simple partial seizure?

A simple partial seizure involves a focal neurological symptom that can be sensory (for example, auditory or visual hallucinations), motor, or psychomotor. Consciousness is always retained.

What happens in a complex partial seizure?

The initial focus of abnormal discharge spreads, so that the patient experiences loss of consciousness and postictal (postseizure) confusion. Symptoms can include coordinated motor activity, mental distortion, and sensory hallucinations.

Where do complex partial seizures originate?

The majority originate in the temporal lobe.

What part of the brain is involved in a generalized tonic-clonic (grand mal) seizure?

The entire cerebral cortex

Name and describe the typical phases of a grand mal seizure.

Tonic phase—loss of consciousness, rigidity, loss of bowel and bladder control

Clonic phase—jerking movements of the entire body

Can a partial seizure progress into a grand mal seizure?

Yes. This is known as partial seizure with secondary generalization.

What is status epilepticus?

Continuous seizures not separated by any periods of regained consciousness. This condition is a medical emergency.

What are the characteristics of absence (petit mal) seizures?

They usually occur in children 2 to 12 years of age.

They are characterized by a very brief few seconds loss of consciousness. The child will stop whatever he or she is doing and stare or have some facial twitching.

Following the attack, the child immediately becomes alert and is seldom even aware that it has occurred.

What are the characteristics of febrile seizures?

They occur in children.

They usually last less than 10 min.

The child has a fever, but there is no apparent infection or other defined cause for the seizure.

What are the characteristics of myoclonic seizures?

They are sudden, short episodes of either local or generalized muscle contractions.

They can occur at any age.

They are associated with a variety of rare hereditary neurodegenerative disorders.

Define epilepsy.

Epilepsy is a group of chronic syndromes characterized by recurrent seizures with periods of consciousness.

What percentage of the population is affected by epilepsy?

About 1%

What are the major pharmacological treatment options for seizures?

Phenytoin
Carbamazepine/oxcarbazepine
Phenobarbital
Primidone
Valproic acid
Topiramate
Ethosuximide
Benzodiazepines
Tiagabine
Vigabatrin
Gabapentin
Lamotrigine
Zonisamide (See Figure 14-1).

PHENYTOIN (DILANTIN)

What are the therapeutic uses of phenytoin?

Phenytoin is effective in treating tonic-clonic seizures and partial seizures but not absence seizures. It is also used in the treatment of status epilepticus after the preliminary administration of **diazepam**.

What is the mechanism of action?

Phenytoin binds to Na^+ channels and prolongs their inactivated state.

Describe the absorption and metabolism of this drug.

Oral absorption is slow. **Phenytoin** undergoes hydroxylation by the hepatic cytochrome P450 system. At high doses, the hydroxylation system becomes saturated; it is therefore important to watch for toxicity.

What are the toxic effects?

Gingival hyperplasia
Diplopia, nystagmus
Megaloblastic anemia secondary to
    interference with folate metabolism

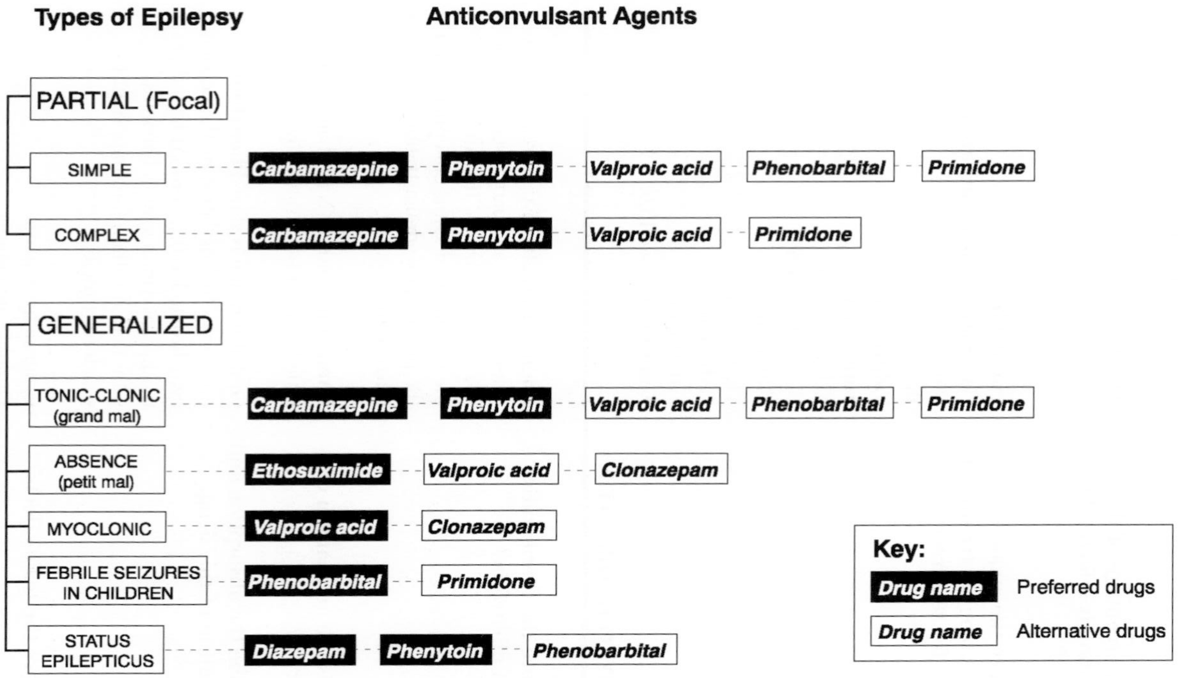

Types of Epilepsy

Anticonvulsant Agents

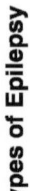

PARTIAL (Focal)

| SIMPLE | Carbamazepine | Phenytoin | Valproic acid | Phenobarbital | Primidone |
| COMPLEX | Carbamazepine | Phenytoin | Valproic acid | Primidone |

GENERALIZED

TONIC-CLONIC (grand mal)	Carbamazepine	Phenytoin	Valproic acid	Phenobarbital	Primidone
ABSENCE (petit mal)	Ethosuximide	Valproic acid	Clonazepam
MYOCLONIC	Valproic acid	Clonazepam
FEBRILE SEIZURES IN CHILDREN	Phenobarbital	Primidone
STATUS EPILEPTICUS	Diazepam	Phenytoin	Phenobarbital

Key:

| **Drug name** | Preferred drugs |
| Drug name | Alternative drugs |

Figure 14–1. Therapeutic indications for anticonvulsant agents. (Adapted and redrawn with permission from Howland RD, Mycek MJ [Harvey RA, Champe PC, eds.]. *Lippincott's Illustrated Reviews: Pharmacology,* 3rd ed. Baltimore: Lippincott Williams & Wilkins, 2006, p. 172.)

Hirsutism

Diminished deep tendon reflexes in the extremities

CNS depression

Endocrine disturbances—diabetes insipidus, hyperglycemia, glycosuria, osteomalacia

Name three drugs that increase the plasma concentration of phenytoin.

1. **Chloramphenicol**
2. **Isoniazid**
3. **Cimetidine**

Name one drug that is well known to decrease the plasma concentrations of phenytoin.

Carbamazepine

Is phenytoin teratogenic?

Yes. It produces fetal hydantoin syndrome, which is characterized by prenatal growth deficiency and mental deficiencies. There is also an increased incidence of congenital malformations, such as cleft palate and heart malformations.

CARBAMAZEPINE (TEGRETOL)/OXCARBAZEPINE (TRILEPTAL)

What is the therapeutic use of carbamazepine?

It is the drug of choice for treating partial and tonic-clonic seizures. It is also the drug of choice for treating trigeminal neuralgia.

What is its mechanism of action?

It prolongs the inactivated state of Na^+ channels.

What are the absorption and metabolism of this drug?

Carbamazepine is absorbed slowly when given orally and is metabolized by the P-450 system.

Which drugs inhibit the metabolism of carbamazepine?

Erythromycin
Isoniazid
Propoxyphene
Verapamil
Cimetidine

What are carbamazepine's adverse effects?

Acute intoxication can lead to respiratory depression, stupor, or coma.

Severe liver toxicity. Patients need frequent liver function tests while receiving this drug.

Aplastic anemia

Agranulocytosis

Patients frequently complain of drowsiness, ataxia, nystagmus, and vomiting.

How does oxcarbazepine differ from carbamazepine?

Oxcarbazepine has a slightly different chemical structure than carbamazepine, which helps minimize its side effects. **Oxcarbazepine** also does not induce the cytochrome P-450 system as much as carbamazepine. It does, however, have a mechanism of action and antiepileptic activity similar to those of carbamazepine.

PHENOBARBITAL (LUMINAL)

What is the classification of this drug?

It is a barbiturate.

State its mechanism of action.

Potentiation of GABA-mediated synaptic inhibition. The mechanism of action is not completely clear, but it is thought to prolong the opening of Cl^- ion channels.

What are phenobarbital's therapeutic uses?

1. It is the drug of choice for treating febrile seizures; it is also used to treat grand mal seizures in children.
2. It is good for treating partial seizures and tonic-clonic seizures; however, its sedative effects have reduced its use as a primary agent.

How is phenobarbital absorbed and metabolized?

The drug is well absorbed orally; 75% of it is metabolized in the liver. It is a potent inducer of the cytochrome P-450 system. The metabolic by-products are excreted in the urine.

State phenobarbital's adverse effects.

Sedation
Nystagmus
Psychotic reactions
Hypersensitivity reactions—Stevens-
    Johnson syndrome

PRIMIDONE (MYSOLINE)

What drug is primidone structurally related to?

It is related to **phenobarbital** and it works the same way as **phenobarbital**.

When is this drug used?

Primidone is an alternative choice for adults who have partial seizures (both simple and complex) and generalized tonic-clonic seizures.

How is this drug metabolized?

Primidone is converted to phenylethyl-malonamide (PEMA) and to **phenobarbital** in the liver.

What are its adverse effects?

This drug's toxic effects are very similar to those of **phenobarbital**:
Sedation
Ataxia
Nausea
Vomiting
Drowsiness

VALPROIC ACID (DEPAKENE)

What are the indications for use of this drug?

Valproic acid is the most effective agent for treating myoclonic seizures. It is also used in the treatment of absence seizures.

How does this drug work?

It prolongs the inactivated state of Na^+ channels. It may also increase GABA concentrations in the brain.

What is the route of administration?

Valproic acid is well absorbed orally. Once absorbed, approximately 90% of the drug is bound to plasma proteins.

How is it metabolized?	The drug is extensively metabolized in the liver by the cytochrome P-450 system. However, it does not induce the enzymes of this system, as do **carbamazepine** and **phenytoin**. Approximately 3% of the drug is excreted unchanged.
Does valproic acid block the metabolism of other drugs?	Yes. It can increase the plasma levels of other drugs such as **phenobarbital** or **phenytoin**.
What side effects should you watch for when administering valproic acid?	Hepatotoxicity. This drug may cause a fulminant hepatitis, which can be fatal. Therefore liver enzymes should be monitored. GI distress; nausea and vomiting Sedation Tremor
Should pregnant women be given valproic acid?	No! The incidence of neural tube defects is very high if this drug is taken during the first trimester of pregnancy.

TOPIRAMATE (TOPAMAX)

How does this drug work?	**Topiramate** has several sites of action. It blocks glutamate receptors and Na+ channels. It also potentiates the action of GABA.
When should topiramate be prescribed?	As an adjuvant in the treatment of partial or generalized tonic-clonic seizures
How toxic is topiramate?	Generally the side affects are mild. They include fatigue, ataxia, and dizziness. Renal stones have also been reported. Pregnant women, however, should not use topiramate because of its teratogenic nature.

ETHOSUXIMIDE (ZARONTIN)

What is this drug used for?	**Ethosuximide** is the drug of choice for treating absence seizures.
What is its mechanism of action?	**Ethosuximide** inhibits Ca^{2+} influx through T-type channels in the thalamic neurons.
How is this drug absorbed and metabolized?	It is well absorbed orally. The majority of the drug is metabolized by the cytochrome P-450 system in the liver. It does not induce P-450 enzyme synthesis.
State the toxic effects.	Dizziness Agitation GI distress Confusion Blood dyscrasias such as leukopenia, aplastic anemia, and thrombocytopenia may occur in extremely sensitive patients. Skin reactions such as Stevens-Johnson syndrome have also been reported.

BENZODIAZEPINES

See *Chapter 11—Anxiolytics, Hypnotics, and Sedatives,* for further details about benzodiazepines.

Give three examples of benzodiazepines that are used for antiepileptic purposes.	1. **Diazepam** (Valium) 2. **Clonazepam** (Klonopin) 3. **Clorazepate** (Tranxene)
What is the therapeutic use of these drugs?	Intravenous diazepam is the drug of choice for initiating treatment of status epilepticus. **Clonazepam** can be used for treating myoclonic or absence seizures in children. **Clorazepate** may be used for partial seizures in combination with other drugs.

State the adverse effects of benzodiazepines.	The benzodiazepines, when used correctly, have relatively minor side effects, but you should watch for the following: Drowsiness Respiratory depression Cardiac depression

TIAGABINE (GABITRIL)

When would you use this drug?	For the treatment of partial seizures with or without secondary generalization
How does it work?	Increases GABA concentrations in the synapse by blocking GABA reuptake
What are the side effects to watch for?	Dizziness GI upset Tremor

LEVETIRACETAM (KEPPRA)

How does this drug work?	Its mechanism of action is unclear. No evidence has emerged that it works on either voltage gated channels or GABA receptors.
When would you use this drug?	As an adjuvant for partial seizures. It does not interact with other seizure medications and therefore is a good choice for combination therapy.
What adverse effects does it have?	The most common effects include drowsiness, asthenia, and dizziness.

GABAPENTIN (NEURONTIN)

State the therapeutic use of this drug.	**Gabapentin** is used to treat partial seizures with and without secondary generalization. This drug is used in adults in combination with other antiseizure drugs. Gabapentin has also been found useful for the treatment of neuropathic pain.
What is the mechanism of action?	Gabapentin has been found to promote the release of GABA.
What is the metabolism of this drug?	It is excreted unchanged in the urine.
State the toxic effects.	Ataxia Somnolence Headache

LAMOTRIGINE (LAMICTAL)

What is the therapeutic role of lamotrigine?	It is used to treat partial seizures, generalized tonic-clonic seizures, and absence seizures.
What is its mechanism of action?	**Lamotrigine** blocks sustained repetitive firing by blocking voltage-dependent Na^+ channels.
Name the site of metabolism.	This drug is metabolized in the liver.
What are the toxic effects of lamotrigine?	Dizziness Blurred vision Rarely life-threatening skin disorders such as Stevens-Johnson syndrome and toxic epidermal necrolysis
How does the drug compare to zonisamide?	Zonisamide can also cause renal stones.

ZONISANDE (ZONEGRAN)

How does this seizure medication work?	It blocks voltage gated Na^+ channels and T-type calcium currents.
When would this drug be prescribed?	As an adjustment drug in the therapy of partial seizures and generalized seizures.
What are its toxic effects?	Most commonly somnolence, ataxia, and headache. Rarely can cause renal stones.

15   Drugs Used to Treat CNS Degenerative Disorders

PARKINSON'S DISEASE

What is Parkinson's disease?

A movement disorder that has the following four cardinal characteristics:
1. Resting tremors
2. Muscle rigidity
3. Bradykinesia
4. Abnormal posture and gait

What is the pathophysiology of this disease?

The disorder is thought to occur because of a loss of dopamine in the nigrostriatal pathway (Figure 15-1). The loss of dopamine disrupts the delicate balance between the cholinergic and dopaminergic systems within the striatum and basal ganglia.

What are the pharmacological treatment options?

1. Dopamine agonists—**levodopa/carbidopa, bromocriptine, pergolide, pramipexole, ropinirole**
2. MAO inhibitors—**selegiline**
3. **Amantadine**
4. Antimuscarinic agents
5. Catechol-O-Methyltransferase (COMT) inhibitors—**entacapone, tolcapone**

Can these drugs cure?

No! Pharmacologic treatments can offer only temporary relief; they neither reverse nor arrest the disease process.

**Sites of inhibition (-) or
excitation (+) in the striatum
and substantia nigra**

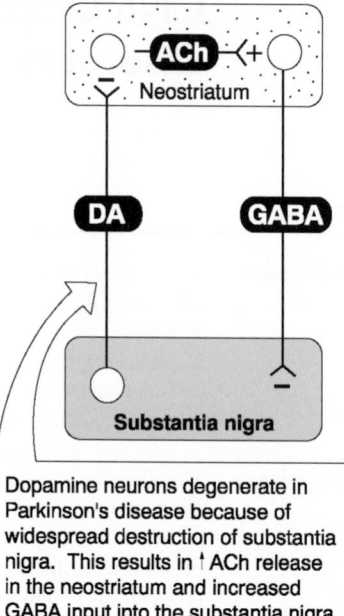

Figure 15–1. Effects of dopaminergic neuron loss in Parkinson's disease. DA = dopamine; GABA = γ-aminobutyric acid; ACh = acetylcholine. (Redrawn with permission from Mycek MJ, Harvey RA, Champe PC [Harvey RA, Champe PC, eds.]. *Lippincott's Illustrated Reviews: Pharmacology,* 2nd ed. Philadelphia: Lippincott-Raven Publishers, 1997, p. 84.)

What is the treatment strategy?	The ultimate goal is to reestablish the balance between dopamine and acetylcholine in the brain. This can be accomplished by either (1) increasing dopamine in the nigrostriatal system or (2) reducing the cholinergic output of the striatum.

LEVODOPA (LARODOPA)

What is it?	This metabolic precursor of dopamine is a first-line drug in the therapy for Parkinson's disease.

What is the advantage of using a precursor to dopamine?

Dopamine itself does not cross the blood-brain barrier. However, **levodopa** is transported into the brain and subsequently converted to dopamine in the basal ganglia.

What are the disadvantages of using this drug alone?

Large doses of **levodopa** are required if it is used alone because this drug is decarboxylated in the periphery to dopamine. **Levodopa** is typically used in combination with another drug, such as **carbidopa**.

What are the pharmacokinetics of levodopa?

This drug is absorbed well from the GI tract. However, if it is ingested with high-protein meals, its transport across the blood-brain barrier is impaired because of competition from neutral amino acids.

What is the on-off phenomenon?

Because **levodopa** has an extremely short half-life, plasma levels may drop suddenly. This may cause sudden immobility, tremors, and cramps. The development of rapid changes in clinical response to the drug is known as the on-off phenomenon.

What drugs should NOT be given with levodopa?

Nonselective monoamine oxidase inhibitors—This combination will result in excess dopamine in the periphery, which could lead to a life-threatening hypertensive crisis.

Pyridoxine—This drug diminishes the effectiveness of **levodopa** because it increases peripheral breakdown of the drug.

Antipsychotics—these drugs block dopamine receptors and can actually cause parkinsonian-like symptoms

What are the adverse effects of levodopa?

Nausea, vomiting, arrhythmias, and postural hypotension—due to the conversion of **levodopa** dopamine in the periphery

Dyskinesia, hallucinations, restlessness, and confusion—due to overstimulation of central dopamine receptors

CARBIDOPA (LODOSYN)

What is it?

A dopamine decarboxylase inhibitor that does not cross the blood-brain barrier

Why use it?

When administered with **levodopa**, **carbidopa** reduces the metabolism of dopamine in the periphery and therefore increases the availability of dopamine to the CNS. The addition of carbidopa reduces the amount of **levodopa** needed for therapy. It also reduces the *peripheral* side effects of **levodopa**, such as nausea and vomiting.

What is the efficacy of levodopa/carbidopa (Sinemet) treatment?

Two-thirds of persons who follow this regimen show some remission of symptoms (especially bradykinesia) in the first 2 years of treatment. Treatment efficacy declines as the disease progresses. This occurs because levodopa requires some healthy dopaminergic neurons to be effective.

BROMOCRIPTINE (PARLODEL)

What is it?

Bromocriptine is an ergotamine derivative that acts as a dopamine receptor agonist at D_2 receptors. It is a second-line drug after **levodopa**.

What are its therapeutic uses?

Bromocriptine is used in conjunction with **levodopa**. It may allow reduction in the maintenance dosage of **levodopa** and therefore reduce the occurrence of side effects associated with long-term **levodopa** use. **Bromocriptine** has very little effect on parkinsonian symptoms when used alone; however, when used in conjunction with **levodopa**, it helps relieve rigidity and tremor. It has minimal effects on bradykinesia.

In addition to being used to treat Parkinson's disease, it is the drug of choice to treat cases of hyperprolactinemia (✎ common board question).

What are the adverse effects of this drug?

Hallucination and delirium occur more often with **bromocriptine** than with **levodopa**

Nausea and vomiting

Cardiac arrhythmia, postural hypotension

Erythromelalgia—a condition characterized by red, painful, and swollen feet or hands

PERGOLIDE (PERMAX)

How does pergolide work?

Like **bromocriptine**, it is an ergot derivative; however, it is a dopamine agonist at both D_1 *and* D_2 receptors.

What role does it have in the treatment of Parkinson's disease?

It is usually used in combination with **levodopa** and anticholinergic drugs.

What are the adverse effects?

Confusion

Hallucinations

Orthostatic hypotension

Urinary tract infections

PRAMIPEXOLE (MIRAPEX) AND ROPINIROLE (REQUIP)

How do these drugs work?

They are **non-ergot** agonists at dopamine (D_2) receptors. They can be used as first-line therapy or as an adjunct to **levodopa** treatment.

How do they differ from bromocriptine and pergolide?

Unlike **bromocriptine** and pergolide, they can be initiated at therapeutic levels quickly rather than by a slow increase, and they also cause fewer GI side effects.

What side effects should you monitor?	Patients taking these drugs can exhibit dyskinesia, insomnia or somnolence, dizziness, and orthostatic hypotension.
How are they eliminated?	Both are excreted through the kidney. **Ropinirole** is much more extensively metabolized than **pramipexole.**

SELEGILINE (ELDEPRYL)

What is its mechanism of action?	**Selegiline** selectively inhibits monamine oxidase B (MAO-B), which metabolizes dopamine. Monoamine oxidase A (MAO-A), however, is not affected unless extremely high doses of **selegiline** are given.
What is its therapeutic use?	Because it decreases the metabolism of dopamine in the periphery, **selegiline** increases dopamine levels in the brain. The effects of **levodopa** are enhanced when it is used in conjunction with **selegiline**; however, there is a threat of hypertensive crisis when this drug is administered in high dosages.

AMANTADINE (SYMMETREL)

What is this drug's classification?	**Amantadine** is an antiviral agent used to treat influenza.
What is its mechanism of action?	The exact mechanism is unknown. **Amantadine** appears to either enhance the release of dopamine from surviving nigral neurons or inhibit the reuptake of dopamine at synapses.
What is its therapeutic use?	**Amantadine** may improve bradykinesia, tremor, and rigidity when used along with **levodopa**. It is usually effective for only a few weeks but seems to be more effective than anticholinergic agents.
What are the toxic effects of this drug?	Restlessness, agitation, confusion Orthostatic hypotension Peripheral edema Livedo reticularis (skin rash)

ANTICHOLINERGIC AGENTS

Name three examples of this class of drugs.

The three most commonly used anticholinergics are:
1. **Benztropine** (Cogentin)
2. **Biperiden** (Akineton)
3. **Trihexyphenidyl** (Artane)

Why use them?

These drugs help reduce the cholinergic output of the striatum (see Figure 15-1). Again, this is another method to restore balance between dopamine and acetylcholine within the nigrostriatal system.

What is their therapeutic efficacy?

These drugs are much less efficacious than **levodopa**. They are commonly used adjuvantly in parkinsonian therapy. They primarily help reduce tremor, rigidity, bradykinesia, and akinesia; secondary symptoms such as drooling are also reduced.

What are their adverse effects?

The following are caused by decreased parasympathetic response:
Sedation
Urinary retention
Dry mouth
Constipation
Mental confusion

COMT INHIBITORS

ENTACAPONE AND TOLCAPONE

What is their mechanism of action?

Both of these drugs work by blocking the peripheral conversion of **levodopa** to 3-O-methyldopa (3OMD) by COMT. 3OMD normally competes with **levodopa** for active transport into the CNS; when its production is decreased, the net effect is increased uptake of **levodopa** into the CNS.

Are they approved for first-line therapy?	No. They are used only as adjuncts to **levodopa/carbidopa** therapy.
What are their adverse effects?	Toxicities are related to increased concentrations of **levodopa**. They include diarrhea, orthostatic hypotension, dyskinesias, sleep disorders, and hallucinations. **Tolcapone** also can cause hepatic necrosis; therefore, frequent monitoring of patient liver enzymes is crucial.

ADDITIONAL CNS DISORDERS

What is drug-induced parkinsonism?	Parkinsonian symptoms can be caused by potent antipsychotic agents such as **haloperidol** because they block dopamine receptors.
What is the treatment for drug-induced parkinsonism?	There are three treatment options: 1. Lower the drug levels. 2. Change the drug to a less potent one. 3. Use an anticholinergic agent.
Define Huntington's disease.	A genetic disorder due to a single defect on chromosome 4
What are the symptoms?	Individuals who have this disease display depression, cognitive decline and/or chorea.
What is the pathophysiology?	This disease is thought to occur because of diminished γ-aminobutyric acid (GABA) functions in the basal ganglia (caudate and putamen). Usually fatal over a course of 15–30 years.
What is the treatment?	Treatment is symptomatic and only partially successful. Dopamine blockers such as **haloperidol** (Haldol) or **tetrabenazine** are used to treat this disorder. **Fluoxetine** is used to treat depression and irritability.
What is Tourette's syndrome?	A disease characterized by abnormal tics and facial movements

What is the treatment?

Clonidine (Catapres). **Haloperidol** has also been used.

Define Alzheimer's disease (AD).

AD is a neurodegenerative condition marked by a loss of cognitive function and eventually mobility. The pathologic hallmarks are senile plaques, loss of cortical neurons and neurofibrillary tangles.

What are the treatment options for AD?

1. Acetylcholinesterase inhibitors
2. NMDA receptor antagonist

Name four anticholinesterase inhibitors.

Donepezil (Aricept)
Rivastigmine (Excelon)
Galantamine (Razadyne)
Tacrine (Cognex)

How do they work?

By inhibiting the enzyme acetylcholinesterase, they increase the amount of acetylcholine available for CNS functions such as memory.

How are they administered?

Orally

What are their side effects?

Tacrine, unlike the others, causes marked hepatotoxicity and therefore is not used widely. In general the drugs cause nausea, vomiting, diarrhea, and cramping.

Name an NMDA receptor antagonist and explain its role in AD.

Memantine (Namenda) helps improve cognitive abilities by protecting CNS neurons from the excitotoxic effects of glutamate, which is believed to contribute to the pathophysiology of AD.

Does it have any toxic effects?

In general it is well tolerated. Headache, dizziness, and confusion can occur.

16

Anesthetics

What are the two major classes of anesthetic agents?

General and local

Describe the routes of administration and primary actions of each of these two classes.

General anesthetics are given either as **inhaled** or **intravenous** agents; they primarily have CNS effects.

Local agents are injected at the operative site to block nerve conduction.

GENERAL ANESTHETICS

What are the stages of general anesthesia?

There are four stages:

Stage I: Analgesia—Reduced sensation of pain; the patient remains conscious and conversational.

Stage II: Excitement—Delirium and combative behavior ensue; there is an increase in blood pressure and respiratory rate.

Stage III: Surgical anesthesia—The patient is unconscious and regular respiration returns; there is muscle relaxation and decreased vasomotor response to painful stimuli.

Stage IV: Medullary paralysis—Respiratory drive decreases and vasomotor output diminishes; death may quickly ensue.

How do the pharmacokinetics of anesthetics affect these stages?

With slow-onset agents (for example, ether), all four stages are discernible. Faster-acting agents allow for quicker progression through the stages.

What is induction of anesthesia?

The time from administration of a general anesthetic to the achievement of surgical anesthesia

What does induction depend on?	How fast the anesthetic reaches the CNS
How are the complications of anesthetic induction avoided?	An ultra-fast-acting, short-lived agent (such as propofol) is given IV so that the patient will rapidly progress through the first and second stages of anesthesia.
What is recovery?	Simply the reverse of induction
What does recovery depend on?	How quickly the anesthetic is removed from the CNS
For inhaled anesthetics, what five factors influence the rate of induction?	1. Solubility 2. Pulmonary ventilation 3. Partial pressure of the inhaled agent 4. Alveolar blood flow 5. Arteriovenous concentration gradient
Describe how solubility affects the rate of induction.	The blood-gas partition coefficient is an index of solubility; a low coefficient implies relative insolubility. An agent with a **low solubility** requires fewer molecules to raise the partial pressure of the agent in the blood; thus, the equilibrium between alveolar partial pressure and arterial partial pressure is achieved rapidly, which leads to a **faster induction**. Recovery is likewise hastened when the anesthetic agent is discontinued (Figure 16–1).
How does pulmonary ventilation affect the rate of induction?	The rate and depth of ventilation (the minute ventilation) affects the rate of increase in partial pressure of the anesthetic in the blood. An increase in the minute ventilation results in an increased amount of agent. This effect is most important for agents with low solubility because they require greater amounts of agent to achieve equilibrium.

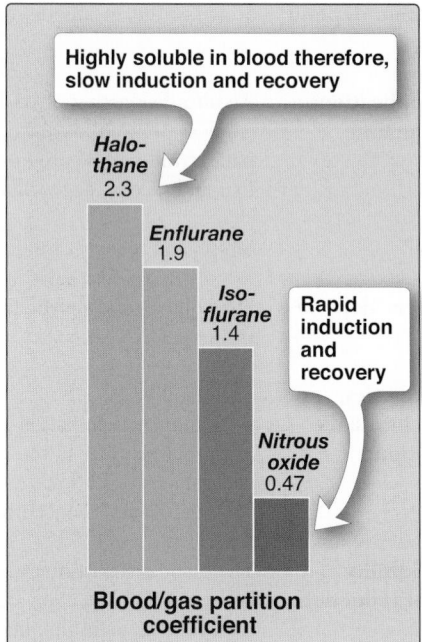

Figure 16–1. Blood/gas partition coefficients for some inhalation anesthetics. (Adapted with permission from Howland RD, Mycek MJ [Harvey RA, Champe PC, eds.]. *Lippincott's Illustrated Reviews: Pharmacology,* 3rd ed. Baltimore: Lippincott Williams & Wilkins, 2006, p 129.)

Describe how partial pressure of the inhaled agent affects the rate of induction.	An increased concentration in the inhaled air mixture leads to greater concentration at the alveoli and thus increases the arterial partial pressure of the agent. In clinical practice, a greater concentration is given initially to speed induction, and then it is reduced to a maintenance level.
How does alveolar blood flow affect the rate of induction?	Increased flow allows for more rapid uptake of the agent and quicker effect on the CNS.
Describe how the arteriovenous concentration gradient affects the rate of induction.	This depends on the uptake of the agent by tissue. A high rate and extent of tissue uptake will decrease the venous concentration of the anesthetic. As a result, it will take a longer time for the

anesthetic concentration of arterial and venous blood to equilibrate.

What factors influence tissue uptake of an anesthetic?

Anesthetic uptake is influenced by many of the same factors that influence transfer from lung to blood: tissue-blood partition coefficients, rates of blood flow to the tissues, and concentration gradients are all important factors. Highly perfused tissues (brain, heart, liver, kidneys, and splanchnic bed) will exert the greatest influence on arteriovenous concentration. Skin and muscle undergo slow diffusion because these tissues are less richly perfused and thus exert less of an effect on arteriovenous concentration.

What is the molecular mechanism of action for general anesthetics?

The mechanism is not clear. All anesthetics have the common property of increasing the threshold of action potentials and inhibiting the rapid increase in membrane permeability to sodium ions. The effect of these changes is not known. Recent studies, however, indicate that $GABA_A$ receptors play a role in the mechanism of general anesthetics.

INHALED AGENTS

Name seven inhaled agents.

1. **Halothane**
2. **Enflurane**
3. **Isoflurane**
4. **Desflurane**
5. **Sevoflurane**
6. **Methoxyflurane**—discontinued from the U.S. market for severe renal and hepatotoxicity
7. **Nitrous oxide**

How is the potency of inhaled anesthetics defined and measured?

Using the concept of **MAC**

What is MAC?

MAC is the *minimum alveolar concentration* of an anesthetic necessary to eliminate movement among 50% of patients challenged by a standardized skin incision. It is commonly expressed as the percent of gas in a mixture required to achieve the desired effect.

How does MAC relate to potency?

The greater the MAC of an agent, the greater the concentration needed to provide anesthesia. Thus, an agent with a high MAC has a low potency (nitrous oxide) and an agent with a low MAC has high potency (halothane) (Figure 16–2).

How does lipid solubility relate to potency?

The more lipid-soluble an anesthetic is, the lower the concentration of anesthetic needed to produce anesthesia. Highly lipid soluble drugs therefore will have high potency.

How can the MAC of any inhaled agent be reduced?

By using the agent in conjunction with another inhaled agent, analgesics, or sedative hypnotics.

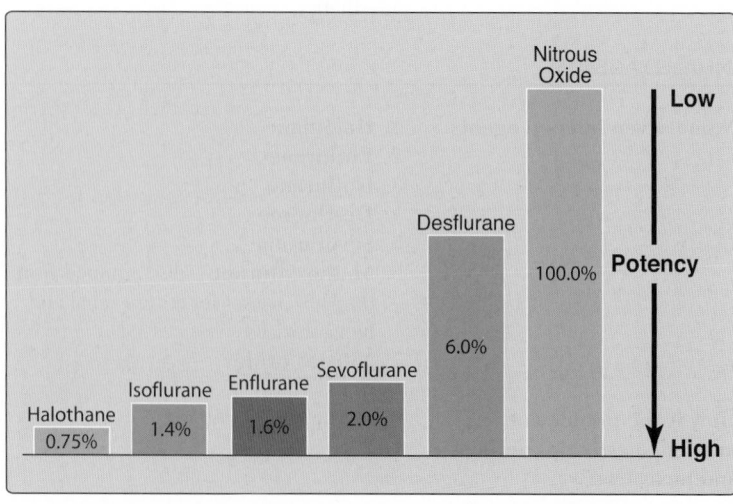

Figure 16–2. Relationship of MAC percentages and potency.

Halothane

Describe this drug.	The first of the halogenated volatile anesthetics to be developed, halothane has been largely replaced by more modern agents.
What is its clinical indication?	It is still used in the pediatric population because of its pleasant odor and lack of hepatotoxicity.
Is this drug metabolized?	Approximately 20% is eliminated by metabolism; the remainder is eliminated unchanged in expired air.
What is halothane's MAC?	0.75%
What are the cardiovascular effects of halothane?	Halothane sensitizes the myocardium to the effects of catecholamines (thus increasing the risk of arrhythmia), decreases heart rate and cardiac output, and leads to lowered blood pressure and peripheral resistance.
Are there any toxic effects?	Hepatotoxicity—**halothane hepatitis,** a fulminant hepatic necrosis—has been associated with halothane. Cardiac arrhythmias, hypotension. Malignant hyperthermia—halothane can induce malignant hyperthermia especially when used in combination with muscle relaxant succinylcholine.
What is malignant hyperthermia?	A potentially fatal reaction to any of the halogenated inhaled anesthetics, which results in hyperthermia, metabolic acidosis, tachycardia, and accelerated muscle contraction
How is this condition treated?	With **dantrolene** and cessation of the offending agent

Enflurane

What are its clinical indications?	Rapid induction and maintenance of general anesthesia
Is this drug metabolized?	Approximately 2% of the agent is metabolized to a fluoride ion, which is then excreted by the kidney. The rest is eliminated unchanged in the expired air.
What is enflurane's MAC?	1.6%
What are this drug's cardiovascular effects?	Enflurane is similar to halothane in that it decreases heart rate, blood pressure, and peripheral resistance. Although it has less of a sensitizing effect on the myocardium than does halothane, enflurane can nevertheless produce cardiac arrhythmia.
Describe the toxic effects.	The fluoride ion resulting from enflurane's metabolism can be nephrotoxic. A decrease in the kidney's concentrating ability after prolonged exposure to enflurane has been observed in patients with preoperative kidney insufficiency.

Isoflurane

What are the clinical indications?	Maintenance of general anesthesia
Is this drug metabolized?	Isoflurane is minimally metabolized; almost all of the drug is eliminated unchanged in the expired air.
What is its MAC?	1.4%
What are the cardiovascular effects?	Coronary casodilation Does not affect cardiac output Can lower blood pressure and reduce peripheral vascular resistance profoundly Does not sensitize the myocardium to catecholamines Does not induce arrhythmia

Are there any toxic effects?	Potential for malignant hyperthermia, respiratory depression, airway irritant

Desflurane

Describe this drug's clinical indications.	General anesthesia for outpatient surgery because of rapid onset and recovery
Does this drug undergo metabolism?	Desflurane is eliminated unchanged in the expired air.
What is its MAC?	6%
What are desflurane's cardiovascular effects?	Its profile very similar to that of isoflurane.
Are there toxic effects?	Potential for malignant hyperthermia, airway irritation

Sevoflurane

What are the clinical indications?	General anesthesia especially in children because it is not irritating to the airway.
Does sevoflurane undergo metabolism?	A small percentage of this agent is metabolized to fluoride ion; the remainder is eliminated unchanged in the expired air.
What is this drug's MAC?	2%
Describe sevoflurane's cardiovascular effects.	It has a cardiac profile similar to that of both desflurane and isoflurane.
Are there any toxic effects?	Although metabolism of sevoflurane produces a fluoride ion, it does not affect renal function as enflurane does. It has been hypothesized that because sevoflurane is not metabolized in the kidney (as enflurane is), toxic effects do not occur.

Nitrous Oxide ("Laughing Gas")

What are the clinical indications?	Induction of general anesthesia, used in outpatient dentistry in combination with oxygen to provide sedation and significant analgesia.

How is this drug administered?

Because of its low potency, nitrous oxide is usually used in conjunction with other anesthetics (either inhaled or intravenous) for effective general anesthesia.

Is nitrous oxide metabolized?

No. It is eliminated through the lungs.

What is its MAC?

100%—Even if 100% nitrous oxide were given to patients, surgical anesthesia would not be achieved (and profound hypoxia would result!).

Are there cardiovascular effects?

Nitrous oxide affects the cardiovascular system minimally.

Name a major contraindication to the use of nitrous oxide.

If nitrous oxide is administered to patients who have closed air cavities (e.g., pneumothorax), the gas will diffuse into the cavity and increase the pressure within it.

What special considerations should be taken into account during the recovery phase?

Care must be taken to adequately oxygenate the patient, because nitrous oxide will diffuse from the blood into the alveoli so quickly that it entirely replaces oxygen, which results in a **diffusion hypoxia.**

What are the toxic effects?

Nitrous oxide is relatively safe. The most important thing to watch for is hypoxia caused by suppressed ventilation. It is neither nephrotoxic or hepatotoxic.

INTRAVENOUS AGENTS

What are the classes of intravenous anesthetics?

Barbiturates, benzodiazepines, opioids, and dissociative agents

Ultra-Short-Acting Barbiturates

Thiopental

What is the clinical indication for this drug?

Thiopental is used for the induction of anesthesia in combination with inhaled anesthetics. It has a rapid onset of action, with unconsciousness occurring 15 to 30 seconds after administration. It does not have significant analgesic activity.

What is this drug's mechanism of action?

Thiopental binds to the **γ-aminobutyric acid A** ($GABA_A$) receptor, which results in prolonged opening of the chloride channel. The neuron's membrane is thus hyperpolarized, causing a reduction of neuronal excitability.

What phenomenon is responsible for this drug's fast onset of action and short duration?

Thiopental has **high lipid solubility** and thus crosses the blood-brain barrier very quickly. However, the drug just as quickly diffuses out of the brain and other highly vascularized organs and is rapidly redistributed to muscle, fat, and other body tissues, which accounts for its short duration of action.

Is thiopental metabolized?

Yes. Metabolism (in the liver) occurs much more slowly than does redistribution. Nearly 99% of the drug is metabolized; thus, after large doses (especially continuous infusions), recovery can be very slow.

What are the cardiovascular effects?

Thiopental reduces blood pressure and cardiac output but does not affect peripheral resistance.

Describe the respiratory effects.

Thiopental depresses the respiratory center of the brain and blunts the response to CO_2 and hypoxia. This effect on cerebral blood flow makes **thiopental** a desirable agent in patients who have cerebral edema.

What are this drug's effects on cerebral blood flow?

It decreases cerebral blood flow and oxygen consumption by the brain.

Are there any side effects?

Thiopental may induce laryngospasm and bronchospasm. It may also exacerbate acute intermittent porphyria by inducing the synthesis of hepatic δ-aminolevulinic acid synthase (**thiopental** has precipitated porphyric crisis).

Benzodiazepines—Midazolam, Diazepam, Lorazepam

See *Chapter 11—Anxiolytics, Hypnotics, and Sedatives,* for further information on the benzodiazepines.

Describe the clinical indication for these drugs.

Benzodiazepines are used for preoperative sedation, intraoperative sedation for procedures not requiring analgesia (colonoscopy, cardioversion, and so forth), and as part of **balanced anesthesia** (using several agents simultaneously to obtain surgical anesthesia).

What is the mechanism of action?

Benzodiazepines bind GABA receptors, which results in reduced neuronal excitability. These drugs have a much slower onset of action than do the barbiturates.

Why is midazolam used as a preanesthetic medication?

This drug produces antegrade amnesia (loss of memory of events after administration of the drug), which calms the patient.

Why is midazolam also the preferred benzodiazepine for induction and maintenance of anesthesia?

Midazolam has a shorter onset of action, greater potency, and more rapid elimination than other benzodiazepines.

What are the side effects of benzodiazepines?

Alone, these drugs can cause moderate circulatory and respiratory depression. If used with opioids, cardiovascular collapse and respiratory arrest can occur.

Are there other uses for these drugs?
They are used to control seizures and in the alcohol withdrawal process to control symptoms.

Is there a benzodiazepine antagonist?
Flumazenil antagonizes the CNS depression caused by benzodiazepines.

Opioids—Fentanyl, Morphine

What are the clinical indications for these drugs?
Opioids are used as general anesthetics in patients undergoing cardiac surgery or other major surgeries for which cardiac reserve is limited. They have excellent analgesic properties.

Why is fentanyl used more often than morphine?
It has a greater potency and less impact on respiratory drive than does **morphine**.

Are there any side effects?
IV opioids can cause chest wall rigidity, which makes ventilation more difficult. Postoperative respiratory depression can occur.
Intraoperative awareness with unpleasant postoperative recall may occur.

Is there an opioid antagonist?
Naloxone reverses the respiratory and CNS effects of opioids.

What is Innovar?
Innovar is a combination of **fentanyl** and **droperidol**. When used with nitrous oxide, Innovar produces neuroleptanesthesia (combined analgesia and amnesia).

Other Agents

Propofol (Diprivan)

Describe this drug's clinical indications.
Induction of anesthesia

What are the pharmacologic characteristics of this drug?
Ultra-fast-acting drug with pharmacodynamics similar to that of thiopental

High lipid solubility

Very quick distribution to highly vascularized sites (e.g., the brain)

Rapid diffusion back into the blood, with subsequent redistribution

Why is propofol preferred over thiopental for induction of anesthesia?

Rate of onset very similar to that of **thiopental.**

Recovery is quicker, with patients able to ambulate sooner than with other IV anesthetics.

Patients report less nausea and emesis.

No cumulative effect from **propofol** administration or delayed recovery after prolonged infusion

How is propofol metabolized?

It is rapidly metabolized by liver and other extrahepatic enzymes (10 times more quickly than **thiopental**).

What are the side effects?

Hypotension

Negative inotropic effects

Pain at the site of injection (most commonly encountered side effect)

Apnea

Does propofol have any other uses?

Propofol is often used in the critical care setting as a continuous infusion to provide prolonged sedation.

Ketamine

Describe the clinical indications.

Ketamine, because of its unique cardiovascular effects, is used in trauma cases where cardiovascular support is necessary. It is also used in children undergoing painful procedures (dressing changes of burns) or to facilitate cooperation during radiographic procedures.

What is the mechanism of action?

Ketamine produces a **dissociative anesthesia** characterized by catatonia, amnesia, and analgesia without actual loss of consciousness.

What are the cardiovascular effects?	**Ketamine** is unique in that it produces cardiovascular stimulation, with heart rate, arterial blood pressure, and cardiac output all usually significantly increased. This drug stimulates the sympathetic nervous system, which causes the release of catecholamines.
Is ketamine used in head trauma cases?	No, because it increases cerebral blood flow, oxygen consumption, and intracranial pressure.
What are the side effects?	**Ketamine** can cause an emergence phenomenon consisting of disorientation, sensory and perceptual illusions, and vivid, often unpleasant dreams.
What can be done to reduce the incidence of this phenomenon?	Use of **diazepam** 5 to 10 min before **ketamine** administration
Are there other routes of administration?	Yes. **Ketamine** can be given intramuscularly as well as intravenously.

LOCAL ANESTHETICS

What are the two types of local anesthetics?	The two classes are determined by the bond linking the lipophilic portion of the molecule with the hydrophilic component—either an **ester** or **amide** bond.
Name the ester anesthetics.	**Cocaine** **Benzocaine** **Procaine** **Tetracaine**
Name the amide anesthetics.	**Lidocaine** **Mepivacaine** **Bupivacaine** **Prilocaine**
How does the metabolism of the ester and amide anesthetics differ?	Esters are more rapidly metabolized by blood and tissue esterases, which gives them shorter half-lives. Amides are

metabolized by hepatic microsomal enzymes, which results in a longer half-life.

What is the mechanism of action of local anesthetics?

These agents block nerve conduction by inhibiting the voltage-gated sodium channels of the neuronal membrane.

Which nerve fibers are most sensitive to local anesthetics?

Small, unmyelinated fibers that conduct pain, temperature, and autonomic activity are affected first. With increasing concentrations of anesthetic, pain fibers (C and A fibers) are first affected, then sensory fibers (A fibers), and last motor neurons (A fibers).

What are the clinical indications?

Local anesthetics are used for surface anesthesia, nerve blocks, and spinal and epidural anesthesia. Lidocaine is also a potent antiarrhythmic.

How is the duration of action of local anesthetics increased?

Adding epinephrine to local anesthetics reduces blood flow to the anesthetized area, thus decreasing the absorption of the drugs and enhancing their duration of action.

Are there any side effects?

Systemic effects of local anesthetics occur with high doses of the drug:

CNS disturbances—light-headedness, sensory disturbances, convulsions, coma, and even death at high doses

Cardiovascular effects—myocardial depression and hypotension except for cocaine, which causes vasoconstriction and hypertension

17

CNS Stimulants

**What is the definition of a
CNS stimulant?**

A CNS stimulant is a drug that increases
motor activity, causes excitement, and
decreases feelings of fatigue. CNS
stimulants include the methylxanthines,
nicotine, and the amphetamines.

METHYLXANTHINES

What are methylxanthines?

A group of psychomotor stimulants
including:
Caffeine
Theophylline
Theobromine (found in cocoa but of little
    clinical interest)

**How do methylxanthines
work?**

Research indicates that methylxanthines
increase cyclic guanosine monophosphate
(cGMP) and cyclic adenosine
monophosphate (cAMP) by **inhibiting
phosphodiesterase** and **blocking
adenosine** receptors.

CAFFEINE

**What are the physiological
effects of caffeine?**

Caffeine affects a number of organ
systems within the body:
CNS—Caffeine increases motor activity
    and alertness.
Cardiovascular—Caffeine increases
    heart rate and contractility.
Smooth muscle—Caffeine and its
    derivatives relax the smooth muscles
    of the bronchioles.
Genitourinary—Caffeine can act as
    weak diuretic and increase urinary
    output of Na^+, Cl^-, and K^+.
Gastrointestinal—Caffeine stimulates
    secretion of HCl from the gastric
    mucosa. Therefore patients who have

peptic ulcer disease should be
counseled to avoid caffeine.

What are the adverse effects
of chronic caffeine use?

At low doses—Insomnia and agitation
can occur.
At higher doses (8 to 10 g)—Emesis,
convulsions, and even cardiac
arrhythmias can occur.

Do methylxanthines cross
the placenta?

Yes, and they are secreted into the
mother's milk. Patients should be advised
to avoid them during pregnancy and
while nursing.

THEOPHYLLINE

See *Chapter 28—Drugs Used to Treat Asthma, Coughs, and Colds*, for
additional discussion of theophylline.

What is the therapeutic role
of theophylline?

Theophylline can be used in the
treatment of asthma, but currently it is
not being used frequently because it has
a very narrow therapeutic index and is
not as effective as the newer β agonists.

NICOTINE

How are the physiological
effects of nicotine related to
the dose?

In low doses, nicotine causes ganglionic
stimulation by depolarization. At high
doses, it causes ganglionic blockade.

What are the physiological
actions of nicotine on the
central nervous system?

At low doses—arousal, relaxation, and
improved attention
At high doses—central respiratory
paralysis caused by disruption of
medullary function

How does nicotine affect the
peripheral nervous system?

At low doses—increase in blood pressure
and heart rate; constriction of blood
vessels
At high doses—decrease in blood
pressure and activity of the GI and
GU tract due to parasympathetic
ganglionic blockade

What are nicotine's therapeutic uses?

As an ingredient of a transdermal patch or chewing gum, low-dose **nicotine** is used to help with smoking cessation.

Can it be used in pregnancy?

No because it readily crosses the placenta and is secreted into the mothers milk.

What is nicotine's route of administration?

Absorption occurs through the oral mucosa, inhalation, and transdermally.

What are its adverse effects?

CNS—irritability and tremors
Peripheral—intestinal cramps, diarrhea, and increased heart rate and blood pressure

What withdrawal symptoms do nicotine addicts experience?

A craving for tobacco accompanied by irritability, restlessness, anxiety, and gastrointestinal pain

AMPHETAMINES

Name three examples of this drug class.

1. **Methylphenidate** (Ritalin)
2. **Methamphetamine** (Methedrine)— "speed"
3. **Dextroamphetamine** (Dexedrine)

How do these drugs work?

Amphetamines work by releasing neuronal stores of catecholamines, especially norepinephrine and dopamine.

What are the physiological actions of these drugs?

Euphoria
Decrease in fatigue
Increase in blood pressure
Increase in rate of respiration
Decrease in appetite

What is their clinical use?

Attention deficit hyperactivity disorder (ADHD)—**Methylphenidate** is used to alleviate this problem.
Appetite control—Amphetamines decrease appetite by blocking the receptors in the lateral hypothalamus.
Narcolepsy

What is the route of administration?	Oral
Where are amphetamines metabolized and excreted?	Metabolized in the liver and excreted in the urine
Does physiological and psychological dependence occur with amphetamine use?	Yes. Amphetamines can be very addictive.
What are the adverse effects of these drugs?	Amphetamines, like **caffeine** and **nicotine**, affect multiple organ systems: **Central nervous system**—insomnia, irritability, convulsions; chronic use can lead to a psychotic state resembling schizophrenia **Gastrointestinal tract**—anorexia, nausea, diarrhea **Cardiovascular system**—palpitations, angina, arrhythmias, hypertension
Amphetamines are contraindicated with what group of drugs?	The monoamine oxidase (MAO) inhibitors
How is amphetamine overdose managed?	**Chlorpromazine** is beneficial in amphetamine overdose because it blocks the α receptors, which are responsible for the CNS changes and hypertension.

18   Alcohol and Other Drugs of Abuse

ALCOHOL

Name three types of alcohol.

1. Ethanol
2. Methanol
3. Ethylene glycol
This chapter focuses mostly on ethanol use.

What is ethanol's mechanism of action?

Ethanol is a CNS depressant that works through γ-aminobutyric (GABA) receptors to enhance GABA-mediated synaptic transmission.

What is ethanol initially metabolized into?

Acetaldehyde

Which enzymes are responsible for the first steps in the metabolism of ethanol?

1. **Alcohol dehydrogenase**—a nicotinamide adenine dinucleotide (NAD)–dependent enzyme that metabolizes alcohol at a fixed rate of approximately 7 to 10 g/hr. This enzyme must follow zero-order kinetics because of a limited supply of the NAD cofactor. The enzyme is found primarily in the liver and GI tract.
2. **Microsomal ethanol oxidizing system (MEOS)**—Found mainly in the liver, this enzyme increases in activity with chronic ethanol exposure. This increase may account for the tolerance that develops with regular ethanol use.

What is acetaldehyde further metabolized into?

Acetaldehyde is converted into acetic acid by aldehyde dehydrogenase.

Are there therapeutic indications for ethanol use?	Yes:

1. **Methanol overdose**
2. **Ethylene glycol overdose**—Ethanol is used in this circumstance because it preferentially binds to alcohol dehydrogenase and therefore prevents the formation of toxic metabolites from either methanol or ethylene glycol (Figure 18–1).
3. Recent research indicates that one alcoholic drink (red wine) a day may reduce the risk of coronary artery disease.

What are the *acute* effects of ethanol intoxication?

Euphoria, disinhibition, slurred speech
Reduced visual acuity
Ataxia
Relaxation of vascular and uterine smooth muscle
Blood levels of alcohol greater than 300 mg/dL can lead to loss of consciousness and decreased myocardial action.
Blood levels of alcohol greater than 400 mg/dL can be fatal.

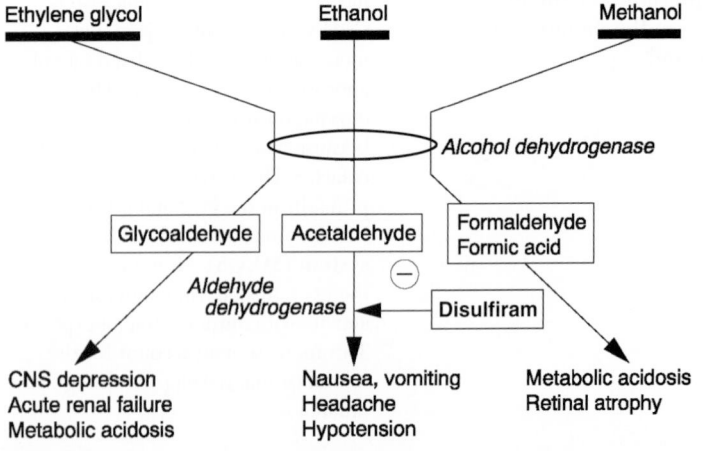

Figure 18–1. Toxic metabolites of alcohols. Ethanol, a preferred substrate for alcohol dehydrogenase, is used in methanol and ethylene glycol poisoning to slow the production of toxic metabolites from these alcohols.

What are the *chronic CNS* effects of alcoholism?

A deficiency of thiamine associated with chronic alcohol use can lead to Wernicke-Korsakoff syndrome. This disease is characterized by ophthalmoplegia, ataxia, and confusion.

What are the *chronic peripheral* effects of alcoholism?

Decreased liver and pancreatic function—Hepatitis, cirrhosis and pancreatitis may develop.
GI irritation, inflammation, and bleeding
Gynecomastia and testicular atrophy in men due to the cirrhotic liver's inability to metabolize estrogen
Hypertension
Dilated cardiomyopathy
Although alcohol is not considered to be a direct carcinogen, alcohol consumption can lead to an increased risk of GI cancer.

Why is it unsafe for pregnant women to drink alcohol?

Ethanol use during pregnancy may lead to **fetal alcohol syndrome**, which includes mental retardation, growth deficiencies, microcephaly, and malformations of the face and head.

What are "the DTs"?

Delirium tremens—tremor, anxiety, tachycardia, delusions, and agitation. These symptoms are experienced by chronic alcohol users who are suddenly deprived of ethanol.

What is disulfiram used for?

Disulfiram (Antabuse), an **aldehyde dehydrogenase inhibitor,** is used adjunctively in some alcohol treatment programs. Patients who drink while taking disulfiram will experience nausea, hypotension, and vomiting. These adverse symptoms encourage avoidance of ethanol (Figure 18–1).

Which drugs are well known to cause a disulfiram-type reaction when used in conjunction with alcohol?

Metronidazole, the cephalosporins, and **procarbazine**

What is the management of alcohol toxicity?	In the acute phase, the patient is stabilized with supportive therapy such as fluids, thiamine, and electrolyte balancing. Long-term detox may include a long-acting sedative (i.e., diazepam) with gradual tapering of the dose.

PHENCYCLIDINE (PCP)

What is it?	Phencyclidine or PCP, also known as "angel dust," is a **dissociative anesthetic** (analgesia and catatonia without loss of consciousness) that blocks N-methyl, D-aspartic acid (NMDA) receptors (i.e., glutamate receptors). It is also a ketamine analogue.
What is this drug's mechanism of action?	It blocks serotonin (5-hydroxytryptamine [5-HT]) uptake.
What are the central physiologic actions of PCP?	PCP causes a schizophrenia-like psychosis involving distortion of time, space, and body image. Extremely high doses can cause seizures and coma.
What are the peripheral physiological effects of PCP?	Increased blood pressure and heart rate Limb numbness Ataxia Hypersalivation Nystagmus

LSD

What is it?	Lysergic acid diethylamide
How does it work?	It interacts with 5-HT receptors in the midbrain.
What are the physiological actions of LSD on the CNS?	Visual hallucinations and flashbacks Arousal Excitation Disturbed perception Disturbed mood Panic

What are the peripheral physiological effects?	Mydriasis Tachycardia Flushing, lacrimation, salivation Increased blood pressure
What drug can block the hallucinatory effects of LSD?	**Haloperidol**

MARIJUANA

What is it?	Marijuana's s active component is Δ-9 THC (tetrahydrocannabinol), which is derived from the flowering tops of the hemp plant (*Cannabis sativa*).
What are marijuana's effects on the CNS?	Sedation Euphoria Decreased psychomotor activity Impaired judgment, memory, and time sense
What peripheral physiological effects does marijuana have?	Increased heart rate and blood pressure Injected (red) conjunctiva Dry mouth Bronchodilation Increased appetite
Does marijuana have any clinical indications?	Yes. **Dronabinol** is a pharmaceutical preparation of Δ-9 THC that is used to treat anorexia related to terminal conditions and as an antiemetic in chemotherapy.

COCAINE

What is cocaine's mechanism of action?	Cocaine blocks the reuptake of norepinephrine, serotonin, and dopamine (5-HT) into presynaptic nerve terminals. This blockade results in enhanced activity of these neurotransmitters.

What physiological changes occur as a result of cocaine use?

Cocaine causes mydriasis; increases heart rate, alertness, and self-confidence; and induces a temporary state of euphoria by stimulating the limbic system.

What are the signs of overdose?

Excitation
Hallucinations and psychosis
Seizures
Hypertension
Respiratory depression
Arrhythmias secondary to coronary
    vasospasm
Coma

Does cocaine have any clinical use?

Yes. It is sometimes used as a local anesthetic and vasoconstrictor during ENT procedures.

OTHER DRUGS OF ABUSE

Are there additional drugs that can be abused?

Almost any drug has the potential for abuse. Only a few of the classic drugs of abuse have been mentioned in this chapter; others, such as caffeine, amphetamine, and nicotine, are discussed in detail in *Chapter 17—CNS Stimulants.* Also, benzodiazepines and opioids are each discussed separately in *Chapter 11—Anxiolytics, Hypnotics, and Sedatives* and *Chapter 19—Opioid Analgesics and Antagonists.*

19 Opioid Analgesics and Antagonists

What are opioids?

The term *opioid* refers to all agonists and antagonists with morphine-like activity as well as to naturally occurring and synthetic opioid peptides.

Give three examples of naturally occurring opioids.

1. Enkephalins
2. Endorphins
3. Dynorphins

Where do opioids act?

Primarily on the CNS—more specifically, on three main classes of opioid receptors:
1. Mu (μ) receptors
2. Kappa (κ) receptors
3. Delta (δ) receptors
These receptors are located throughout the CNS, including the cortex, thalamus, brainstem, and spinal cord.

Describe the effects of μ, κ, and δ receptors.

μ receptors—responsible for producing spinal/supraspinal analgesia, euphoria, respiratory depression, miosis, and constipation

κ receptors—responsible for producing spinal analgesia, sedation, dysphoria, and miosis

δ receptors—responsible for producing supraspinal/spinal analgesia

How do opioids help reduce the sensation of pain?

They cause hyperpolarization of nerve cells, and inhibit both nerve firing and presynaptic transmitter release.

Which drugs are considered opioid agonists?

Morphine
Meperidine
Methadone
Fentanyl
Heroin
Hydromorphone

Which drugs are considered moderate or weak agonists?	**Codeine** **Propoxyphene** **Oxycodone** **Hydrocodone** **Buprenorphine**
Which drugs are considered agonists/antagonists and partial agonists?	**Pentazocine** **Nalbuphine** **Butorphanol** **Buprenorphine**
Which drugs are considered opioid antagonists?	**Naloxone** **Naltrexone**
How do all of these drugs differ in potency when compared to morphine?	See Table 19–1.

Table 19–1. Selected Opioid Analgesics: Comparison with Morphine

		Related Potency to Morphine (Approx.)[a]	Duration of Analgesia
Fentanyl (Sublimaze)	MORE POTENT ↑	100×	1–1.5 hr
Buprenorphine (Buprenex)		25–50×	4–8 hr
Hydromorphone (Dilaudid)			4-5 hr
Butorphanol (Stadol)			3–4 hr
Morphine (Roxanol, MS Contin)		*1×*	*4–5 hr*
Pentazocine (Talwin)	LESS POTENT ↓		3–4 hr
Meperidine (Demerol)			2–4 hr
Codeine		1/7×	3–4 hr
Propoxyphene (Darvon)			4–5 hr

[a] Varies by route of administration

OPIOID AGONISTS

MORPHINE (ROXANOL, MS CONTIN)

What is it?

A drug derived from the poppy plant, *Papaver somniferum.* It is the prototypical opioid.

What receptors does morphine act on?

Morphine shows strong affinity for μ receptors and varying affinities for δ and κ receptors.

What are morphine's physiological actions?

Histamine release and hormonal actions (increased prolactin, decreased GRH, CRH, CH, FSH, ACTH)

Emesis

Contraction of smooth muscle in the biliary tract as well as the bladder and ureter

Cardiovascular changes—There is very little cardiovascular change at normal dosages; orthostatic hypotension, however, may occur.

Decreased cough reflex, **D**ecreased GI motility, **D**ecreased uterine tone, and **D**epression of mental functioning (sedation)

Respiratory depression—Fatalities can occur at high doses. Increased CO_2 levels can dilate cerebral vasculature and cause increased ICP.

Euphoria

Analgesia—Opioids are the most potent drugs available for relief of pain.

Miosis

Morphine gives you one "**HEC**k of a **DREAM.**"

What two physiological effects of morphine are not affected by tolerance?

Miosis and constipation

How is this drug used therapeutically?

Analgesia
Diarrhea (loperamide)
Relief of cough

Relief of acute pulmonary edema
(primarily in the past)

What is the route of administration?

Multiple routes can be taken: IV, PO, SQ, or IM

Describe the pharmacokinetics of morphine and most other opioids.

They are well absorbed orally (except for **morphine**), metabolized by the liver (usually to the glucuronide conjugates), and subsequently eliminated in the urine.

Can opioids be used in pregnancy?

Morphine and other opioids can cross the placental barrier and cause respiratory depression and, with chronic use, dependency in the fetus.

Are there any adverse effects?

Yes. Respiratory depression—be particularly careful of this in patients with cor pulmonale. Other adverse effects include nausea; vomiting; elevation of intracranial pressure, especially in head injury; and urinary retention.

What type of withdrawal symptoms are seen with opioids?

Chills
Diarrhea
Myalgia
Agitation
Anxiety

What important drug interactions exist when using opioids?

Opioids should not be used with anti-psychotics, antidepressants, sedatives, or MAO inhibitors. The combination can lead to death from CNS suppression.

What should I know about the other drugs discussed in this chapter?

They all produce physiological effects and side effects similar to those of **morphine**; therefore, only special traits such as sites of action and unique characteristics are discussed. Remember that **morphine** is the classic opiate.

MEPERIDINE (DEMEROL)

What is the site of action?	This drug binds primarily to μ receptors.
What does meperidine do to the eyes?	It does not produce pinpoint pupils like other opiates, but rather causes the pupils to dilate because of its anticholinergic activity, similar to that of **atropine**.
Describe the adverse effects.	Tremors Muscle twitches Rarely, convulsions
Name an important contraindication to meperidine use.	Never give **meperidine** or other opioids to patients on **MAOIs** because this combination may result in severe respiratory depressions, hyperpyrexia, and convulsions.
What is loperamide (Imodium)?	A **meperidine** analogue used to treat diarrhea

METHADONE (Dolophine)

What is the site of action?	This drug exerts its greatest actions on the μ receptors.
How is methadone administered?	Orally
What is its therapeutic use?	Narcotic detoxification—Because of its long half life (15 to 40 hr), **methadone** can prevent an addict from suffering severe withdrawal symptoms as the body normalizes.

FENTANYL (Sublimaze)

Describe this drug and its site of action.	**Fentanyl** is a synthetic opioid agonist active at the μ receptors.
How is fentanyl used therapeutically?	For anesthesia—alone or in combination with **droperidol** For chronic and postoperative pain

How is fentanyl administered?	IV or transdermally
What are the adverse effects?	Apnea/hypoventilation CNS depression Muscular rigidity

HEROIN (Diacetylmorphine)

What are the pharmacological properties of heroin?	**Heroin** is hydrolyzed into **morphine** and therefore has properties similar to **morphine**'s. **Heroin** is, however, more lipid-soluble and crosses the blood-brain barrier more quickly than does **morphine**.

HYDROMORPHONE (Dilaudid)

State this agonist's site of action.	The μ receptors
How is it used therapeutically?	For moderate pain

MODERATE/WEAK AGONISTS

CODEINE

What is the site of action?	**Codeine** has low affinity for μ receptors.
Describe its pharmacologic actions.	**Codeine** resembles morphine pharmacologically but has milder actions.
How is this drug used therapeutically?	As an antitussive and to relieve mild-to-moderate pain. **Dextromethorphan** is an analogue of **codeine**, which also is used for its antitussive effects. It has very little analgesic or addictive property.
What are codeine's adverse effects?	Dependence and overdose potential Constipation and nausea

TRAMADOL (Ultram)

What is it?	A synthetic **codeine** analog that is a weak μ agonist. Some of its analgesic effects come from its ability to inhibit the uptake of norepinephrine and serotonin.
What is it used for?	Mild to moderate pain relief
What are its adverse effects?	Nausea and vomiting. Unlike the effect of morphine, respiratory depression is minimal.

PROPOXYPHENE (Darvon)

Where is the site of action?	At the μ receptors
How is propoxyphene used therapeutically?	For mild to moderate analgesia
Are there adverse effects?	Convulsions respiratory depression and hallucination

HYDROCODONE (Hycodan)

Describe this agonist's site of action.	The μ receptors
What are the adverse effects?	Histamine release

OXYCODONE (Roxicodone)

What is this agonist's site of action?	The μ receptors
Are there any adverse effects?	The adverse effects are similar to those of **morphine**.

MIXED AGONISTS/ANTAGONISTS AND PARTIAL AGONISTS

PENTAZOCINE (Talwin)

Describe how this drug functions at its dual sites of action.	**Pentazocine** is the prototypical mixed opioid. It acts as an agonist at κ and δ receptors and as a weak antagonist or partial agonist at μ and receptors.
What are its therapeutic uses?	Analgesia—relief of moderate to severe pain
Are there adverse effects?	Psychotomimetic effects (anxiety, nightmares) Nausea, sweating

NALBUPHINE (Nubain)

Describe how this drug functions at its dual sites of action.	It acts as an agonist at the κ receptors and an antagonist at the μ receptors. Available only in injection form.
What are the therapeutic uses?	Analgesia—relief of moderate to severe pain
Are there any adverse effects?	Sedation, sweating, and headache are the most common.

BUTORPHANOL (Stadol)

How does this drug function at its dual sites of action?	It acts as an agonist at the κ receptors and as a weak antagonist at the μ receptors. It is available only in injection form.
Is there a therapeutic use?	Acute pain relief
What are the adverse effects?	Drowsiness Weakness Sweating Nausea

BUPRENORPHINE (Buprenex)

Where is the site of action?	**Buprenorphine** is a partial agonist at μ receptors.
How does buprenorphine function?	It dissociates from the μ receptors *slowly*, which may contribute to its long duration of action and low physical dependence.
Describe this drug's therapeutic indications.	Analgesia in postoperative patients Opiate detoxication Relief of moderate to severe pain
What are the adverse effects?	Similar to those of morphine, but to a much lesser extent—respiratory depression (can not be reversed by naloxone), sedation, and nausea and vomiting
Can opioid agonists be used in combination with other drugs?	Yes. For example, **hydrocodone** is frequently combined with **acetaminophen** (Vicodin), **oxycodone** and **aspirin** (Percodan), **oxycodone** and **acetaminophen** (Percocet).

OPIOID ANTAGONISTS

NALOXONE (NARCAN)

How does this drug work?	**Naloxone** binds all opioid receptors to displace bound opioid agonists.
How is naloxone used therapeutically?	It reverses the acute respiratory depression and coma of opioid overdose.
How quickly does it work?	Within 30 s of IV injection
What is naloxone's duration of action?	From 1 to 2 hr—This is important because *patients may relapse into respiratory depression and coma if repeated dosages of naloxone are not given!*
Are there adverse effects?	Tachycardia and arrhythmias

NALTREXONE (TREXAN)

Describe this drug's mechanism of action.

Naltrexone binds at all opioid receptors.

What is naltrexone's therapeutic use?

It is beneficial for treating opioid dependency because it can be given orally and has a longer duration of action than naloxone (approximately 48 hr).

List the adverse effects.

Hepatotoxicity
Nausea
Sedation
Headache

What happens if naloxone or naltrexone is given in the absence of an opioid agonist?

At most doses there is no physiological effect if an opioid agonist is not present.

Section IV

Cardiovascular System

20

Antihypertensive Drugs

Define hypertension.

Persistent diastolic blood pressure greater than 90 mm Hg and systolic pressure greater than 140 mm Hg

How can hypertension be categorized?

The latest definition of hypertension takes into account presence of risk factors and target-organ damage

Normal: ≤120 systolic and ≤80 diastolic

Prehypertension—Blood pressure usually 120 to 139 systolic or 80 to 89 diastolic mm Hg, although values ≥140/90 mm Hg may be occasionally or intermittently observed and there is no evidence of target-organ damage.

Stage 1—Resting blood pressure between 140-159 systolic or diastolic 90-99.

Stage 2—Sustained resting blood pressure may be ≥160 systolic or ≥100 diastolic

What causes hypertension?

Of patients who have hypertension, 90% have what is known as essential hypertension (i.e., the etiology is unknown). The other 10% have hypertension secondary to other diseases such as renal artery stenosis, pheochromocytoma, Cushing's disease, and coarctation of the aorta. Environmental factors such as sodium intake, obesity, and smoking can also cause hypertension.

What is the most common presenting sign of hypertension?

There is none! When patients are first diagnosed, they are usually asymptomatic.

What are some of the potential complications of hypertension?

Coronary artery disease, cardiac and renal failure, and stroke

What is the hydraulic equation for blood pressure?

Cardiac output × total peripheral vascular resistance = blood pressure

What conclusions can be drawn from this equation?

Drugs that reduce either cardiac output (CO) or peripheral vascular resistance (PVR) will produce a reduction in blood pressure.

What are the major classes of drugs used to treat hypertension?

Sympatholytic agents—Methyldopa, clonidine, guanfacine, α blockers, β blockers, ganglionic blockers, and postganglionic adrenergic neuronal blockers. All of these agents reduce peripheral vascular resistance or cardiac output.

Diuretics—Loop and thiazide diuretics are the most important agents of this antihypertensive drug class.

Vasodilators—Hydralazine, minoxidil, sodium nitroprusside, diazoxide, and calcium channel blockers. These agents reduce PVR.

Angiotensin-converting enzyme (ACE) inhibitors and angiotensin II receptor antagonists— Captopril, enalapril, lisinopril, and **losartan**. These drugs reduce PVR; however, they also reduce blood volume by reducing the secretion of aldosterone.

Figure 20-1 shows the sites of action of the major classes of antihypertensive drugs.

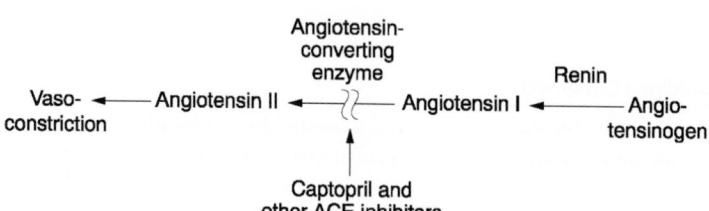

Vasomotor Center
Methyldopa
Clonidine

**Sympathetic Nerve
Terminals**
Guanethidine
Reserpine

β-Receptors of Heart
Propranolol
Other β-blockers

Sympathetic Ganglia
Trimethaphan

**Angiotensin
Receptors
of Vessels**
Losartan

**α-Receptors
of Vessels**
Prazosin
and other
α₁-blockers

Vascular Smooth Muscle
Hydralazine   Verapamil
Minoxidil   and other
Nitroprusside calcium
Diazoxide   channel
               blockers

Kidney Tubules
Thiazides, etc.

**β-Receptors of Juxtaglomerular
Cells That Release Renin**
Propranolol and
other β-blockers

Angiotensin-
converting
enzyme

Renin

Vaso- ← Angiotensin II ← Angiotensin I ← Angio-
constriction   tensinogen

Captopril and
other ACE inhibitors

Figure 20–1. Sites of action of the major classes of antihypertensive drugs. (Redrawn with permission from Katzung BG. *Basic & Clinical Pharmacology,* 9th ed. New York: McGraw-Hill, 2004.)

SYMPATHOLYTIC AGENTS

CENTRALLY ACTING ANTIHYPERTENSIVES

Methyldopa (Aldomet)

What is this drug's mechanism of action?	**Methyldopa** stimulates central presynaptic α_2-adrenergic receptors and inhibits the release of norepinephrine.
What is its primary effect?	The decreased sympathetic outflow results in decreased peripheral vascular resistance. It also creates some reduction in cardiac output.
What is the route of administration?	Oral or intravenous
What is the clinical indication for methyldopa?	Moderate hypertension. **Methyldopa** is often given to patients with renal insufficiency since it does not decrease blood flow to the kidney. It can be used safely in pregnancy.
What are the potential toxicities of methyldopa?	A drug-induced positive Coombs test that is sometimes associated with hemolytic anemia Lactation associated with increased prolactin release Edema Sedation Impotence Dry mouth Hepatitis

Clonidine (Catapres)

Describe this drug's mechanism of action.	Like **methyldopa**, **clonidine** stimulates presynaptic central α_2-adrenergic receptors, which results in diminished central adrenergic outflow. Its antihypertensive effects are due primarily to decreased peripheral vascular resistance. However, it also decreases heart rate and thus cardiac output.

When is this drug used clinically?	For mild-to-moderate hypertension. Usually a second line agent.
What is the route of administration?	Oral, intravenous, or transdermal (for extended use)
What are the adverse effects?	Sedation Dizziness Dry mouth Rebound hypertension after sudden withdrawal from high doses (can be treated with **labetalol** or **nitroprusside**) Bradycardia especially in patients with AV nodal disease
What drug interactions should the physician be concerned about?	**Clonidine** should not be given with tricyclic drugs. This combination may inhibit the actions of **clonidine**.

Guanfacine (Tenex)

What is this drug?	A centrally acting antihypertensive with a mechanism of action and side-effect profile very similar to those of **clonidine**

α BLOCKERS

For more information on α blockers, see *Chapter 9—Adrenergic Antagonists.*

Give some examples of α_1-adrenergic blockers.	**Prazosin** (Minipress) **Terazosin** (Hytrin) **Doxazosin** (Cardura)
How do they work?	They block the α_1-adrenergic receptors.
What are the antihypertensive effects of these drugs?	The antihypertensive effects are mainly related to a decrease in peripheral vascular resistance. These drugs exert minimal effects on cardiac output.
Describe the clinical use for α_1-adrenergic blockers.	Moderate hypertension Benign prostatic hypertrophy (relaxes the smooth muscle in the bladder neck)

What are the adverse effects of prazosin and its synthetic analogues?	Dizziness Orthostatic hypotension—especially after the first dose (first-dose effect) Headache

β BLOCKERS

For more information on β blockers, see *Chapter 9—Adrenergic Antagonists.*

Give some examples of β blockers.	**Propranolol** **Metoprolol** **Atenolol** **Labetalol** (both α and β blocker) **Carvedilol**
Describe the mechanism of action.	Blockade of β_1- and β_2-adrenergic receptors
What is the clinical use?	A β blocker is often one of the first-line agents chosen to treat patients with mild-to-moderate hypertension and a concomitant disease such as angina or chronic heart failure. They are more effective in the white population and in younger individuals. These drugs may be of particular use in high renin states because they reduce renin release. See Figure 20–2.
When should these drugs be avoided?	In patients with peripheral vascular disease, asthma and acute heart failure.
What are the adverse effects?	Sedation Fatigue Bronchoconstriction Impotence May decrease HDL and increase plasma triacylglycerol

GANGLIONIC BLOCKERS

See *Chapter 7—Cholinergic Antagonists,* for more information on ganglionic blockers.

Give two examples of ganglionic blockers.	**Trimethaphan** and **hexamethonium**

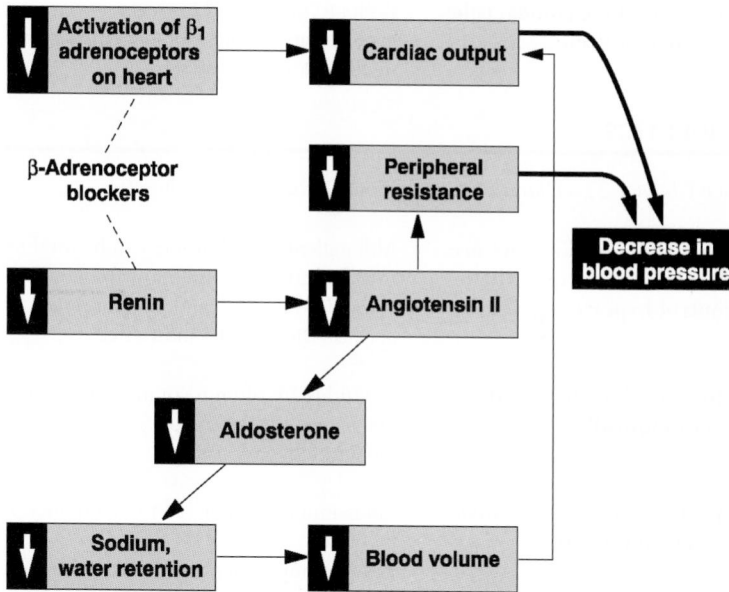

Figure 20–2. Actions of β-adrenergic blocking agents. (Redrawn with permission from Howland RD, Mycek MJ [Harvey RA, Champe PC, eds.]. *Lippincott's Illustrated Reviews: Pharmacology,* 3rd ed. Baltimore: Lippincott Williams & Wilkins, 2006, p. 218.)

What is their clinical use?	These agents are no longer used to treat hypertension because of their severe adverse effects. They are mentioned here because they are of historical importance and sometimes tested on the USMLE ✎.
Describe the adverse effects.	Parasympathetic blockade (urinary retention, blurred vision, and so forth) as well as sympathetic blockade (sexual dysfunction and orthostatic hypotension).

POSTGANGLIONIC ADRENERGIC NEURONAL BLOCKERS

See *Chapter 9—Adrenergic Antagonists,* for more information on these agents.

Give two examples.	**Reserpine** and **guanethidine**
What is the mechanism of action?	These drugs block the release of stored norepinephrine.

| **Describe their clinical role in hypertension.** | Both are rarely used to treat hypertension because of low efficacy and significant adverse effects. |

DIURETICS

See Chapter 23—Diuretics, for additional information on diuretics.

What types of diuretics are chosen most frequently to control hypertension?	Although all oral diuretics can be used to treat hypertension, the most frequently chosen are thiazide and loop diuretics because they are the most effective.
How are diuretics used therapeutically?	Thiazides are often recommended as first line agents for the treatment of mild-to-moderate hypertension
What are some of the toxic effects of diuretics?	Potassium depletion—most common effect Possible impairment of glucose tolerance Possible increase in plasma lipid concentrations

VASODILATORS

HYDRALAZINE (APRESOLINE)

Describe this drug's mechanism of action.	Direct vasodilation of **arteriolar** smooth muscle, which results in decreased PVR. This reduction in resistance is usually followed by reflex tachycardia and fluid retention. β blockers are often coadministered to minimize the sympathetic effects.
How is hydralazine used clinically?	For moderate hypertension and CHF
What are the adverse effects?	Lupus-like syndrome (✎ board question) Cardiovascular effects—hypotension, reflex tachycardia, palpitations, angina Headache Nausea Diarrhea

MINOXIDIL (Loniten)

What is this drug's mechanism of action?	**Minoxidil** is a potent **arterial** vasodilator that works by opening potassium channels, which results in hyperpolarization and relaxation of smooth muscle cells.
How is minoxidil used clinically?	For severe hypertension refractory to other drugs For hair replacement (Rogaine) As with hydralazine, minoxidil is often administered with β blockers and diuretics.
Describe the adverse effects.	Edema due to sodium and water retention Reflex tachycardia Flushing Headache Hypertrichosis (increased hair growth)

SODIUM NITROPRUSSIDE

Describe its mechanism of action.	Sodium nitroprusside releases nitric oxide, which stimulates the enzyme guanylyl cyclase and increases production of intracellular cyclic guanosine monophosphate (cGMP) concentrations. This results in a decrease in intracellular calcium ions and consequent relaxation of vascular smooth muscle (both arterial and venous).
How is sodium nitroprusside used clinically?	For hypertensive emergencies and CHF
What is the route of administration?	Intravenous
What are the adverse effects?	Hypotension Metabolic acidosis Cyanide toxicity—This may occur as a result of cyanide ions produced during metabolism of sodium nitroprusside. (Cyanide toxicity can be treated with

an infusion of rhodanese, an enzyme
that combines cyanide and thiosulfate
to produce thiocyanate, a less toxic
metabolite.)

Thiocyanate toxicity—Symptoms include
weakness, psychosis, muscle spasms,
and convulsions.

DIAZOXIDE

What is its major mechanism of action?	**Diazoxide** prevents arterial smooth muscle contraction by opening potassium channels and stabilizing membrane potentials.
What other action does this drug have?	It prevents insulin release from the pancreas.
State the route of administration.	IV
How is diazoxide used clinically?	For hypertensive emergencies
What are this drug's adverse effects?	Hypotension Reflex tachycardia Hyperglycemia

CALCIUM CHANNEL BLOCKERS

See *Chapter 22—Drugs Used to Treat Congestive Heart Failure,* for
additional information on calcium channel blockers.

Give three examples of calcium channel blockers.	**Nifedipine, verapamil,** and **diltiazem**
Describe the mechanism of action.	Inhibition of calcium influx into smooth muscle cells. **Nifedipine** is the most selective for the peripheral vasculature.
What are the adverse effects of these drugs?	Constipation Headache Dizziness

ACE INHIBITORS

What are they?	ACE inhibitors are angiotensin-converting enzyme inhibitors.
Against which physiological system are ACE inhibitors effective?	The renin-angiotensin-aldosterone system
Explain this system.	Renin is an enzyme that acts on the substrate angiotensinogen and converts it to angiotensin I, which is then converted to angiotensin II in the lungs by ACE (peptidyl-dipeptidase A). Angiotensin II is a potent vasoconstrictor and stimulates the release of aldosterone. Figure 20-3 shows the relationship between the angiotensinogen and kininogen systems.
Give some examples of ACE inhibitors.	**Captopril** (Capoten)—prototype **Lisinopril** (Prinivil, Zestril) **Enalapril** (Vasotec) **Benazepril** (Lotensin)
How do they work?	ACE inhibitors block the conversion of angiotensin I to angiotensin II and also increase levels of bradykinin, which is a potent vasodilator (see Figure 20–3). These drugs do not have much of an effect on cardiac output and heart rate.
For what conditions does a physician prescribe ACE inhibitors?	Mild-to-moderate hypertension CHF (vasodilatory effects) Diabetic nephropathy
Describe the absorption of captopril.	It is well absorbed orally. It does not enter the CNS.
How is captopril eliminated?	Elimination occurs primarily through the urine.
What are the adverse effects of ACE inhibitors?	Dizziness Cough Angioedema

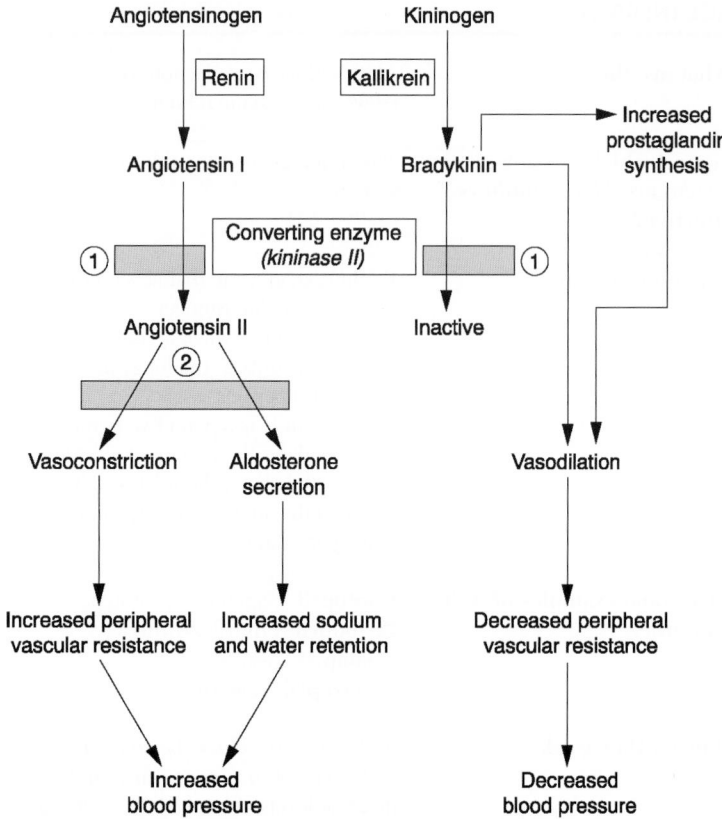

Figure 20–3. Sites of action of ACE inhibitors and receptor blockers. ① = Site of ACE blockade. ② = Site of receptor blockade. (Redrawn with permission from Katzung BG. *Basic & Clinical Pharmacology,* 9th ed. New York: McGraw-Hill, 2004.)

Hyperkalemia
Sudden drop in blood pressure after an initial dose—This can occur in patients who are hypovolemic.
Renal failure in patients who have bilateral renal artery stenosis
Proteinuria
Neutropenia (rare)

Should ACE inhibitors be administered to pregnant women?

No! In the second and third trimesters, there is a risk of fetal hypotension, anuria, and malformations.

What drug interactions should physicians monitor while administering ACE inhibitors?	Nonsteroidal anti-inflammatory drugs (NSAIDs) may reduce the vasodilatory effects of ACE inhibitors, because NSAIDs block the actions of bradykinin.

ANGIOTENSIN II RECEPTOR ANTAGONISTS

Name four angiotensin II receptor antagonists.	**Losartan** (Cozaar), prototype **Valsartan** (Diovan) **Candesartan** (Atacand) **Irbesartan** (Avapro)
Describe the mechanism of action of these drugs.	They block angiotensin II at its receptor site, thus inhibiting both the vasoconstriction and aldosterone-secreting effects of angiotensin II. They do not affect the bradykinin system.
What is the route of administration?	Oral
How are these drugs used clinically?	For mild-to-moderate hypertension
Name three adverse effects of the angiotensin receptor antagonists.	1. Headache 2. Hyperkalemia—especially in patients taking potassium-sparing diuretics 3. Hypotension They do not, however, cause the cough seen with ACE inhibitors.
What are the contraindications?	Like the ACE inhibitors, losartan and valsartan are contraindicated in pregnancy because they may cause fetal malformations, anuria, and hypotension.

SUMMARY

How do physicians choose which antihypertensive medications to use?	Unless the patient has severe hypertension, a single agent will be used initially—usually a diuretic or a β-adrenergic blocker. The specific choice will depend on the patient's other medical conditions. If the hypertension remains uncontrolled, other agents will be added in a stepwise fashion (Figure 20–4).

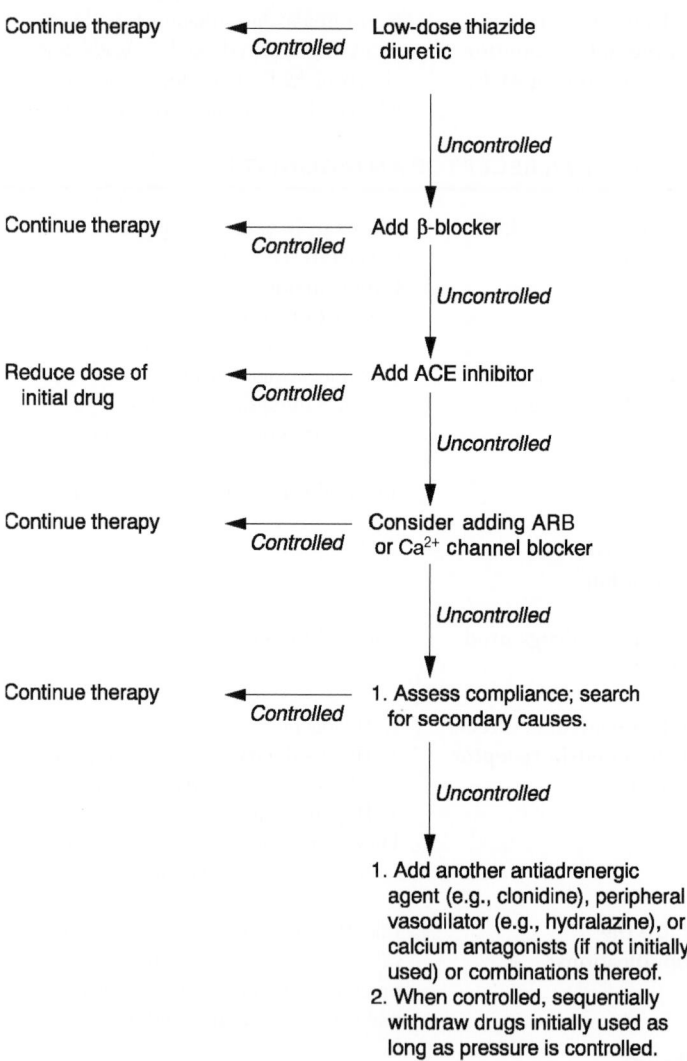

Continue therapy ◄——— *Controlled* ——— Low-dose thiazide diuretic

↓ *Uncontrolled*

Continue therapy ◄——— *Controlled* ——— Add β-blocker

↓ *Uncontrolled*

Reduce dose of initial drug ◄——— *Controlled* ——— Add ACE inhibitor

↓ *Uncontrolled*

Continue therapy ◄——— *Controlled* ——— Consider adding ARB or Ca²⁺ channel blocker

↓ *Uncontrolled*

Continue therapy ◄——— *Controlled* ——— 1. Assess compliance; search for secondary causes.

↓ *Uncontrolled*

1. Add another antiadrenergic agent (e.g., clonidine), peripheral vasodilator (e.g., hydralazine), or calcium antagonists (if not initially used) or combinations thereof.
2. When controlled, sequentially withdraw drugs initially used as long as pressure is controlled.

Figure 20–4. Schematic approach to the treatment of the patient with hypertension in whom a specific form of therapy is not indicated and volume expansion is not present. (Redrawn with permission from Fauci AS, Braunwald E, Isselbacher KJ, et al: *Harrison's Principles of Internal Medicine,* 14th ed. New York: McGraw-Hill, 1997.)

What is malignant hypertension?

Hypertension with associated target-organ vascular damage (i.e., hypertensive encephalopathy, retinal hemorrhage, angina)

How is this condition treated?

In the initial stages, intravenous antihypertensive agents such as diazoxide, labetalol and sodium nitroprusside are used. The goal is not normalization of blood pressure but rather a 25% reduction, because sudden hypoperfusion may result in brain injury. Excess fluid may be removed with loop diuretics or, if necessary, dialysis.

21

Antiarrhythmic Drugs

What is an arrhythmia?

In a normal heart, an impulse originates in the SA node, travels through the atrial muscle into the AV node, through the Purkinje system, and down to the ventricular muscle. Any rhythm that does not start at the SA node or that is not under the usual autonomic control is defined as an arrhythmia.

Why are cardiac arrhythmias significant?

Cardiac arrhythmias are the number one cause of death in the United States, following a myocardial infarction (✎ board question).

How do arrhythmias form?

In one of three ways:
1. **Reentry**—This is the most common cause of arrhythmias (Figure 21–1). The reentry phenomenon occurs when myocardial injury blocks a normally viable conduction pathway. Once initiated, an action potential is usually conducted through several different pathways to the rest of the myocardium; however, if one of the pathways is partially blocked, then by the time the impulse travels through the damaged pathway, the surrounding cells may be in a resting state and ready to be depolarized. If this is the case, then reexcitation of the cardiac tissue will occur.
2. **Enhanced automaticity**—Normally the SA node sets the pace for the heart. If other areas of the heart begin to depolarize more quickly than the SA node, an arrhythmia may result.

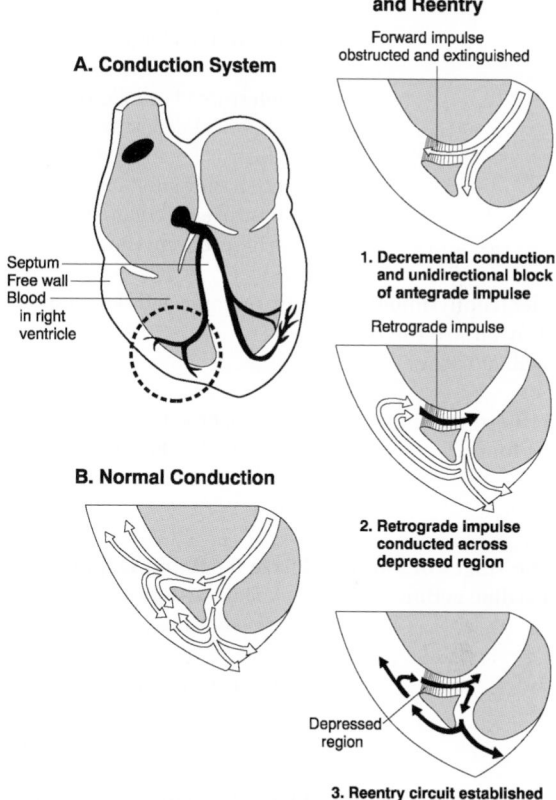

C. Unidirectional Block and Reentry

Forward impulse obstructed and extinguished

A. Conduction System

Septum
Free wall
Blood in right ventricle

1. Decremental conduction and unidirectional block of antegrade impulse

Retrograde impulse

B. Normal Conduction

2. Retrograde impulse conducted across depressed region

Depressed region

3. Reentry circuit established

Figure 21–1. Schematic drawings of the heart showing unidirectional block and reentry—the most common cause of arrhythmias. (A) Conduction system. Circled area (enlarged in the other drawings) shows small bifurcating twig of the Purkinje system where it enters the ventricular wall. (B) The normal passage and fate of an impulse that is conducted down the twig. It splits into two impulses at the bifurcation, and these collide (and extinguish each other) after exciting the ventricular muscle. (C) The sequence of events when the normal impulse finds an areas of unidirectional block (blocked depressed region) in one of the branches. As shown by the path of the impulse in the depressed region (*1*), this weak stimulus is unable to conduct through or to "jump over" the area of block. In contrast, the wave in the undepressed branch is able to excite the entire ventricular wall (*2*). Because the ventricular wall constitutes a large mass of cells, the strong ventricular depolarization is able to jump the depressed region and results in a retrograde impulse *(shown by the black arrows in 2 and 3)*. The retrograde impulse may be propagated if the impulse finds excitable tissue, i.e., the refractory period is shorter than the conduction time. This impulse will then reexcite tissue it had previously passed through, and a reentry arrhythmia will be established in the circuit *(indicated by the black arrows in 3)*. (Redrawn with permission from Katzung BG. *Basic and Clinical Pharmacology,* 7th ed. Stamford, CT: Appleton & Lange, 1998, p. 225.)

3. **Triggered automaticity**—On occasion (during ischemia, digitalis intoxication, or adrenergic stress), a normal cardiac action potential may be interrupted or followed by an abnormal depolarization. These abnormal secondary action potentials occur only after a normal **triggering** upstroke and therefore are called **triggered rhythms**.

From an electrophysiologic standpoint, what are the two types of cardiac tissue?

Fast-response and slow-response

Where are these cardiac tissue types found?

Slow-response tissue is found in the SA and AV nodes. Fast response tissue is found in the myocardium and Purkinje cells.

Describe the stages of a fast-response cardiac action potential.

Phase 0—Rapid Depolarization—Voltage-sensitive Na^+ channels open, which results in a rapid influx of Na^+ ions.

Phase 1—Partial Repolarization—Na^+ channels become inactivated; K^+ channels begin to open, which results in an efflux of K^+ and Cl^- influx.

Phase 2—Plateau—Ca^{2+} influx and K^+ efflux causes a plateau, which is unique to the cardiac action potential.

Phase 3—Rapid Repolarization—K^+ efflux and inactivation of Ca^{2+} channels occur.

Phase 4—Diastolic Depolarization—The resting membrane potential is maintained by K^+ efflux and slow Na^+ and Ca^{2+} influx (Figure 21–2).

How does a slow-response cardiac action potential differ from a fast-response action potential?

The SA and AV nodes have a slow upstroke velocity, a smaller magnitude of action potential, and a brief plateau. There are no fast Na^+ channels, and the action potential is caused by the opening of Ca^{2+} channels (see Figure 21–2).

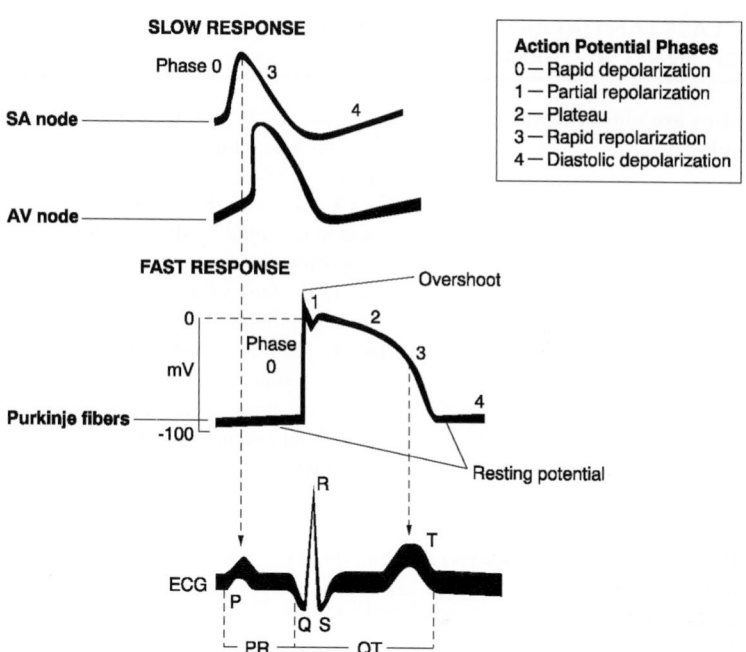

Figure 21–2. Schematic representation of normal cardiac action potentials from different tissues in the heart and their relationship to a standard ECG.

What are some examples of supraventricular arrhythmias?	AV nodal reentrant arrhythmias, atrial fibrillation, atrial flutter, and multifocal atrial tachycardia
What are some examples of ventricular arrhythmias?	Ventricular tachycardia, ventricular fibrillation, and premature ventricular contractions
Generally, what is the mechanism of action of the antiarrhythmic drugs?	Suppression of arrhythmias by blocking either autonomic function or specific ion channels
What are the four classes of antiarrhythmic drugs?	Class I—sodium channel blockers Class II—β-adrenergic blockers Class III—potassium channel blockers Class IV—calcium channel blockers Some drugs, such as **sotalol** and **amiodarone**, will exhibit properties of more than one class. Other drugs, such as **digoxin** and **magnesium sulfate**, do not belong to a particular class.

CLASS I ANTIARRHYTHMICS—SODIUM CHANNEL BLOCKERS

How are class I drugs subdivided?	Into classes I_A, I_B, and I_C based on their effects on the action potential. In general: **Class I_A** increases the duration of the action potential by slowing phase 0 depolarization. **Class I_B** decreases the duration of the action potential by shortening phase 3. **Class I_C** has little effect on the duration of the action potential. Rather, they decrease automatically by increasing threshold potential and thus slowing conduction velocity.

CLASS I_A

Which drugs are considered to be class I_A antiarrhythmics?	Quinidine, procainamide, and disopyramide

Quinidine (Quinidex)

How does quinidine work?	**Quinidine** binds to activated Na^+ channels, which prevents Na^+ influx. This slows the repolarization of phase 0 and decreases the slope of phase 4. Thus, tissues that are frequently depolarizing will be selectively suppressed over tissues that are depolarizing at a normal frequency. This drug property is termed **use-dependent block. Quinidine** also inhibits K^+ currents and increases repolarization time.
What are the clinical indications for administration of quinidine?	Ventricular tachycardia and supraventricular arrhythmias (most commonly, atrial fibrillation and atrial flutter)
What are its effects on ECG?	**Quinidine** prolongs the QT interval.
How is this drug administered?	PO

Where is it metabolized?

In the liver—half-life of 6 to 8 hr

What are the adverse effects of quinidine?

Noncardiac:

GI—Diarrhea, nausea, and vomiting are commonly observed.

Possible cinchonism—a symptom complex that includes blurred vision, dizziness, headache, and tinnitus

Quinidine syncope, characterized by recurrent light-headedness and episodes of fainting

Thrombocytopenic purpura

Cardiac:

Torsades de pointes—a type of arrhythmia with prolongation of the QT interval

Proarrhythmogenic effects—AV block or asystole

Are there drug interactions?

Quinidine increases plasma levels of digoxin and oral anticoagulants.

Phenobarbital and **phenytoin** reduce **quinidine** plasma levels.

Procainamide (Pronestyl)

What are the therapeutic indications for procainamide?

It is used for treating both ventricular and supraventricular arrhythmias.

Describe the metabolite of procainamide.

A portion of **procainamide** is metabolized in the liver to N-acetyl procainamide (NAPA), which has the properties of a class III drug. This metabolite may cause torsades de pointes.

How is procainamide administered?

PO or IV; can cause marked hypotension.

What are the adverse effects?

Lupus-like syndrome (✎ common board question)—Initially, this drug-induced lupus will manifest as a rash and small-joint arthralgia. Renal involvement is unusual.

Pleuritis and pericarditis can also occur.

Toxic effects can cause asystole, hallucination, and psychosis.

Torsades de pointes

Disopyramide (Norpace)

Describe this drug's mechanism of action.	Very similar to that of **quinidine** except that it produces a greater negative inotropic effect and possesses stronger anticholinergic effects
How is disopyramide administered?	IV or PO
In what clinical situations is disopyramide used?	It can be used for treating both ventricular and supraventricular arrhythmias.
Describe the metabolism of this drug.	It is largely excreted in the urine unchanged but a small portion of it is metabolized in the liver.
What adverse effects should you watch for?	Anticholinergic effects—dry mouth, urinary retention, constipation, precipitation of glaucoma Torsades de pointes Heart failure in patients who have left ventricular dysfunction Prostatism

CLASS I$_B$

Which drugs are considered class I$_B$ antiarrhythmics?	**Lidocaine** **Tocainide** **Mexiletine** **Phenytoin**

Lidocaine (Xylocaine)

What ion channels does lidocaine affect?	**Lidocaine** blocks both open and inactivated Na$^+$ channels but exerts greater effects on inactivated channels. It also shortens phase 3 repolarization and decreases the slope of phase.
When do you use this drug?	**Lidocaine** is used for the acute management of ventricular arrhythmias, especially in patients with myocardial infarction. Although this is an old indication, lidocaine has a particular affinity for ischemic muscle. In clinical practice, there is enough evidence to believe that it is not the best; we

therefore use **amiodarone** as our first choice. It is also used as a local anesthetic.

How is lidocaine administered?

IV

Describe the metabolism of lidocaine.

Lidocaine undergoes extensive first pass metabolism in the liver. Dosage must be adjusted in patients who have hepatic dysfunction.

What are the ECG effects?

Usually there is no change in the duration of the PR or QRS interval.

Are there side effects to monitor during administration?

CNS effects—Drowsiness, numbness, slurred speech, and convulsions; nystagmus is an early sign of toxicity. Can induce cardiac arrhythmias.

Tocainide (Tonocard)

What are the therapeutic indications?

Tocainide is used primarily for treating ventricular arrhythmias.

How is it administered?

Orally

What are this drug's adverse effects?

Cardiovascular effects—bradycardia, tachycardia, AV block, hypotension, ventricular tachycardia
Anorexia, nausea
Tremor
Pulmonary fibrosis (rare)
Bone marrow aplasia (rare)

Mexiletine (Mexitil)

What is this drug's clinical use?

It is used to treat ventricular arrhythmias.

How is mexiletine administered?

Orally

What toxicities are important to remember when using mexiletine?

Dizziness, nervousness
Nausea and vomiting
Blood dyscrasias
Nystagmus, thrombocytopenia
Leukopenia, agranulocytosis

Phenytoin (Dilantin)

How is this drug classified?	**Phenytoin** is an anticonvulsant that binds to inactivated Na$^+$ channels and prolongs the inactivated state.
What is the route of administration?	IV or PO
State the therapeutic indications.	Drug of choice for treating digoxin-induced atrial and ventricular arrhythmias
Are there adverse effects?	CNS effects—nystagmus, ataxia Gingival hyperplasia Serious bone marrow and dermatologic reactions can occur.

CLASS I$_C$

Name three drugs considered to be class I$_C$ antiarrhythmics.	1. **Flecainide** 2. **Propafenone** 3. **Moricizine**

Flecainide (Tambocor)

How does this drug work?	**Flecainide** blocks Na$^+$ channels in Purkinje cells, which shortens the duration of the action potential. It also blocks K$^+$ channels in ventricular myocytes, which prolongs the action potential. The net effect is minimal change in action potential duration.
When is flecainide used?	For treating life-threatening ventricular arrhythmias in patients without myocardial structural abnormalities
What toxicities are associated with flecainide?	Proarrhythmogenic effects—The Cardiac Arrhythmia Suppressor Trial (CAST) study showed that **flecainide** increased mortality in patients who recently suffered a MI and had asymptomatic ventricular arrhythmias. Therefore it is used only as a last-line agent. CNS effects—blurred vision, headache Heart block in patients who have conduction system disease

Propafenone (Rythmol)

How is this drug used clinically?	For treating supraventricular and ventricular arrhythmias
What is its mechanism of action?	**Propafenone** possesses a mechanism of action similar to that of **flecainide**, but it exerts β-adrenergic blockade activity as well.
Describe the metabolism of propafenone	Hepatic metabolism. There are slow and fast metabolizers. In slow metabolizers the drug accumulates and causes toxicity. Very important to monitor plasma levels.
State the adverse effects.	Proarrhythmogenic effects β-blockade effects (bronchospasm, bradycardia)

Moricizine (Ethmozine)

How does moricizine work?	Its mechanism of action is similar to that of **flecainide**.
How is this drug used clinically?	**Moricizine** is used for the treatment of severe ventricular arrhythmias.
What are the adverse reactions?	Proarrhythmogenic effects

CLASS II ANTIARRHYTHMICS—β BLOCKERS

See *Chapter 9—Adrenergic Antagonists,* for a more detailed discussion of these agents.

Give some examples of drugs in this group.	**Propranolol, metoprolol, atenolol, esmolol**
At which part of the action potential do these drugs work?	Class II drugs work at diminishing phase 4, thus depressing automaticity and decreasing heart rate.
How are these drugs used clinically?	They are effective in preventing arrhythmias after an MI. Both supraventricular and ventricular tachyarrhythmias respond to β blockers.

ESMOLOL

When is this drug used?	Esmolol is a very short-acting β-adrenergic blocker and is almost always used in the treatment of acute surgical arrhythmias.

CLASS III ANTIARRHYTHMICS—POTASSIUM CHANNEL BLOCKERS

Which drugs fall into this category?	**Sotalol, bretylium, amiodarone, ibutilide, dofetilide**
In general how do these drugs work?	Class III drugs exert their effects by blocking K^+ channels, which, in turn, prolongs phase 3 of the action potential.

SOTALOL

What is its mechanism of action?	**Sotalol** decreases automaticity, slows AV nodal conduction, and prolongs the AV refractory period by K^+ channel blockade and mild blockade of β-adrenergic receptors.
How is this drug used clinically?	It is used to treat ventricular tachyarrhythmias and supraventricular arrhythmias. Sotalol is effective in reducing mortality in patients with these conditions.

BRETYLIUM

State the mechanism of action for bretylium.	It prolongs the ventricular action potential and effective refractory period. It also blocks norepinephrine release.
Describe this drug's clinical use.	**Bretylium** is used for treating refractory ventricular fibrillation and ventricular tachycardia during times of cardiac arrest. It is very rarely used.
What are the adverse effects?	Postural hypotension

AMIODARONE (CORDARONE)

What is it?	A drug structurally related to thyroid hormone
Describe its mechanism of action.	**Amiodarone** exhibits properties of class I to IV drugs but predominantly has class III actions.
What are its clinical uses?	This drug is used for treating refractory atrial flutter/fibrillation and ventricular tachyarrhythmia.
How is amiodarone administered?	Orally or IV
What are the adverse effects of amiodarone?	Interstitial pulmonary fibrosis CNS—tremor, ataxia Hepatocellular necrosis Photosensitivity Corneal microdeposits Thyroid dysfunction (hypo- or hyperthyroidism) Blue skin discoloration caused by iodine accumulation Because of these side effects, patients will have liver function tests (LFTs), pulmonary function tests (PFTs), and thyroid function tests (TFTs) checked prior to initiating treatment and monitored regularly.

IBUTILIDE (CORVERT)

What are its clinical indications?	Treatment of atrial flutter and fibrillation
How is it administered?	IV
What are its toxic effects?	Inducing torsades de pointes

DOFETILIDE (TIKOSYN)

What are its clinical indications?	Maintaining sinus rhythm in patients with atrial flutter or fibrillation
Are there any adverse effects?	Inducing torsades de pointes

CLASS IV ANTIARRHYTHMICS—CALCIUM CHANNEL BLOCKERS

Which drugs belong to this group?	**Verapamil, diltiazem,** and **nifedipine**
How do they work?	These drugs block "L"-type calcium channels and decrease both SA node automaticity and AV nodal conduction. More specifically, they decrease the rate of phase 4 spontaneous depolarization and thus increase the effective refractory period. **Verapamil** has the greatest effect on cardiac tissue.
What types of arrhythmias are treated with calcium channel blockers?	Supraventricular arrhythmias (atrial flutter, atrial fibrillation)
What are the major side effects of calcium channel blockers?	Bradycardia CHF Hypotension Dizziness Constipation

For more information on calcium channel blockers, see *Chapter 20—Antihypertensive Drugs.*

OTHER ANTIARRHYTHMIC AGENTS

DIGOXIN (LANOXIN)

How does this drug work?
Digoxin inhibits the Na^+/K^+-ATPase pump in myocardial cell membranes.

How does digoxin serve as an antiarrhythmic?
It increases the refractory period and decreases the conduction time of the AV node.

How is digoxin used therapeutically?
For treating supraventricular arrhythmias and congestive heart failure

What are the toxicities to watch for?
Atrial or ventricular dysrhythmias (most commonly atrial tachycardia)

What is the treatment for digoxin toxicity?
Digoxin antibodies

See *Chapter 22—Drugs Used to Treat Congestive Heart Failure*, for a more detailed discussion of cardiac glycosides.

MAGNESIUM SULFATE

How does magnesium sulfate prevent arrhythmia?
The mechanism is not completely clear, but it is thought to stabilize cardiac cell membranes.

When do you use this drug?
For treating torsades de pointes

What are the adverse effects?
Bradycardia
Respiratory paralysis
Flushing
Headache

ADENOSINE (ADENOCARD)

How does adenosine work?

It activates acetylcholine-sensitive K^+ channels, especially in the SA and AV nodes. This increase in K^+ conductance results in a shortening of action potential duration, hyperpolarization and decreased automaticity.

How is it administered?

IV only

Describe adenosine's clinical role.

It is a beneficial drug for diagnosing and terminating paroxysmal supraventricular tachyarrhythmias because of its limited toxicities and rapid onset.

What are the adverse effects?

Flushing
Dyspnea
Chest pain
Headache

22

Drugs Used to Treat Congestive Heart Failure

The pharmacology of many of the drugs mentioned in this chapter is discussed in greater detail in other chapters of this book. Please note the cross-references.

Define congestive heart failure (CHF).	CHF results when cardiac output is inadequate for the metabolic demands of the body.
What are some of the most common causes of CHF?	Myocardial infarction (MI) Hypertension (HTN) Arrhythmia Valvular disease Arteriosclerotic heart disease These conditions either impair the ability of cardiac muscle to contract (MI, arrhythmia) or increase the workload imposed upon the heart (HTN).
Name some of the physical signs of CHF.	Left-sided heart failure results in pulmonary edema and dyspnea. Right-sided heart failure results in liver congestion and peripheral edema.
Describe the compensatory physiological mechanisms that occur in heart failure.	Increased sympathetic tone, which results in tachycardia and greater peripheral vascular resistance. Reduced renal blood flow, which stimulates aldosterone and increases salt and water retention. Myocardial hypertrophy

Name three major pharmacological approaches for the treatment of CHF.

1. Improve myocardial contractility
2. Reduce preload (which decreases myocardial oxygen demands)
3. Reduce afterload. Remember that cardiac output = heart rate × stroke volume. Stroke volume is dependent on preload, afterload, and contractility.

What are the pharmacological options for treating patients who have CHF?

Cardiac glycosides
Bipyridine derivatives
β-adrenergic agonists
Vasodilators
Diuretics
Angiotensin-converting enzyme (ACE) inhibitors
β-adrenergic blockers

CARDIAC GLYCOSIDES

Name three cardiac glycosides.

1. **Digoxin** (Lanoxin)
2. **Digitoxin** (Crystodigin)
3. Ouabain (no longer in use)
Digoxin is by far the most widely used form because of its favorable pharmacokinetics.

Where do cardiac glycosides originate?

They are extracts of the foxglove plant, *Digitalis lanata.*

Describe how glycosides work.

Cardiac glycosides inhibit the Na^+, K^+-ATPase pump on cardiac cell membranes, which results in increased intracellular Na^+. This increase in intracellular Na^+ reduces the electrochemical gradient that drives the extrusion of intracellular Ca^{2+} by the Na^+/Ca^{2+} exchanger (Figure 22–1). The resulting accumulation of intracellular Ca^{2+} is stored in the sarcoplasmic reticulum and, when released, causes increased myocardial contractility.

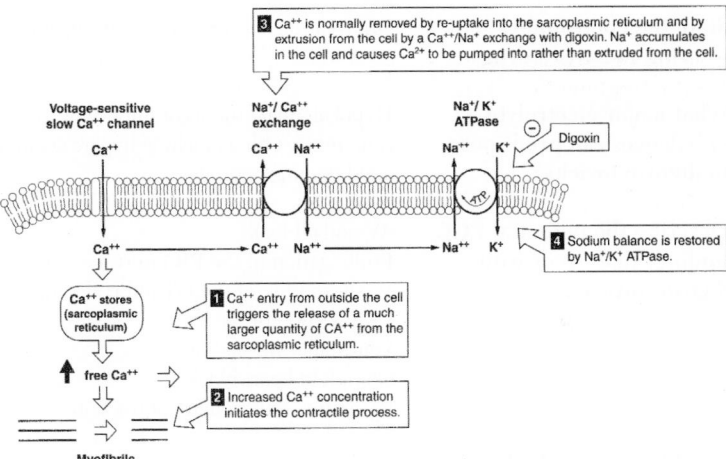

3 Ca^{++} is normally removed by re-uptake into the sarcoplasmic reticulum and by extrusion from the cell by a Ca^{++}/Na^+ exchange with digoxin. Na^+ accumulates in the cell and causes Ca^{2+} to be pumped into rather than extruded from the cell.

Voltage-sensitive slow Ca^{++} channel

Na^+/Ca^{++} exchange

Na^+/K^+ ATPase

Digoxin

Ca^{++}

Ca^{++} Na^{++}

Na^{++} K^+

$Ca^{++} \longrightarrow Ca^{++}$ $Na^{++} \longrightarrow Na^{++}$ K^+

4 Sodium balance is restored by Na^+/K^+ ATPase.

Ca^{++} stores (sarcoplasmic reticulum)

1 Ca^{++} entry from outside the cell triggers the release of a much larger quantity of CA^{++} from the sarcoplasmic reticulum.

↑ free Ca^{++}

2 Increased Ca^{++} concentration initiates the contractile process.

Myofibrils

Figure 22–1. Normal ion movements during the contraction of cardiac muscle. (Adapted with permission from Howland RD, Mycek MJ [Harvey RA, Champe PC, eds.]. *Lippincott's Illustrated Reviews: Pharmacology,* 3rd ed. Baltimore: Lippincott Williams & Wilkins, 2006, p. 184.)

How does digoxin differ from digitoxin with respect to the route of administration, half-life, percent of plasma-bound protein, and metabolism?

	Digoxin	Digitoxin
Route of administration	PO, IV, IM	PO
Half-life	36–48 hr	4–8 days (the longer name has the longer half-life)
% plasma-bound protein	20–30	90–95
Metabolism	Renal	Hepatic

What are the clinical indications for the administration of digoxin?

Congestive heart failure—No longer a first-line agent. It is currently reserved for patients who are symptomatic despite having maximal therapy with ACE Inhibitors, β blockers, and diuretics.

Atrial flutter and fibrillation—Digoxin slows the conduction velocity and increases the refractory period at the AV node.

State the contraindications to using these two drugs.

Bradycardia and ventricular fibrillation

What major electrolyte imbalances can predispose to digoxin toxicity?

Hypokalemia—the most important to remember. Others include hypercalcemia and hypomagnesemia.

Describe the potential ECG findings that occur with digoxin toxicity.

AV nodal block
Prolongation of the PR interval, shortening of the QT interval, and inversion of the t wave
Ventricular fibrillation
Complete heart block
Premature ventricular contraction

In addition to arrhythmias, patients with digoxin toxicity have what symptoms?

Nausea and vomiting
Diarrhea
Headache
Fatigue
Blurred vision
Hallucinations
Altered color perception (yellow-green hue)
Rarely, gynecomastia

How do you treat digoxin toxicity?

By discontinuing use of the drug
By correcting any electrolyte imbalances
Antiarrhythmics (**lidocaine**)
If necessary, by using digoxin antibodies that bind to and inactivate the drug
Cardiac pacer: last resort

Are there any important drug interactions to be aware of?

Quinidine, amiodarone, and **verapamil** all reduce plasma clearance of digoxin and can precipitate **digoxin** toxicity. Loop and thiazide diuretics can deplete K^+ and cause digoxin toxicity.

Has digoxin been shown to reduce mortality?

No. Unlike ACE inhibitors or β blockers, **digoxin** reduces only symptoms, not mortality.

BIPYRIDINE DERIVATIVES

Name two bipyridine derivatives.	**Amrinone** (Inocor) and **milrinone** (Primacor)
What is their mechanism of action?	They inhibit phosphodiesterase, which leads to increased levels of cyclic adenosine monophosphate and intracellular calcium. This subsequently results in increased contractility. Bipyridines also cause vasodilation.
Describe the route of administration.	Both of these drugs are given intravenously only.
What is their clinical role?	Bipyridines are rarely used today because of their adverse effects. In the past they were used to treat acute heart failure.
What are the major toxicities of amrinone and milrinone?	Arrhythmias Gastrointestinal disturbances Hepatotoxicity Thrombocytopenia—**amrinone** only

β-ADRENERGIC AGONISTS

Name two β-adrenergic agonists used in the treatment of CHF.	**Dobutamine** (Dobutrex) and **dopamine**
What is their mechanism of action?	By stimulating β-adrenergic receptors, they increase cardiac contractility.
How are these drugs used clinically?	They are used to treat **acute** heart failure only; they are not indicated for chronic therapy.

See *Chapter 8—Adrenergic Agonists,* for further information about β agonists.

VASODILATORS

Which vasodilators are considered appropriate for the treatment of CHF?	Nitrates (discussed in *Chapter 24—Antianginal Drugs*) Hydralazine (Apresoline; discussed in *Chapter 20—Antihypertensive Drugs*) ACE inhibitors
What is the reasoning behind using vasodilators?	Vasodilators reduce both preload (through venodilation) and afterload (through arterial dilation).

See *Chapter 20—Antihypertensive Drugs,* for further information on vasodilators.

DIURETICS

Give some examples of diuretics used in CHF.	**Furosemide, hydrochlorothiazide,** and **spironolactone**
How do diuretics work in the treatment of congestive heart failure?	These agents reduce preload by minimizing salt and water retention. They also reduce afterload by decreasing plasma volume. See *Chapter 23—Diuretics,* for a detailed discussion of these agents. **Furosemide** is useful in acute CHF, while **spironolactone** is more commonly used in chronic CHF.

ACE INHIBITORS

Give some examples of these drugs.	**Quinapril** **Enalapril** **Captopril** **Lisinopril**
Why are ACE inhibitors used in the management of CHF?	Ace inhibitors provide several benefits to patients who have heart failure: They reduce peripheral resistance by causing vasodilation. They minimize salt and water retention by reducing aldosterone levels.

> They reduce cardiac remodeling. (The term "tissue remodeling" refers to slow structural tissue changes. These include proliferation of connective tissue cells as well as growth of abnormal myocytes.)
>
> ACE inhibitors have been shown to reduce mortality.

If ACE inhibitors are not well tolerated by the patient, what can be used as a potential substitute?

An angiotensin receptor blocker (ARB) such as **Losartan**.

See *Chapter 20—Antihypertensive Drugs,* for a detailed discussion of ACE inhibitors.

β-ADRENERGIC BLOCKERS

Name two β blockers approved for treatment of chronic CHF.

Carvedilol, Metoprolol

What role do they play in CHF?

Although it may seem paradoxical to use β-adrenergic blockers in the treatment of CHF, recent clinical trials have shown that mortality is reduced with their use. β-adrenergic blockers seem to help by preventing the adverse effects of chronic sympathetic output and reducing remodeling of the heart.

When should physicians employ β-adrenergic blockers?

These agents should be used only when the patient is **hemodynamically stable**; they should never be used during acute heart failure.

See *Chapter 9—Adrenergic Antagonists,* for further information about β antagonists.

23   Diuretics

What are diuretics?   Diuretics are drugs that increase the volume of urine flow.

How do diuretics work?   In general, diuretics affect ion transport in the nephron. Clinically useful diuretics primarily inhibit **Na$^+$ reabsorption.** Water is then carried along passively in order to maintain an osmotic equilibrium.

What are their principal sites of action?   Proximal convoluted tubule (PCT)
Thick ascending limb of loop of Henle
Distal convoluted tubule (DCT)
Collecting duct
See Figure 23–1.

Major Locations of Ion and Water Exchange in the Nephron

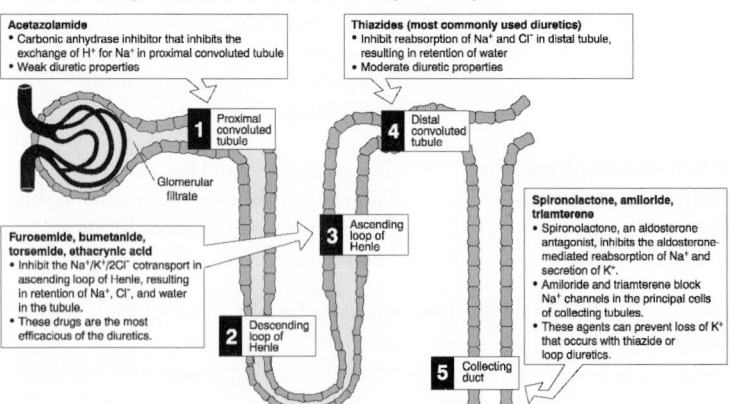

Acetazolamide
* Carbonic anhydrase inhibitor that inhibits the exchange of H$^+$ for Na$^+$ in proximal convoluted tubule
* Weak diuretic properties

Thiazides (most commonly used diuretics)
* Inhibit reabsorption of Na$^+$ and Cl$^-$ in distal tubule, resulting in retention of water
* Moderate diuretic properties

Furosemide, bumetanide, torsemide, ethacrynic acid
* Inhibit the Na$^+$/K$^+$/2Cl$^-$ cotransport in ascending loop of Henle, resulting in retention of Na$^+$, Cl$^-$, and water in the tubule.
* These drugs are the most efficacious of the diuretics.

Spironolactone, amiloride, triamterene
* Spironolactone, an aldosterone antagonist, inhibits the aldosterone-mediated reabsorption of Na$^+$ and secretion of K$^+$.
* Amiloride and triamterene block Na$^+$ channels in the principal cells of collecting tubules.
* These agents can prevent loss of K$^+$ that occurs with thiazide or loop diuretics.

1 Proximal convoluted tubule
2 Descending loop of Henle
3 Ascending loop of Henle
4 Distal convoluted tubule
5 Collecting duct

Glomerular filtrate

Figure 23–1. Major locations of ion and water exchange in the nephron, showing sites of action of the diuretic drugs. (Redrawn with permission from Howland RD, Mycek MJ [Harvey RA, Champe PC, eds.]. *Lippincott's Illustrated Reviews: Pharmacology,* 3rd ed. Baltimore: Lippincott Williams & Wilkins, 2006, p 258.)

Why is knowing the sites of action important?

This knowledge helps predict:
1. The magnitude and pattern of diuresis
2. The side effects of the medication
3. The pattern of electrolyte loss

Name the five major classes of diuretics.

1. Carbonic anhydrase inhibitors
2. Loop diuretics
3. Thiazide diuretics
4. Osmotic diuretics
5. Potassium-sparing diuretics

CARBONIC ANHYDRASE INHIBITORS

What is the function of carbonic anhydrase?

Carbonic anhydrase is an enzyme that catalyzes the following reaction:

$$CO_2 + H_2O \rightleftarrows H_2CO_3$$

How does a carbonic anhydrase inhibitor produce diuresis?

The H^+ ion produced by the spontaneous breakdown of H_2CO_3 is usually exchanged for Na^+ and is also used to combine with HCO_3^- in the lumen of the PCT. Without the H^+ there is decreased reabsorption of Na^+ and HCO_3^-; this results in diuresis.
See Figure 23–2.

How efficient is the diuresis produced by a carbonic anhydrase inhibitor?

It is relatively weak because other sites further along in the nephron can compensate for the increased Na^+ load.

Name the prototype carbonic anhydrase inhibitor.

Acetazolamide (Diamox)

What is the route of administration?

Oral or IV. **Acetazolamide** analogues such as **dorzolamide** can be given topically for use in the eye.

What are the clinical uses of acetazolamide?

Glaucoma—**Acetazolamide** decreases production of aqueous humor.
To correct a metabolic alkalosis
Mountain sickness—**Acetazolamide** is occasionally used as prophylaxis against mountain (altitude) sickness.

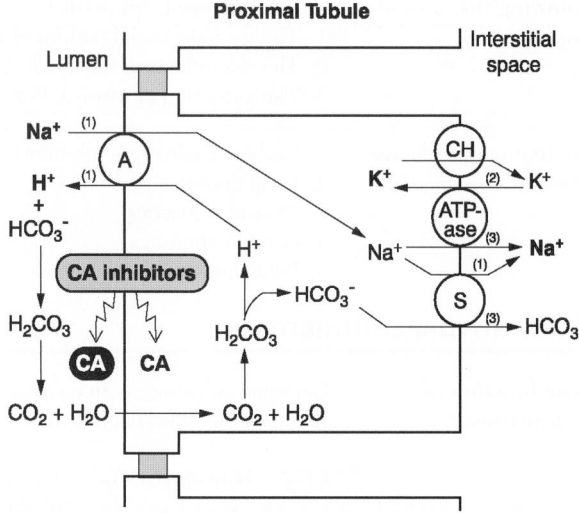

Figure 23–2. NaHCO$_3$ reabsorption in the proximal tubule and mechanism of diuretic action of carbonic anhydrase (CA) inhibitors. A = antiporter; S = symporter; CH = ion channel. (The actual reaction catalyzed by carbonic anhydrase is OH$^-$ + CO$_2$ $\rightleftarrows$ HCO$_3^-$; however, H$_2$O $\rightleftarrows$ OH$^-$ + H$^+$, and HCO$_3$ + H$^+$ $\rightleftarrows$ H$_2$CO$_3$, so that the net reaction is H$_2$O + CO$_2$ $\rightleftarrows$ H2CO$_3^-$.) Numbers in parentheses indicate stoichiometry. (Redrawn from Goodman LS, Gilman AG [eds.]. The *Pharmacological Basis of Therapeutics,* 7th ed. New York: Macmillan, 1985, p 693. Used with permission of The McGraw-Hill Companies.)

Epilepsy—in combination with other antiepileptic drugs.

What are this drug's adverse effects?

Paresthesias and drowsiness are fairly common.

Hyperchloremic metabolic acidosis caused by loss of bicarbonate.

Potassium depletion caused by the sodium load and increased flow rate past the DCT.

Renal calculus—the alkalinization of the urine can cause the precipitation of calcium salts.

Acetazolamide is a sulfonamide derivative and therefore can cause problems similar to those of other sulfonamides, such as allergic reactions.

LOOP DIURETICS

Name the loop diuretics.	**Furosemide** (Lasix), **ethacrynic acid** (Edecrin), and **bumetanide** (Bumex)
What are the mechanism of action and site of action of these drugs?	Loop diuretics work by blocking the $Na^+/K^+/2Cl^-$ cotransport system in the thick ascending limb of the loop of Henle.
Why are the loop diuretics also called "high-ceiling diuretics?"	Because they have the highest efficacy of all diuretics.
Why are they the most efficacious diuretics?	25% to 35% of NaCl is normally reabsorbed at the ascending loop of Henle. Sites downstream along the nephron (distal convoluted tubule and collecting duct) cannot fully compensate if Na^+ reabsorption in the loop of Henle is blocked.
How do loop diuretics affect Ca^{2+} metabolism?	Loop diuretics increase the Ca^{2+} content of the urine (Figure 23–3).
What are the clinical uses of loop diuretics?	Pulmonary edema, CHF, or other states that require a rapid reduction in blood volume Acute hypercalcemia, hyperkalemia, and acute renal failure
What is the route of administration?	IV or oral
What are the adverse effects?	Volume depletion Ototoxicity—especially when used in conjunction with an aminoglycoside Hyperuricemia Hypokalemia Hypomagnesemia Hypocalcemia Hyperchloremic metabolic alkalosis Interstitial nephritis—Loop diuretics are sulfonamide derivatives.

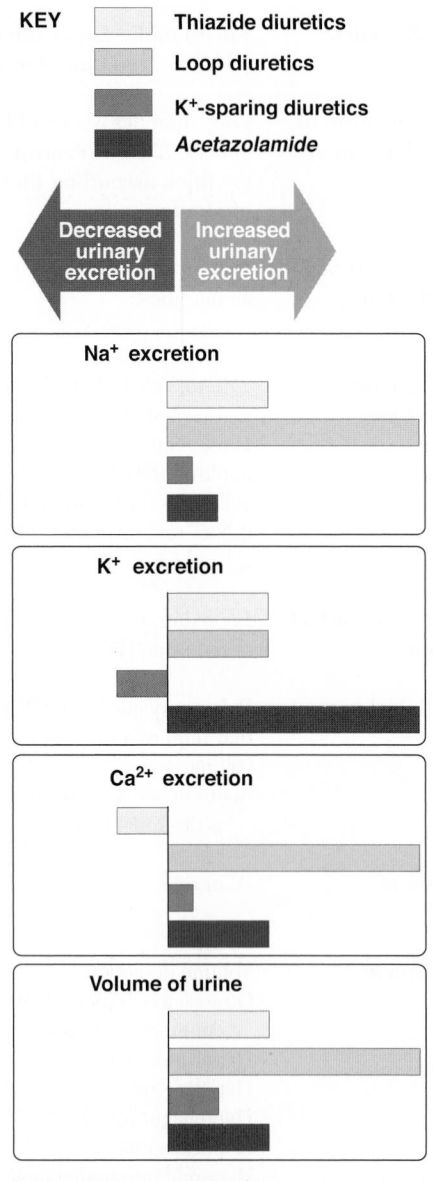

Figure 23–3. Summary of relative changes in urinary composition induced by diuretic drugs.

THIAZIDE DIURETICS

What are they?	Sulfonamide derivatives related structurally to the carbonic anhydrase inhibitors
Give some examples.	**Chlorothiazide**—prototype **Hydrochlorothiazide** (HydroDIURIL) **Metolazone** (Zaroxolyn) and **Indapamide** (Lozol)—are considered thiazide analogues because they differ slightly in structure but share a similar mechanism of action.
Where do they work?	All thiazides work in the early segment of the distal convoluted tubule.
How do they work?	They block **Na^+/Cl^- cotransport on the luminal side of the distal convoluted tubule.**
How effective are thiazides?	They are only moderately effective because most of the filtered Na^+ is absorbed before it reaches the DCT.
What are the uses of thiazides?	They are used to treat: Hypertension Congestive heart failure Nephrosis Hypercalciuria Nephrogenic diabetes insipidus— Thiazides have the ability to produce a slightly hyperosmolar urine and thus diminish polyuria.
Which thiazides are most effective?	All thiazides are equally effective; they differ only in potency.
How do thiazides affect plasma Ca^{2+} levels?	Thiazides, unlike loop diuretics, decrease Ca^{2+} levels in the urine, which results in **increased** Ca^{2+} levels in the blood.

What are the side effects of thiazide diuretics?	Hypokalemia—most common Hyponatremia Hypochloremic metabolic alkalosis Hyperuricemia Hyperglycemia Hyperlipidemia Hypercalcemia

OSMOTIC DIURETICS

What are the most commonly used osmotic diuretics?	**Mannitol** and **urea**
What is their mechanism of action?	Osmotic diuretics are freely filterable substances; once they become a component of the luminal fluid, they create an osmotic effect to pull in water along the entire nephron but especially at the PCT and collecting duct. These agents are not effective in excreting Na^+ like other diuretics.
What are the clinical uses of these drugs?	Osmotic diuretics are mainly used in a hospital setting to treat increased intracranial and intraocular pressure and acute renal failure.
What is the route of administration?	These drugs must be given IV; other modes of administration will cause cathartic diarrhea.
What are the toxicities associated with osmotic diuretics?	Hypovolemia Hypernatremia Can cause pulmonary edema because they rapidly enter the extracellular compartment and pull water out of cells

POTASSIUM-SPARING DIURETICS

Give examples of this class of drugs.	**Spironolactone** (Aldactone) **Amiloride** (Midamor) **Triamterene** (Dyrenium)

What is their mechanism of action?

They work by inhibiting the passage of sodium from the luminal fluid into the principal cells of the late distal convoluted tubule and cortical collecting tubule. Subsequently, this prevents the movement of K^+ from these cells into the luminal fluid. See Figure 23–3.

What is the efficacy of these drugs?

Weak. They are used today primarily in conjunction with another diuretic such as a thiazide in order to limit K^+ wasting.

What is spironolactone?

This drug is a synthetic steroid that is a competitive antagonist for the mineralocorticoid aldosterone. It binds to aldosterone receptor sites and prevents the formation of mediator proteins that stimulate the Na^+/K^+ pump.

What are the clinical indications for the use of spironolactone?

Primary hyperaldosteronism (Conn's syndrome)

Edematous states caused by secondary aldosteronism, especially cirrhosis, nephrotic syndrome, and congestive heart failure

Are there problems associated with administration of spironolactone?

Gynecomastia and impotence in males, owing to **spironolactone**'s structural similarity to progesterone

Irregular menstrual cycle in females

How does spironolactone differ from triamterene and amiloride?

Amiloride and **triamterene** work independently of aldosterone by directly blocking the Na^+ channels; therefore, these agents can be used even in cases of hypoaldosteronism such as Addison's disease. In contrast, **spironolactone** requires elevated levels of aldosterone to have an effect.

What are the adverse effects of potassium-sparing drugs?

Hyperkalemia—most important effect to watch for

Metabolic acidosis—because of an intracellular shift of H^+ ions

Rarely, **triamterene** causes leg cramps and forms renal stones.

24

Antianginal Drugs

What is the definition of angina pectoris?

Sudden substernal chest pain caused by coronary blood flow that is insufficient to meet the oxygen demands of the myocardium

Identify the three types of angina.

1. Classic (stable) angina—chest pain occurring upon **exertion** that is usually due to an atheromatous lesion
2. Unstable angina—angina that suddenly becomes worse or that occurs at rest
3. Prinzmetal's (variant) angina—a form of angina that results from coronary vasospasm

Which type accounts for most angina cases?

Classic angina accounts for approximately 90% of cases.

What percentage of patients who have unstable angina progress to an MI?

10%–20%

What is the treatment strategy for angina?

Because angina is caused by O_2 demand greater than O_2 supply (Figure 24–1), there are two treatment options:
1. Increase oxygen delivery
2. Decrease cardiac oxygen demand

What does myocardial oxygen demand depend on?

Preload—diastolic filling pressure
Afterload—peripheral vascular resistance
Heart rate
Wall tension

Name four major classes of drugs used to treat angina.

1. Nitrates
2. Calcium channel blockers
3. β blockers
4. Aspirin

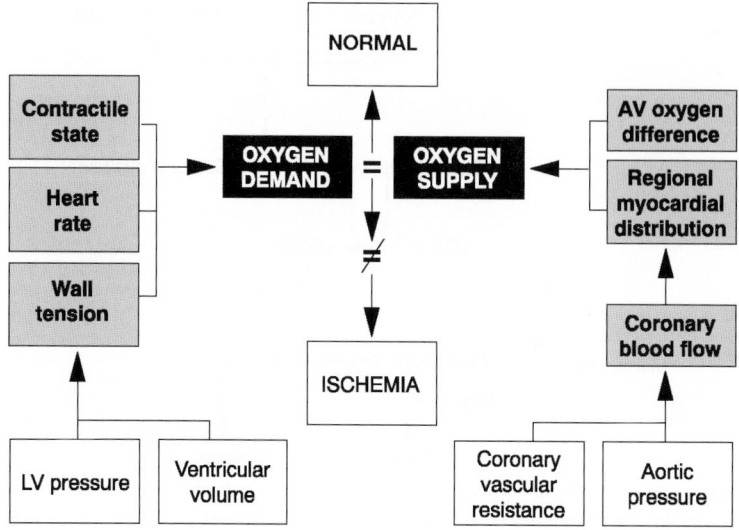

Figure 24–1. Ischemic episodes: an imbalance in the myocardial oxygen supply-demand relationship. (Redrawn with permission from Ross RS. Pathophysiology of coronary circulation. *Br Heart J* 1971;33:173–184.)

Why is aspirin useful in treating angina?

Because of its ability to inhibit platelet aggregation, aspirin has been shown to reduce mortality in patients who have unstable angina. (Aspirin is discussed further in *Chapter 35—Anti-inflammatory Drugs and Acetaminophen.*)

NITRATES

How do nitrates relieve angina?

Nitrates relax vascular smooth muscle through conversion into nitric oxide (NO) and subsequent elevation of intracellular cyclic guanosine monophosphate (cGMP) levels. The increased activity of cGMP ultimately leads to dephosphorylation of myosin light chains and smooth muscle relaxation (Figure 24–2).

What is the principal physiological effect of low doses of nitroglycerin?

Dilation of the **veins**, which causes a diminished preload and reduced cardiac workload

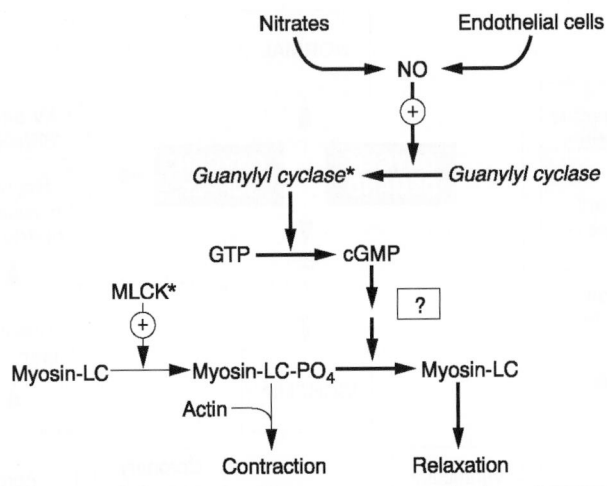

Figure 24–2. Mechanism of action of nitrates, nitrites, and other substances that increase the concentration of nitric oxide (NO) in smooth muscle cells. MLCK* = activated myosin light chain kinase; guanylyl cyclase* = activated guanylyl cyclase; ? = unknown intermediate steps. Steps leading to relaxation are shown with *heavy arrows*. (Redrawn with permission from Katzung BG: *Basic and Clinical Pharmacology,* 7th ed. Stamford, CT: Appleton & Lange, 1998, p 181.)

What happens at higher doses of nitrates?	Arterioles become dilated, which leads to a decrease in peripheral resistance and blood pressure.
Give three examples of nitrates and their routes of administration.	1. **Nitroglycerin**—sublingual (Nitrostat), transdermal (Nitro-Dur), oral (Nitro-Bid), and IV 2. **Isosorbide dinitrate**—oral 3. **Amyl nitrate**—inhaled, rarely used
What is the pharmacokinetics of nitroglycerin?	An extensive first-pass metabolism of nitroglycerin (90%) occurs in the liver. Therefore it is common to give the drug sublingually or through the use of a transdermal patch.
What are the therapeutic uses of nitroglycerin?	Acute anginal attacks—Use the sublingual form of **nitroglycerin** because its onset of action is seconds to minutes.

Prevention of attacks—Use the oral or transdermal form of **nitroglycerin**.

Does tolerance develop to nitrates?

Yes—therefore it is important to have nitrate-free periods during long-term use.

What are the toxicities of nitrates due to vasodilation?

Postural hypotension
Reflex tachycardia
Dizziness
Throbbing headaches due to meningeal artery dilation
Hot flushes

When are nitrates contraindicated?

Nitrates should not be used in conjunction with drugs used to treat erectile dysfunction, such as **sildenafil** (Viagra). The combination can cause extreme hypotension.

Name another important use for nitrates other than angina.

They are used in the treatment of cyanide poisoning (see *Chapter 52— Toxicology*).

CALCIUM CHANNEL BLOCKERS

Give three examples of this drug class.

1. **Nifedipine** (Procardia)
2. **Verapamil** (Calan)
3. **Diltiazem** (Cardizem)

What is the mechanism of action?

All three drugs inhibit the influx of Ca^{2+} into cardiac and smooth muscle cells by blocking voltage-dependent "L-type" calcium channels, thereby reducing smooth muscle and cardiac contractility. The degree of blockade is proportional to the degree of stimulation of these calcium channels.

What are the therapeutic uses?

Calcium channel blockers are the drugs of choice for Prinzmetal's angina. They can also be used for chronic stable angina, migraine, hypertension, supraventricular arrhythmias, and Raynaud's syndrome.

What are the special traits of verapamil?

Of the three calcium channel blockers, **verapamil** has the most inhibitory effect on cardiac conduction, especially at the atrioventricular (AV) node. It also tends to increase digoxin levels. (Remember **V** for **V**entricle.)

What is the site of action for nifedipine?

It mainly causes vasodilation of the arterioles and therefore causes the greatest decrease in blood pressure. Unlike **verapamil**, it has little effect on cardiac conduction or heart rate. (Remember: **N**ifedipine—**N**o major effect on heart)

What are the special traits of diltiazem?

Diltiazem is an intermediate drug compared with **verapamil** and **nifedipine**. It has moderate effects on cardiac conduction and the vasculature.

How can Ca^{2+} channel blockers be administered?

IV, PO, or sublingually

List the possible toxic effects of the calcium channel blockers.

Headache
Dizziness
Flushing
Constipation
Peripheral edema

More serious complications:
Congestive heart failure
AV node blockage (Verapamil)

β BLOCKERS

See *Chapter 9—Adrenergic Antagonists,* for a detailed discussion of β blockers.

What is the role of β blockers in angina?

They help to reduce the frequency and severity of classic (exertional) anginal attacks by decreasing (1) heart rate, (2) contractility, and (3) blood pressure, thus reducing myocardial oxygen demand.

They also help to reduce mortality in patients who progress to a myocardial infarction.

What are the contraindications to the use of these drugs?

Patients who have variant angina, asthma, diabetes, and peripheral vascular disease should not be given β blockers. Use Ca^{2+} channel blockers as an alternative.

How do you decide which β blocker to use?

All can be effective, but **atenolol, timolol,** and **metoprolol** are three of the most commonly used because they are cardioselective.

Can anti-anginal drugs be used in combination?

Yes. Because the different classes of agents work through different mechanisms, they can be used together to produce added benefits. Nitrates and β blockers, for example, can be used effectively together to reduce exertional angina. **β blockers help prevent the reflex tachycardia that occurs with nitrates.**

25

Anticoagulant, Fibrinolytic, and Antiplatelet Drugs

Define the term "thrombus."

A thrombus is a clot that forms within the heart or a blood vessel.

What causes a thrombus?

A pathological condition of the vascular system, such as endothelial damage or vascular stasis, that initiates a complex series of interactions between platelets, endothelial cells, and the coagulation cascade (Figure 25–1).

What are the two major pathways of the coagulation cascade and what activates each?

The two pathways are distinct yet interconnected.

1. The **extrinsic system** is initiated by vascular damage, the release of tissue thromboplastin, and the activation of clotting factor VII.
2. The **intrinsic system** is initiated by the activation of clotting factor XII (Figure 25–2).

Name two drugs commonly used to anticoagulate a patient.

1. **Heparin**
2. **Warfarin** (Coumadin)

HEPARIN

What type of chemical compound is heparin?

Heparin is a highly acidic straight-chain glycosaminoglycan.

Does heparin exist normally within the body?

Yes, heparin is normally found in a complex with histamine in mast cells. Its physiological role has yet to be completely elucidated.

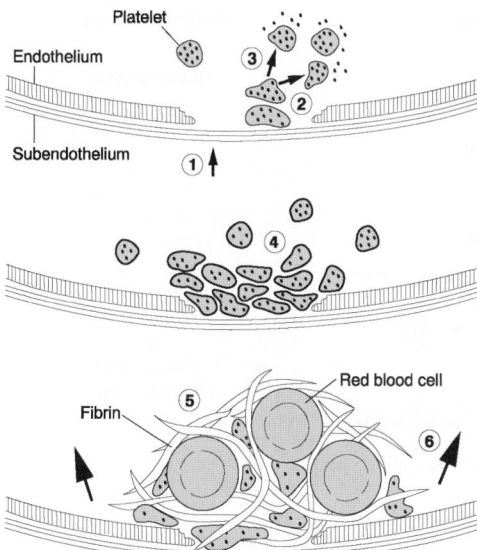

Figure 25–1. Summary of thrombogenesis. ① Endothelial injury releases tissue factor and exposes subendothelial connective tissues. ② Platelet adherence and plasma clotting system are triggered. ③ Granule release and prostaglandin generation begin. ④ Platelet aggregation induced by released ADP and vasoconstriction (5HT, thromboxanes) result in primary (temporary) hemostatis plug. ⑤ Thrombin, thromboxanes, and endoperoxides promote release reaction and irreversible aggregation; amorphous platelet mass and trapped red cells are enmeshed in fibrin to form definitive (permanent) hemostatic plug. ⑥ Endothelial plasminogen activator and plasma antithrombin check rapid clotting. (Time scale: Steps 1 to 4 = seconds to minutes; steps 5 to 6 = several minutes.) (Adapted with permission from Cotran RS, Jumar V, Robbins SL. *Robbins Pathologic Basis of Disease,* 5th ed. Philadelphia: Saunders, 1994.)

How does heparin work?

Antithrombin III is a naturally occurring α_2-globulin that binds to and inactivates clotting factors IIa, IXa, Xa, XIa, and XIIa. This process is normally very slow; **heparin** binds to antithrombin III and accelerates the reaction a thousandfold.

What is heparin's major indication?

Because of its rapid onset of action, **heparin** is used whenever immediate initiation of anticoagulation is needed; for example, in treating pulmonary embolism, deep venous thrombosis, and acute myocardial infarction.

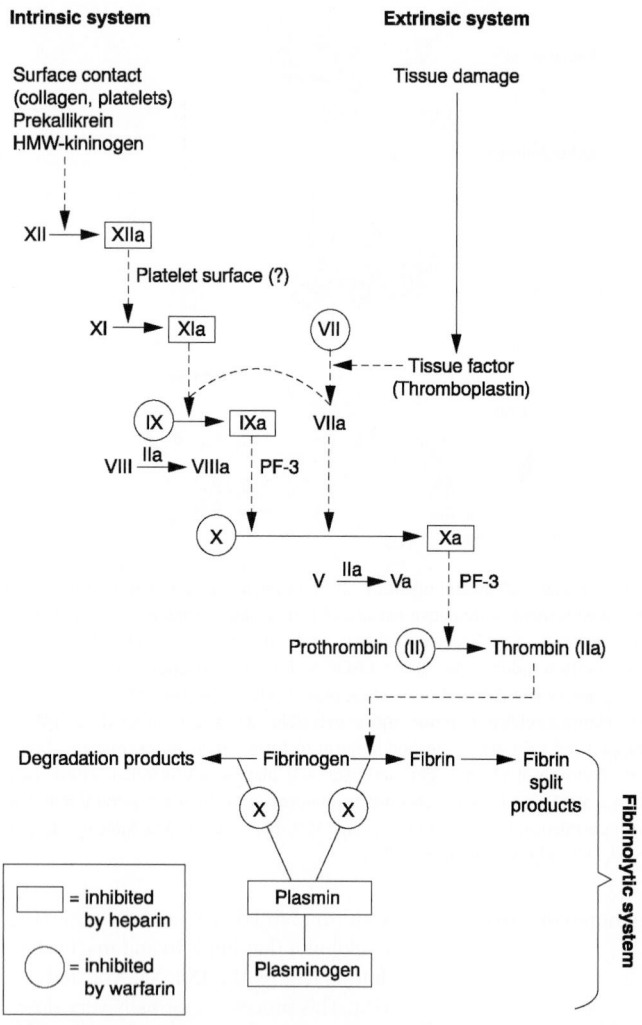

Figure 25–2. The intrinsic pathway is initiated when blood comes in contact with the negatively charged deendothelialized vascular surface. Factor XII is activated, and, in a sequential reaction, factors XI and IX are activated. On the platelet surface, factors IXa and VIII interact with calcium and activate factor Xa. In the extrinsic pathway, tissue thromboplastin is released after vessel wall injury activates factor VII, which in turn activates factor X. Then, on the platelet surface, factors Xa and Va interact with calcium and catalyze the conversion of prothrombin to thrombin. Thrombin converts fibrinogen to fibrin monomers and activates factor XIII, which in turn is converted to fibrin polymers in the developing clot. Note that factor VII from the extrinsic pathway may activate factor IX in the intrinsic pathway. (Adapted and redrawn with permission from Cotran RS, Jumar V, Robbins SL. *Robbins Pathologic Basis of Disease,* 5th ed. Philadelphia: Saunders, 1994.)

What other uses does heparin have?

Heparin can also be used prophylactically to prevent postoperative embolisms.

What are the limitations of heparin?

Heparin stops the expansion of thrombi and prevents the formation of new thrombi. However, it does not dissolve existing thrombi.

What is the route of administration?

Heparin must be given either subcutaneously or intravenously. Intramuscular injections must be avoided because of potential hematoma formation.

What lab measure is used to monitor the actions of heparin—prothrombin time (PT) or activated partial thromboplastin time (PTT)?

PTT. Prolonged times of 1.5 to 2 times normal are considered therapeutic.

How is this drug metabolized?

By the liver

Is heparin safe to use in pregnant women?

Yes—with qualifications. The drug will not cross the placenta. **Heparin** is probably the preferred anticoagulant for pregnant women, but *it is not risk free.* Approximately 13% to 20% of pregnant women who use this drug experience outcomes such as stillbirths and prematurity. Therefore *use **heparin** cautiously,* especially during the last trimester.

What adverse effects should you watch for in administering heparin?

Hemorrhage—This is the most important effect to watch for.

Hypersensitivity reaction—Watch for chills, fever, or urticaria.

Thrombocytopenia—After approximately a week of **heparin** administration, patients may develop **heparin**-induced antiplatelet antibodies.

Alopecia and osteoporosis—associated with long-term use

How do you counteract the effects of heparin?

Use **protamine sulfate** (✎ common board question)

What are the contraindications to the administration of heparin?

Heparin should be avoided in patients who have had any of the following:
A hypersensitivity reaction
A bleeding disorder
Surgery of the brain, eye, or spinal cord
Intracranial hemorrhage
Infective endocarditis

What is low-molecular-weight (LMW) heparin?

Unlike regular **heparin**, which is a large molecule consisting of several polymers, **LMW heparin** is smaller and weighs less, approximately 2000 to 6000 daltons. Regular heparin weighs 5000 to 30,000 daltons (mean 12,000 daltons).

Give an example of a LMW heparin.

Enoxaparin (Lovenox), the most widely used

What are the important differences between regular and LMW heparin?

1. **LMW heparin** has a greater bioavailability and longer half-life.
2. **LMW heparin** is less likely to induce thrombocytopenia.
3. **LMW heparin** can be administered without constant laboratory monitoring because there is more of a consistent dose–response relationship for **LMW heparin** than regular **heparin**. This makes it especially useful for outpatient therapy.

LEPIRUDIN (REFLUDAN)

What is it?

A drug made through recombinant DNA technology. It is a derivative of **hirudin**, a compound found in the salivary glands of the medicinal leech.

How does it work?

It binds to the catalytic site of thrombin and prevents its thrombogenic activities.

When is it used?

It is indicated for patients who experience **heparin**-induced thrombocytopenia.

Does it have any toxicities?   Yes. It can cause bleeding.

WARFARIN (COUMADIN)

How is warfarin different from heparin?

Warfarin is administered orally, has a delayed onset of action, and crosses the placenta. See Table 25–1 for more details.

What is warfarin's mechanism of action?

Warfarin interferes with the synthesis of vitamin K (by inhibiting the enzyme **vitamin K epoxide reductase**), which is needed for γ-carboxylation of clotting factors II, VII, IX, and X..

Describe warfarin's onset of action.

Compared with heparin, **warfarin** has a delayed onset of action (usually 8 to 12 hr) that relates to the half-life of preformed vitamin K–dependent clotting factors.

When would you use this drug?

When long-term anticoagulation is needed, as for patients with atrial fibrillation, for prevention of stroke, and for patients with a mechanical heart valve

Table 25–1: Heparin Versus Warfarin: Key Points

	Heparin	Warfarin
Structure	Large, positively charged polymer	Small lipid-soluble molecule
Mechanism of action	Activates antithrombin III	Impairs synthesis of vitamin K factors II, VII, IX and X.
Crosses placenta?	No	Yes, teratogenic
Route of administration	IV, SC	Oral
Onset of action	Rapid	Slow
Overdose treatment	Protamine sulfate	Vitamin K and fresh frozen plasma
Monitoring	PTT	PT

What lab value is used to monitor the effects of warfarin?	Prothrombin time (PT)
Can you use this drug in pregnant women?	No! The drug has teratogenic effects.
How is warfarin metabolized?	It is metabolized in the liver by the cytochrome P-450 system.
What drugs potentiate the actions of warfarin?	Drugs that inhibit the cytochrome P-450 system. Examples include: Alcohol **Cimetidine** (Tagamet) Disulfiram Phenylbutazone
What is the principal toxicity of warfarin?	Hemorrhage. Other toxicities include a dermal vascular necrosis, which can occur early in therapy. This is due to a deficiency of protein C, a vitamin K–dependent endogenous anticoagulant.
How do you reverse the actions of warfarin?	Administer vitamin K or fresh frozen plasma and allow 24 hr for full reversal.

FIBRINOLYTICS

Give three examples of fibrinolytics.	1. **Streptokinase** (Streptase) 2. **Urokinase** (Abbokinase) 3. **Tissue plasminogen activator** (Alteplase)
What is the function of the fibrinolytic system?	It provides a mechanism for the degradation of fibrin clots.
What is the role of plasmin in the fibrinolytic system?	Plasmin is a serine protease that digests fibrin into fibrin split products and therefore dissolves thrombi. Plasminogen is the precursor of plasmin (Figure 25–2).
Do fibrinolytics distinguish between beneficial hemostatic plugs and unwanted thrombi?	No—This is a disadvantage of the fibrinolytics.

What are the contraindications to fibrinolytic therapy?	Intracranial hemorrhage, recent surgery, GI bleeding, aneurysm
How are all fibrinolytics administered?	IV

STREPTOKINASE

Where does streptokinase come from?	**Streptokinase** is an extracellular protein derived from purified culture broth of group C β-hemolytic streptococci.
When do you use it?	Rarely used currently, **streptokinase** was used in cases where rapid clot dissolution is needed, such as acute myocardial infarction, occluded access shunts and arterial thrombosis.
How does streptokinase work?	**Streptokinase** itself has no enzymatic ability; it must first bind plasminogen. The streptokinase-plasminogen complex then catalyzes the rapid conversion of uncomplexed plasminogen into plasmin. The complex also degrades free fibrinogen as well and thus induces a systemic lytic state.
What are the toxicities of streptokinase?	Systemic bleeding
	Drug allergy, which may result in rashes or fever

UROKINASE (ABBOKINASE)

How does urokinase work?	Unlike **streptokinase**, which must first bind with plasminogen, **urokinase** is capable of directly converting plasminogen to plasmin.
What are its therapeutic uses?	**Urokinase** is effective in treating coronary artery thrombosis and pulmonary embolism.
What are the adverse effects?	Bleeding complications

TISSUE PLASMINOGEN ACTIVATOR (ALTEPLASE)

Classify tissue plasminogen activator (TPA).

It is a serine protease that is obtained through recombinant DNA technology.

What is the major advantage of TPA over other thrombolytics?

In theory, it binds to and activates plasminogen bound to fibrin clots rather than free plasminogen, thus decreasing the risk of systemic bleeding. Currently, it is the most widely used fibrinolytic.

What are the indications for this agent?

TPA is used for the treatment of acute myocardial infarction or nonhemorrhagic stroke. It is effective only when given within 1 to 3 hr of the incident.

State its adverse effects.

Bleeding complications, especially cerebral hemorrhage, are the most important adverse effects to watch for.

How do you reverse the actions of streptokinase, urokinase, and TPA?

Use **aminocaproic acid** (Amicar). It binds to plasmin and plasminogen and thus blocks plasmin from binding to fibrin.

ANTIPLATELET DRUGS

What is the role of antiplatelet drugs in clot formation?

They delay clot formation by inhibiting platelet aggregation. This is particularly important in clots that form in the arterial circulation. This delay can be measured in the lab (bleeding time).

ASPIRIN

See *Chapter 35—Anti-inflammatory Drugs and Acetaminophen*, for more detailed information on aspirin.

What is aspirin's mechanism of action?

Aspirin *irreversibly* inhibits thromboxane A_2 synthesis by blocking the enzyme cyclooxygenase. Thromboxane A_2 is critical for platelet aggregation. Because the blockade is irreversible, the effects of **aspirin** on platelets will last until new platelets are created (several days).

What is aspirin's role in anticoagulating a patient?

One **aspirin** a day has been shown to be beneficial in preventing clot formation. It is currently part of the usual treatment protocol for patients who have had transient ischemic attacks or myocardial infarctions. It is not helpful in acute situations such as a sudden pulmonary embolism.

State aspirin's adverse effects.

Nausea
Gastrointestinal bleeding
Rash
Reversible hepatic dysfunction

TICLOPIDINE (TICLID)

Describe the mechanism of action.

Like thromboxane A_2, adenosine diphosphate (ADP) is another important mediator in platelet aggregation. **Ticlopidine** irreversibly binds to ADP receptors located on platelets and thus prevents platelet cross-linking (Figure 25–3).

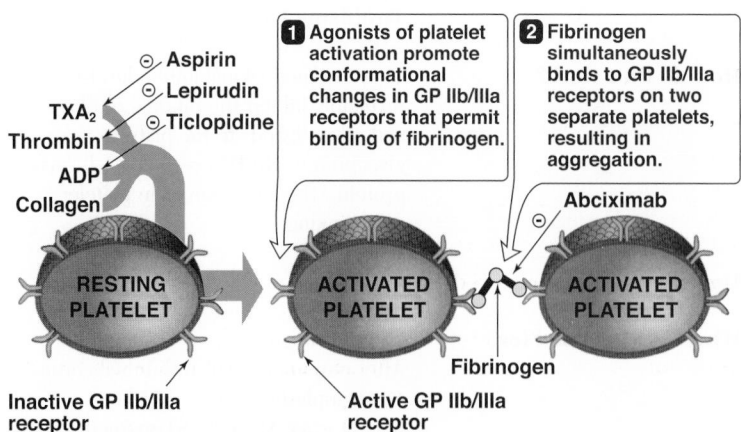

Figure 25–3. Summary of antiplatelet and antithrombin agents. (With permission from Mycek MJ, Harvey RA, Champe PC [Harvey RA, Champe PC, eds.]. *Lippincott's Illustrated Reviews: Pharmacology*, Millennium Edition (updated 2nd ed). Baltimore: Lippincott Williams & Wilkins, 2000, p 447.)

What are its uses?	**Ticlopidine** reduces the risk of thrombotic stroke. Because **ticlopidine** is associated with the risk of neutropenia and agranulocytosis, reserve its use for patients who cannot take **aspirin** or **clopidogrel**.
What are the adverse effects of this drug?	Neutropenia in a small percentage of patients Gastrointestinal complaints (diarrhea, nausea) Skin rash Bleeding complications Agranulocytosis

CLOPIDOGREL (PLAVIX)

What is it?	**Clopidogrel** is a drug similar to **ticlopidine**. It has the same mechanism of action. It has one important difference, however: it does not induce the neutropenia seen with **ticlopidine**. For this reason it has largely replaced **ticlopidine**.

GLYCOPROTEIN IIB AND IIIA INHIBITORS

Name three examples of a IIb/IIIa inhibitor.	**Abciximab** (Reopro) **Eptifibatide** (Integrilin) **Tirofiban** (Aggrastat)
How do they work?	They are monoclonal antibodies that reversibly inhibit the binding of fibrin and other ligands to the platelet glycoprotein IIb/IIIa receptor cell surface protein, which is involved in platelet cross-linking.
How are they administered?	IV
What are they used for?	Unstable angina After percutaneous transluminal coronary angioplasty Non Q-wave MI, non–ST-segment-elevation MI
How long do their effects last?	Abciximab: 24–48 hr Eptifibatide and Tirofiban: 2–4 hr.

What are their toxicities?   Bleeding and chronic use can cause thrombocytopenia.

DIPYRIDAMOLE (PERSANTINE)

What is dipyridamole's mechanism of action?

The mechanism of action is uncertain, but **dipyridamole** is thought to interfere with platelet function by increasing cyclic adenosine monophosphate (cAMP), either by blocking uptake of adenosine or by inhibiting phosphodiesterase. This subsequently leads to decreased thromboxane A_2 synthesis.

What are its uses?

Dipyridamole is used to prevent thrombosis in patients who have artificial heart valves. It is also used to image regions of myocardium at risk for ischemia (**dipyridamole**-thallium scans).

What are dipyridamole's adverse effects?

Dizziness
Angina
Abdominal pain
Headache
Rash

26

Antihyperlipidemic Drugs

Coronary heart disease (CHD) is responsible for a large proportion of deaths in the United States each year. Hyperlipidemia, which leads to atherosclerosis, is one of the most significant risk factors for the development of CHD, stroke, and other vascular diseases.

What is treatment of hyperlipidemia based on?

According to the guidelines of the National Cholesterol Education Program, the decision to treat is based on several factors. Low-density lipoprotein (LDL) levels are just one of them. Others include triglyceride levels, HDL levels, age, gender, family history, and past medical history.

What is a lipoprotein?

A macromolecule made of protein that transports lipids within the body

Name the major lipoproteins.

Chylomicrons
High-density lipoprotein (HDL)
Very-low-density lipoprotein (VLDL)
Low-density lipoprotein (LDL)—
    derived from VLDL in the plasma
Intermediate-density lipoprotein (IDL)
Figure 26–1 illustrates their physiological roles.

What causes hyperlipidemias?

Hyperlipidemias can be organized into two categories, primary and secondary, based on their causes:
1. **Primary hyperlipidemias** are caused by genetic defects and/or environmental factors (Table 26–1).
2. **Secondary hyperlipidemias** result from other metabolic disorders such as diabetes, hypothyroidism, renal disease, and alcoholism.

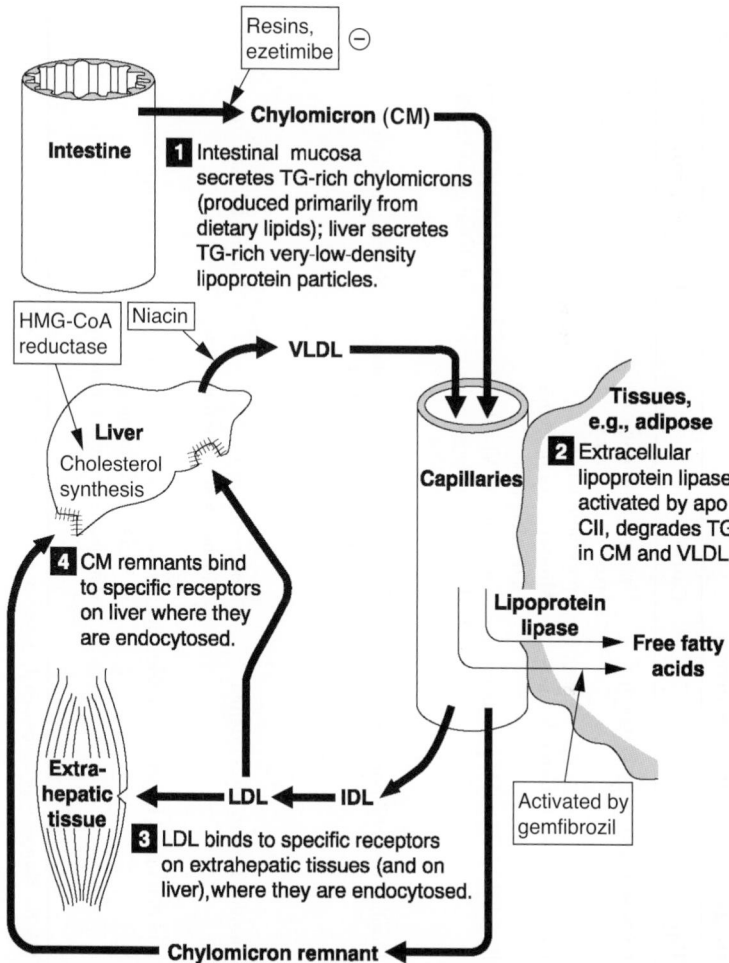

Figure 26–1. Metabolism of plasma lipoproteins. CM = chylomicron; TG = triacylglycerol; VLDL = very low density lipoprotein; LDL = low-density lipoprotein. IDL = intermediate-density lipoprotein. (Redrawn and adapted with permission from Mycek MJ, Gertner SB, Perper MM [Harvey RA, Champe PC, eds.]. *Lippincott's Illustrated Reviews: Pharmacology*, 2nd ed. Philadelphia: Lippincott-Raven Publishers, 1997, p. 208.)

Table 26–1. Pharmacological Management of Lipid Disorders

Laboratory Findings	Type		Cause	Drug Therapy
↑ Chylomicrons	Familial hyperchylomicronemia	I	Deficiency of lipoprotein lipase or deficiency of apoprotein CII	Gemfibrozil to prevent pancreatitis if chylomicrons > 400 mg/dL
↑ LDL	Familial hypercholesterolemia	IIa	Absence of or defective LDL receptors	HMG-CoA reductase inhibitor, niacin, resin
↑ LDL	Familial combined hyperlipidemia	IIb	↑ secretion of VLDL (biochemical cause unknown)	Niacin, HMG-CoA reductase inhibitor, gemfibrozil, resin
↑ VLDL ↓ HDL ↑ IDL	Familial dysbetalipoproteinemia	III	↑ production or ↓ utilization of IDL (defect in apoEII)	Niacin, gemfibrozil
↑ Chylomicrons ↓ LDL ↓ HDL ↑ VLDL	Familial hypertriglyceridemia	IV	↑ secretion of VLDL (biochemical cause unknown)	Niacin, bile acid resins
↓ HDL ↑ VLDL	Familial mixed hypertriglyceridemia	V	↑ production or ↓ removal of VLDL and chylomicrons (biochemical cause unknown)	Drug therapy if necessary
↑ Chylomicrons				

(Adapted from Gallia G, Hann CL, Hewson WH. *The Pharmacology Companion*. La Jolla, CA: Alert & Oriented Publishing Company, 1997. p. 145.)

What are the treatment options?	Diet and exercise management—always the first intervention
	Decrease bile and cholesterol absorption from the gut—bile acid–binding resins, ezetimibe
	Decrease hepatic cholesterol synthesis— HMG-CoA reductase inhibitors
	Increase peripheral clearance of lipoproteins— fibric acid derivatives
	Decrease secretion of hepatic VLDLs— niacin

BILE ACID–BINDING RESINS

What are they?	Bile acid resins are positively charged ammonium polymers used in the treatment of hypercholesterolemia.
Give examples.	**Cholestyramine** (Questran) **Colestipol** (Colestid) **Colesevelam** (Welchol)
What is their mechanism of action?	Resins act by binding negatively charged bile acids in the small intestine, forming insoluble complexes that are then excreted in feces. Loss of bile acids stimulates the liver to increase conversion of stored cholesterol into new bile acids. As more intracellular cholesterol is used to make bile acids, there is a compensatory increase in hepatic LDL receptors. The net effect is a decrease in serum LDL and cholesterol.
What are the adverse effects of bile acid resins?	May cause GI discomfort (constipation, bloating, gritty taste)
	May impede absorption of fat-soluble vitamins and other drugs and vitamins (e.g., vitamin K, **chlorothiazide**, anticoagulants, **digitalis**)
	Can increase triglyceride levels

EZETIMIBE (ZETIA)

What is it?	**Ezetimibe** is a drug that has a unique mechanism of action: it inhibits cholesterol absorptions by enterocytes of the small intestine. Ultimately this leads to a decrease of LDL and triacylglycerol levels.
When is it used?	While it can be used alone, it is most often used in combination with the statins. The combination of **ezetimibe** and a statin has been shown to lower total cholesterol by 25% more than a statin alone.
What are its adverse effects?	Overall, it has a safe profile. The most common adverse effects are tiredness and stomach pain. Rarely, allergic reactions have been reported.

HMG-COA REDUCTASE INHIBITORS

What is the route of administration?	PO
Give examples of these drugs.	**Lovastatin** (Mevacor) **Simvastatin** (Zocor) **Pravastatin** (Pravachol) **Fluvastatin** (Lescol) **Atorvastatin** (Lipitor) —shown to be most effective in large clinical trials Remember to look for the suffix "-statin."
What is HMG-CoA reductase?	The rate-determining enzyme in the synthesis of cholesterol. It converts HMG-CoA to mevalonic acid (Figure 26–2)
What is the effect of reductase inhibitors on hyperlipidemia?	HMG-CoA reductase inhibitors decrease cholesterol synthesis in the liver, which leads to an increase in LDL receptors on the surface of hepatocytes and a decrease in plasma VLDL/LDL.

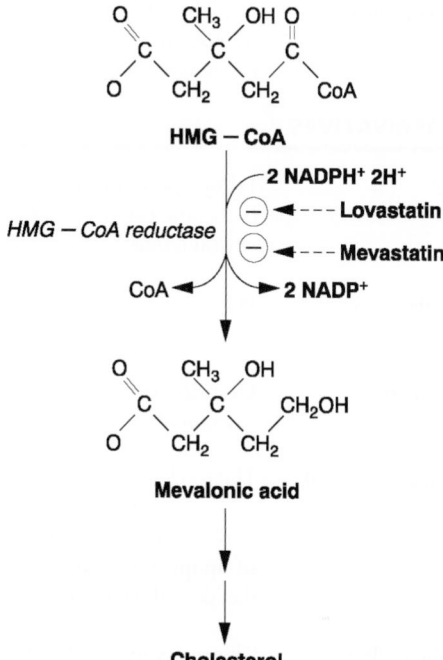

Figure 26–2. Inhibition of HMG-CoA reductase by lovastatin and mevastatin. (Redrawn with permission from Mycek MJ, Harvey RA, Champe PC [Harvey RA, Champe PC, eds]: *Lippincott's Illustrated Reviews: Pharmacology*, 2nd ed. Philadelphia: Lippincott-Raven Publishers, 1997, p. 214.)

	They are the most widely used class of antihyperlipidemic drugs because of their effectiveness in lowering LDL and total cholesterol levels.
What are the adverse effects?	Increased hepatic transaminase levels Myopathy Rarely, patients may experience rhabdomyolysis with statin therapy.
What other drugs should generally not be prescribed to a patient taking HMG-CoA reductase inhibitors?	Fibric acid derivatives Cyclosporine Niacin Erythromycin The incidence of myopathy associated with rhabdomyolysis increases when a reductase inhibitor is used with these drugs

Can pregnant women use statin drugs?	No. They have been shown to be teratogenic and therefore should be avoided in pregnancy.

FIBRIC ACID DERIVATIVES

What are they?	Fibric acid derivatives are ethyl esters that cause catabolism of VLDLs and chylomicrons.
By what route are they administered?	PO
Give examples of these drugs.	**Gemfibrozil** (Lopid) and **clofibrate** (Atromid-S)
What is their mechanism of action?	The mechanism of action is not well understood; however, it is believed that fibric acid derivatives **increase the activity of lipoprotein lipase,** a plasma enzyme that degrades chylomicrons and VLDLs.
For what are these drugs used?	They are very effective for hypertriglyceridemia, in which VLDLs predominate. Useful for Type III hyperlipidemia.
What are the adverse effects?	GI problems (nausea) may occur. Gallstone formation Skin rash is common with **gemfibrozil**. Clofibrate has been associated with an increase in hepatobiliary and gastrointestinal neoplasms and therefore is seldom used. These drugs also potentiate the effects of anticoagulant drugs.
Can you ever use fibric acid derivatives with HMG-CoA reductase inhibitors for added benefits?	When these drugs are used in combination, the risk of rhabdomyolysis usually outweighs the benefits.
Are these drugs safe to use in pregnancy?	No

NIACIN (NICOTINIC ACID)

What is it?	Pyridine-3-carboxylic acid, a part of the vitamin B complex (formerly known as vitamin B_3). **Niacin** is different from **nicotinamide**, which has no efficacy in the treatment of hypercholesterolemia.
What is niacin's clinical use?	Treatment of elevated LDL and/or elevated triglycerides, with or without decreased HDL.
What are niacin's mechanisms of action?	1. It decreases lipolysis in adipose tissue, which in turn reduces circulating free fatty acids. Without the free fatty acids, hepatic secretion of VLDLs is slowed. 2. It increases the activity of lipoprotein lipase. 3. Stimulates mild-to-moderate increases in HDL. This is an important effect that can be very beneficial to patients who have high levels of LDL/VLDL in combination with low levels of HDL.
What are its adverse effects?	A cutaneous flush accompanied by pruritus is one of the most common problems; aspirin can alleviate this. Liver toxicity—This must by monitored by liver function tests at least every 6 months. Hyperglycemia Hyperuricemia—avoid if possible in patients with history of gout Nausea Constipation

27

Agents Used to Treat Anemia

Define anemia.

A red blood cell count, hemoglobin, or hematocrit concentration that is below normal plasma levels. Conditions that increase plasma volumes, such as pregnancy, will cause a relative anemia, not a true anemia.

Name the major categories of anemia.

Microcytic anemia
Normocytic anemia
Macrocytic or megaloblastic anemia

IRON

What type of anemia is caused by iron deficiency?

A hypochromic microcytic anemia

What are the two major causes of iron deficiency?

1. GI bleeding
2. In women, menstrual blood loss
Iron deficiency can also be caused by pregnancy and by periods of rapid growth in children.

How is iron distributed in the body?

Most of the iron present within the body is in hemoglobin. Iron is also bound to transferrin (a transport protein) and stored as ferritin and hemosiderin.

What are the reasons for administering iron?

Iron deficiency anemia is the only indication for the use of iron.

What form of iron is administered?

Iron is most commonly given as ferrous sulfate by mouth.

What are the toxicities of iron?

Gastrointestinal disturbance from irritation is the most common symptom. If the dose is sufficiently high, necrotizing gastroenteritis, shock, metabolic acidosis, and even death can occur.

How do you treat acute iron intoxication?	Immediate treatment is necessary and usually consists of removal of unabsorbed tablets from the stomach as well as administration of a chelating agent known as deferoxamine.
How do you manage chronic iron intoxication?	A chronically elevated plasma level of iron secondary to diseases such as hemochromatosis is treated with regular phlebotomy.

CYANOCOBALAMIN (VITAMIN B$_{12}$)

What is the function of vitamin B$_{12}$?	Vitamin B$_{12}$ is a cofactor in the transfer of one-carbon units, which is a step necessary in the synthesis of DNA.
What is necessary for the absorption of vitamin B$_{12}$?	Presence of intrinsic factor, which is produced by the parietal cells of the stomach
Is vitamin B$_{12}$ stored within the body?	Yes. Vitamin B$_{12}$ is stored in the liver.
What are the three most common causes of B$_{12}$ deficiency?	1. Pernicious anemia (absence of intrinsic factor) 2. Total gastrectomy 3. Disorders of the distal ileum
What symptoms are caused by vitamin B$_{12}$ deficiency?	Vitamin B$_{12}$ deficiency causes **megaloblastic anemia** and tabes dorsalis, which is a neurological disease characterized by degeneration of the posterior spinal columns.
What is its therapeutic use?	Vitamin B$_{12}$ is used for the treatment of naturally occurring pernicious anemia and anemia caused by gastric resection.
What is the route of administration?	Parenteral injections, because vitamin B$_{12}$ deficiency is most commonly caused by poor absorption

What is its toxicity?	There are no known adverse effects.

FOLIC ACID

What is the physiological function of folic acid?	Folic acid is necessary for the transfer of one-carbon fragments in the synthesis of purine and pyrimidine bases.
What are its clinical indications?	Folic acid is used in the treatment of **megaloblastic anemia**. It is important to rule out vitamin B_{12} deficiency before administering folic acid as sole therapy because folic acid will not remedy any coexisting neurological deficits.
Other than for treating anemia, when is folic acid important?	Folic acid is critical during pregnancy. Without it there is a markedly increased risk of neural tube defects.
Is folate stored in the body as much as vitamin B_{12} is?	No. The body's folate supply will run out in just 3 months, whereas vitamin B_{12} supplies last much longer.
What are the most common causes of folate deficiency?	Inadequate dietary intake Pregnancy Drugs such as phenytoin or oral contraceptives (they can interfere with folate absorption)
How is folic acid administered?	It is usually given orally.
What is the toxicity of folic acid?	Orally administered folic acid is usually not toxic.

ERYTHROPOIETIN (EPOGEN)

What is erythropoietin?	A glycoprotein normally produced in the cortex of the kidney
When do you use it?	**Erythropoietin** is used for the treatment of anemias associated with end-stage renal failure and bone marrow failure secondary to cancer chemotherapy or AIDS.

How is it administered?   By subcutaneous injection

What is its toxicity?   The only toxicity is associated with an excessive increase in red blood cell count, which can cause thrombosis and hypertension.

Section V

Respiratory System

28

Drugs Used to Treat Asthma, Coughs, and Colds

ANTIASTHMATIC DRUGS

What is asthma?

Asthma is a chronic inflammatory disease of the tracheobronchial airways characterized by airflow obstruction and hyperreactivity to a variety of stimuli.

Name the causes of airway obstruction in asthma.

Inflammation of the bronchial wall
Constriction of the bronchiolar smooth muscle
Increased mucous secretion

How does asthma clinically manifest?

Shortness of breath
Coughing
Wheezing
Use of accessory muscles of respiration
Chest tightness

What precipitates an asthma attack?

There are three principal triggers of exacerbations:
1. Allergens—These agents induce mast cell release of inflammatory mediators, such as histamine, leukotrienes, and chemotactic factors, which promote bronchiolar spasm and mucosal thickening.
2. Infections—Viral upper respiratory tract infections are particularly problematic. In children it is common for asthmatic episodes to follow these infections.
3. Psychological factors—These can play a significant role, although they are often not readily recognized.

List the pharmacological options for asthma therapy.	Sympathomimetic agents (β_2-adrenergic agonists) Corticosteroids Anticholinergics Leukotriene inhibitors Methylxanthines—theophylline **Cromolyn sodium** and **nedocromil**
Which of these drugs are considered safe to use in pregnant women?	All of them—pregnant women with asthma can be treated as aggressively as nonpregnant asthmatic patients.

SYMPATHOMIMETIC AGENTS

How do β_2-adrenergic agonists work?	They work by increasing intracellular concentrations of cyclic adenosine monophosphate (cAMP). This results in the relaxation of bronchial smooth muscle and subsequently bronchodilation.
Name five β_2-adrenergic agonists that are commonly used for asthma therapy.	1. **Albuterol** (Proventil) 2. **Metaproterenol** (Alupent) 3. **Pirbuterol** (Maxair) 4. **Terbutaline** (Brethaire) 5. **Salmeterol** (Serevent) —Long acting, **not for acute symptoms**
How are β_2-adrenergic agonists usually administered?	Most of these drugs are inhaled, which minimizes their systemic side effects because β_2 agonists are poorly absorbed into the circulation via the lungs.
What is their clinical role?	Because they are rapid in onset, β_2-adrenergic agonists are the *drugs of choice* for acute relief of bronchospasm. **Salmeterol** is used mainly for prophylaxis of symptoms.
Are there adverse effects of inhaled bronchodilators?	Yes. The most common are tremor and tachycardia. Tolerance can also develop with excessive use.

CORTICOSTEROIDS

How do steroids work in the treatment of asthma?	They inhibit the synthesis of arachidonic acid by phospholipase A_2. Consequently, various inflammatory mediators such as leukotrienes, cytokines, and prostaglandins are inhibited (Figure 35–1).
When are corticosteroids used in asthma management?	For both acute and maintenance asthma management: Acute exacerbations—Systemic steroids are used primarily when the attack is severe. Maintenance therapy—Inhaled corticosteroids are used once or twice a day. They help reduce the need for B_2 agonists.
Name five inhaled steroids used in the management of chronic asthma.	1. **Beclomethasone** (Vanceril) 2. **Flunisolide** (Aerobid) 3. **Triamcinolone** (Azmacort) 4. **Fluticasone** (Flovent) 5. **Budesonide** (Pulmicort)
What are the adverse effects of inhaled corticosteroids?	They are much more limited than those of systemic steroids. Adverse effects include cough, oral thrush, and dysphonia.
What are the adverse effects of systemic corticosteroids such as prednisone?	The list is long and includes abnormalities in glucose metabolism, increased appetite, weight gain, hypertension, and adrenal suppression. These symptoms can be minimized by limiting systemic therapy to a few days. (Systemic corticosteroids are further discussed in *Chapter 32—Corticosteroids and Inhibitors.*)

ANTICHOLINERGICS

How do anticholinergics work?	Parasympathetic stimulation causes bronchial constriction and mucous secretion. Anticholinergics are used to

block these responses and maintain bronchial dilation of the airway.

Name an anticholinergic agent used to treat asthma.

Ipratropium (Atrovent), an inhaled anticholinergic

What are its clinical uses?

Treatment of asthma and chronic obstructive pulmonary disease. It is not used as commonly as in the past.

What side effects may patients experience while using ipratropium?

Dry mouth and sedation. The drug has very few side effects owing to poor systemic absorption.

LEUKOTRIENE INHIBITORS

Describe how leukotriene inhibitors work.

They either block the synthesis of leukotrienes from arachidonic acid or block the leukotriene receptor.

Give three examples of leukotriene inhibitors and state the mechanism of action of each.

1. **Zileuton** (Zyflo)—inhibits 5-lipoxygenase, which catalyzes the formation of leukotrienes from arachidonic acid.
2. **Zafirlukast** (Accolate)—LTD_4 receptor antagonist
3. **Montelukast** (Singulair)—LTD_4 receptor antagonist

What is the route of administration for all three?

PO

What is the clinical role of these drugs in asthma?

They prevent bronchoconstriction and airway inflammation. Leukotriene inhibitors are used for chronic maintenance therapy of mild asthma; **they are not beneficial in acute bronchospasm.**

What are the adverse effects of these drugs?

Overall they have a very safe profile.
Zileuton—Some cases of elevated liver enzymes have been reported.
Zafirlukast and **Montelukast**—Rarely, patients develop a vasculitis and systemic eosinophilia resembling Churg-Strauss syndrome.

METHYLXANTHINES—THEOPHYLLINE

What is theophylline and how does it work?	**Theophylline** is a methylxanthine derivative that inhibits phosphodiesterase, the enzyme responsible for the metabolism of cAMP to AMP. Increased levels of cAMP result in bronchodilation. **Theophylline** also has some anti-inflammatory effects.
What is its role in asthma therapy?	Limited, because it has a very small therapeutic window
Are there any drug interactions with theophylline?	**Cimetidine** and **erythromycin** both increase theophylline plasma levels.
Which drugs decrease plasma levels of theophylline?	**Phenytoin** and quinolones
What are possible complications with theophylline overdose?	The most common are tremor, insomnia, gastrointestinal distress, and nausea. The most dangerous are seizures and arrhythmias. Methylxanthines are discussed further in *Chapter 17—CNS Stimulants.*

CROMOLYN SODIUM AND NEDOCROMIL

What are cromolyn sodium (Intal) and nedocromil (Tilade) and how do they work?	They are effective prophylactic agents that stabilize the membranes of mast cells and prevent the release of inflammatory mediators.
Can these drugs be used for treating acute attacks of asthma?	No. They are effective prophylactic agents. Pretreatment with **cromolyn** or **nedocromil** blocks allergen- and exercise-induced bronchoconstriction.
What are the potential toxicities of cromolyn and nedocromil?	**Cromolyn**—infrequent laryngeal edema, cough, and wheezing **Nedocromil**—unpleasant taste

ACUTE AND LONG-TERM MANAGEMENT OF ASTHMA

What is status asthmaticus?   A life-threatening attack of asthma

How do you treat status asthmaticus?

IV corticosteroids and bronchodilators are first-line therapy, followed by **theophylline**.

Which agent is the drug of choice for long-term treatment of asthma in the outpatient setting?

Current recommendations state that patients with mild, persistent symptoms should be started on an inhaled steroid such as **fluticasone propionate** for routine use. Acute breakthrough attacks are then treated with β_2-adrenergic agonists.

ANTITUSSIVES (COUGH MEDICATIONS)

When would you use antitussives?

Antitussives have a limited role. Coughing is a symptom and, where possible, therapy is directed to its etiology. However, in acute respiratory tract infections where cough disrupts sleep, antitussives may be used.

How do opiates suppress cough?

Opiates decrease the CNS cough center's sensitivity to peripheral stimuli and decrease mucosal secretion. These actions occur at doses lower than those required for analgesia.

Name three opiates used as antitussives.

1. **Codeine**
2. **Hydrocodone**
3. **Hydromorphone**

What is dextromethorphan?   A synthetic derivative of codeine

How does dextromethorphan work?

It suppresses the response of the cough center, but it does not have any analgesic or addictive potential and is less constipating than codeine.

RHINITIS AGENTS

Define rhinitis.	Inflammation of the mucous membranes of the nose
What is its etiology?	Rhinitis is most commonly caused by viruses or by hypersensitivity responses to airborne allergens.
How would you treat this condition?	For allergic rhinitis, try avoidance therapy (avoiding contacts with all known allergens/irritants). If irritant avoidance is not realistically possible or if the rhinitis appears to be caused by a virus, medical options include: Nasal corticosteroids **Cromolyn sodium** Antihistamines α-Adrenergic agonists
Name the corticosteroids commonly used to treat chronic rhinitis.	**Beclomethasone** and **flunisolide**. Chronic rhinitis does not show improvement until 2 weeks after the start of therapy.
How do antihistamines work?	Blockers of H_1 histamine receptors are useful in treating the symptoms of allergic rhinitis caused by histamine release.
Name some antihistamines commonly used in the treatment of rhinitis.	**Diphenhydramine** **Chlorpheniramine** **Cyproheptadine** **Promethazine**
How do α-adrenergic agonists work?	α-Adrenergic agonists constrict dilated arterioles in the nasal mucosa and reduce airway resistance. When administered in aerosol form, these drugs have a rapid onset of action and show few systemic effects.
Give two examples of α-adrenergic agonists used in the treatment of rhinitis.	**Ephedrine** and **pseudoephedrine**

What happens with prolonged use of nasal decongestants?

Rebound nasal congestion often occurs after discontinuation from prolonged use.

Section VI

Endocrine System

29

Hypothalamic and Pituitary Hormones

Define endocrinology.

The study of organs and structures whose function is to secrete hormones into the bloodstream

HYPOTHALAMIC HORMONES

What hormones are secreted from the hypothalamus?

Growth hormone–releasing hormone (GHRH)—GHRH is most often used to stimulate growth hormone (somatotropin) release in patients with short stature.

Somatotropin release-inhibiting hormone (somatostatin)—Somatostatin seems to be a generalized inhibiting hormone that is found in both the GI system and CNS and is known to inhibit the release of insulin, glucagon, and gastrin as well as thyrotropin and growth hormone.

What is octreotide (Sandostatin)?

A synthetic analog of **somatostatin** with a longer half-life and greater potency

What is it used for?

Esophageal variceal bleeds
Acromegaly
To reduce symptoms in hormone-secreting pancreatic and carcinoid tumors

What are its side effects?

Nausea, cramps
Steatorrhea

Gonadotropin-releasing hormone (GnRH)—If given in pulsatile doses to mimic physiological cycling, GnRH stimulates the release of follicle-stimulating (FSH) hormone and luteinizing hormone (LH). If given in a continuous dose, it greatly diminishes gonadotropin release. Drugs such as **leuprolide, goserelin, nafarelin,** and **histrelin** are synthetic analogues of **GnRH** and are administered in a continuous fashion to inhibit **GnRH** in patients with conditions such as prostatic cancer, endometriosis, or precocious puberty.

Corticotropin-releasing hormone (CRH)—CRH stimulates the release of **adrenocorticotropic hormone (ACTH)** from the anterior lobe of the pituitary through activation of cyclic adenosine monophosphate.

Thyrotropin-releasing hormone (TRH)—TRH is a peptide that stimulates the release of thyrotropin from the anterior lobe of the pituitary. It also stimulates the release of prolactin.

Dopamine—acts as a natural inhibitor of prolactin release.

How do these hormones work?

The hypothalamic hormones are all peptides that bind to cell surface membrane receptors.

What are these hormones used for?

To test for pituitary insufficiency
For supplemental therapy
For replacement therapy
Bromocriptine, a analogue of dopamine, is used to treat conditions associated with hyperprolactinemia, such as prolactinoma, acromegaly, and amenorrhea.

Which two hormones are synthesized in the hypothalamus but not secreted from there?

Oxytocin and vasopressin are synthesized in the hypothalamus but are transported to the posterior pituitary, where they are stored or released from the pituitary into the systemic circulation.

PITUITARY HORMONES

ANTERIOR LOBE PITUITARY HORMONES

**What hormones are
synthesized and secreted
from the anterior lobe of
the pituitary
(adenohypophysis)?**

Growth hormone (Somatotropin)
Adrenocorticotropic hormone (ACTH)
Thyroid-stimulating hormone (TSH)
Follicle-stimulating hormone (FSH)
Luteinizing hormone (LH)
Prolactin (PRL) (Figure 29–1)

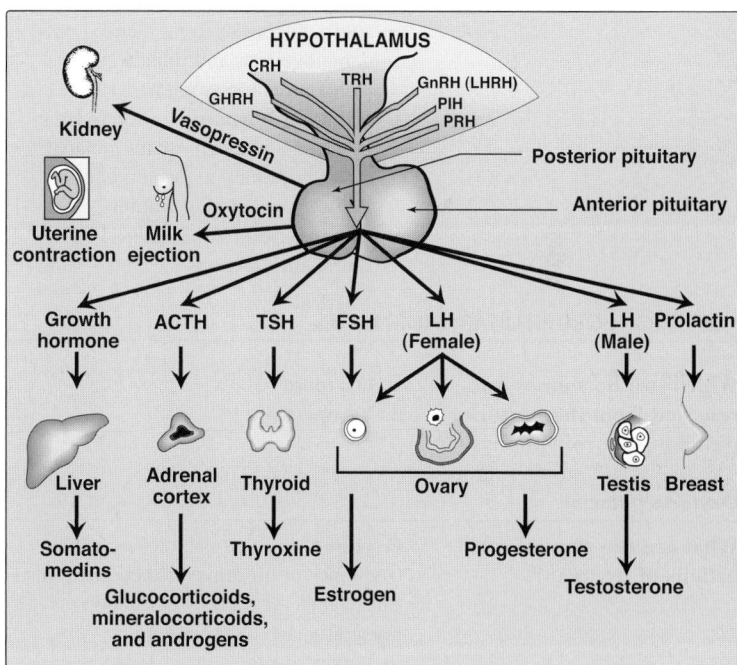

Figure 29–1. Hypothalamic-releasing hormones and actions of anterior pituitary hormones. GRH = growth-hormone–releasing hormone; TRH = thyrotropin-releasing hormone; CRH = corticotropin-releasing hormone; GnRH (LHRH) = gonad-releasing hormone (luteinizing hormone–releasing hormone); PIH = prolactin-inhibiting hormone (dopamine); PRH = prolactin-releasing hormone; ACTH = adrenocorticotropic hormone; TSH = thyrotropin-stimulating hormone; FSH = follicle-stimulating hormone; LH = luteinizing hormone. (Modified with permission from Howland RD, Mycek MJ [Harvey RA, Champe PC, eds.]. *Lippincott's Illustrated Reviews: Pharmacology*, 3rd ed. Baltimore: Lippincott Williams & Wilkins, 2006, p. 272.)

What are the clinical uses of these hormones?

Growth hormone—Somatotropin, made with recombinant DNA technology, is the synthetic form of growth hormone. It is used in the treatment of children with growth hormone deficiency.

Adrenocorticotropic hormone—diagnosis of adrenal insufficiency

Thyroid-stimulating hormone—assessment of thyroid dysfunction (primary vs. secondary hypothyroidism)

Follicle-stimulating hormone—used to treat infertility (stimulates spermatogenesis in men and gametogenesis and follicle development in women)

Luteinizing hormone—used to treat hypogonadism (stimulates gonadal steroid production in men and induces ovulation in women)

Prolactin—never administered for therapeutic reasons

POSTERIOR LOBE PITUITARY HORMONES

Which two hormones are released from the posterior pituitary (neurohypophysis)?

1. **Oxytocin**
2. **Vasopressin**

Oxytocin (Pitocin)

What are the physiological actions of oxytocin?

Oxytocin stimulates the force and frequency of uterine contractions. It also causes milk ejection by contracting myoepithelial cells surrounding mammary alveoli.

State its clinical uses.

Induces and reinforces labor

Controls postpartum and postabortal uterine hemorrhage: administered as an IV

Stimulate milk ejection: given as a nasal spray

State oxytocin's adverse effects.	Hypertensive episodes Uterine rupture

Vasopressin (Pitressin, Antidiuretic Hormone [ADH])

What are vasopressin's mechanisms of action?	**Vasopressin** activates V_1 receptors, which are found in vascular smooth muscle and mediate vasoconstriction. **Vasopressin** also stimulates V_2 receptors in the collecting tubules of nephrons to increase water reabsorption. This results in a more concentrated urine. ADH: **AD**ds **H**ydration to the body.
What are vasopressin's clinical uses?	1. Central but not nephrogenic diabetes insipidus 2. Control of variceal or diverticular colonic bleeding through its vasoconstrictive properties
What are the adverse effects of this drug?	Can decrease coronary circulation Nausea and abdominal cramps Water intoxication Headache

Desmopressin (DDAVP)

What is it?	**Desmopressin** is a long-acting synthetic analogue of **vasopressin** that activates V_2 receptors on the renal tubule cells to increase water permeability and resorption. Unlike **vasopressin**, it has minimal effect on V_1 receptors which mediate vasoconstriction.
What are desmopressin's therapeutic uses?	Drug of choice for central diabetes insipidus Nocturnal enuresis in children Relieves post–lumbar puncture headaches
What are its adverse effects?	Water intoxication Nausea, abdominal pain and cramps Hypotonic hyponatremia at high doses

30

Thyroid and Antithyroid Drugs

Name three major hormones secreted by the thyroid gland.

1. Thyroxine (T_4)
2. Triiodothyronine (T_3)
3. Calcitonin

What are the physiological controls of the thyroid gland?

Thyroid-stimulating hormone (TSH) from the hypothalamus
Thyrotropin-releasing hormone (TRH) from the pituitary
Feedback from T_3 and T_4

What is the basic structure of the thyroid gland?

The thyroid gland is composed of multiple follicles, each of which has a lumen filled with thyroglobulin (colloid), the storage form of thyroid hormone. The follicles are surrounded by parafollicular cells that produce calcitonin.

How are T_3 and T_4 formed?

The tyrosine residues of thyroglobulin are iodinated in the gland to form monoiodotyrosine (MIT) or diiodotyrosine (DIT). T_4 is a combination of two DIT molecules, and T_3 is a combination of one MIT and one DIT molecule (Figure 30–1).

Which is more potent—T_3 or T_4?

T_3 is 10 times more potent than T_4. In fact, most of the systemic effects of the thyroid hormones are due to T_3, because T_4 is converted to T_3 in the peripheral tissues, liver, and kidneys.

How are T_3 and T_4 transported within the body?

Thyroid hormones are largely bound to thyroxine-binding globulin (TBG). Only 0.04% of T_4 and 0.4% of T_3 exist in the free form, and only the free form has metabolic activity.

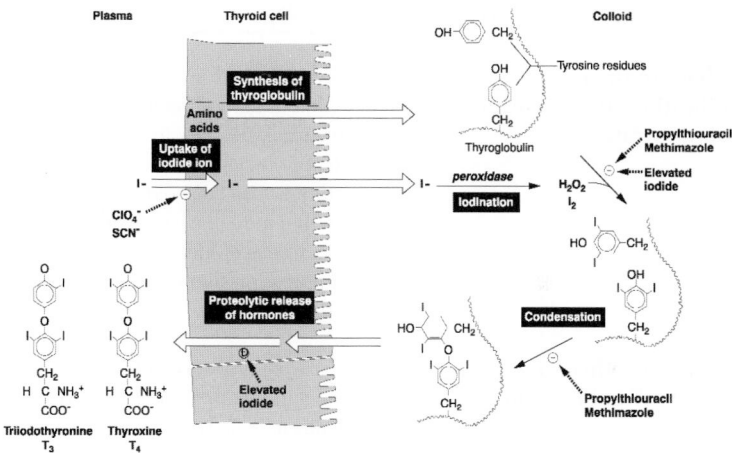

Figure 30–1. Biosynthesis of thyroid hormones. (Redrawn with permission from Mycek MJ, Harvey RA, Champe PC [Harvey RA, Champe PC, eds.]. *Lippincott's Illustrated Reviews: Pharmacology*, 2nd ed. Philadelphia: Lippincott-Raven Publishers, 1997, p 252.)

Where do T₃ and T₄ bind?	The receptors that bind thyroid hormone are located within the nucleus of the cell.

HYPOTHYROIDISM

What are the symptoms of hypothyroidism?	Hypothyroidism affects almost every system in the body. The most common presenting signs, however, are: Fatigue Cold intolerance Weight gain despite reduced appetite Irregular menses In severe cases the skin may show nonpitting edema (myxedema).
What diseases and conditions commonly cause hypothyroidism?	Hashimoto's thyroiditis (an autoimmune disorder) Drugs or radiation exposure Pituitary tumors
What are the treatment options for hypothyroidism?	**Levothyroxine sodium**—drug of choice because of its consistent potency and prolonged duration of action **Liothyronine sodium**

LEVOTHYROXINE SODIUM (T₄—SYNTHROID)

What are the major indications for thyroxine administration?

Hypothyroidism
Prevention of mental retardation in newborns with thyroid deficiency (infantile hypothyroidism)—This condition may be avoided if thyroid supplementation occurs within the first 2 weeks of life.
TSH suppression therapy after treatment for thyroid cancer

How is levothyroxine absorbed and metabolized?

Levothyroxine is absorbed from the small intestine and metabolized in the liver. It has a half-life of 7 days.

What are its adverse effects?

Tachycardia
Heat intolerance
Tremors

LIOTHYRONINE SODIUM (T₃—CYTOMEL)

What are the clinical indications for this drug?

Liothyronine sodium is usually reserved for the treatment of myxedema coma in combination with **levothyroxine**. Symptoms of myxedema coma, which is a medical emergency, include hypothermia, respiratory depression, and unconsciousness. It is most commonly seen in the elderly during winter months.

What are the toxicities of liothyronine?

Similar to those of **levothyroxine,** but **liothyronine** is more cardiotoxic

HYPERTHYROIDISM

What are the symptoms of hyperthyroidism?

In general, the symptoms are the opposite of those seen in hypothyroidism. The most common presenting symptoms are:
Nervousness
Sweating
Hypersensitivity to heat
Weight loss despite increased appetite

What is the most common cause?	Graves' disease, an autoimmune disorder in which a thyroid-stimulating immunoglobulin causes thyrotoxicosis
What are some other causes?	Toxic multinodular goiter Subacute thyroiditis
What are the treatment options?	Propylthiouracil and methimazole Iodine salts Ionic inhibitors Radioactive iodine Surgery

PROPYLTHIOURACIL AND METHIMAZOLE

What are they?	Sulfur-containing molecules known as thioamides
How do they work?	They stop the iodination and coupling of the thyroglobulin molecule. Therefore, MIT and DIT cannot be produced. Without MIT and DIT, it is impossible to produce T_3 and T_4 (see Figure 30–1).
What is the route of administration?	PO
What are the adverse effects?	Agranulocytosis (rare, but the most important effect to watch for) Skin rash (common) Aplastic anemia

IODIDE (IODINE SALTS)

What is the difference between iodine and iodide?	**Iodide** is the ionic form of the element iodine.
Why give iodides?	Giving **iodides** would seem intuitively to exacerbate symptoms of hyperthyroidism. However, **iodides** in large doses actually decrease release of thyroid hormone. This effect, however, is transient and, after a variable period of time, the beneficial effect disappears. **Iodides** also decrease the vascularity and size of the thyroid gland.

In what situations do you use iodides?

Iodides today are not used as sole therapy. Most often they are used before a thyroidectomy or in conjunction with a thioamide and **propranolol** in thyrotoxic crisis.

Give two examples of available iodide preparations.

1. **Lugol's solution**—a mixture of iodine and potassium iodide
2. **Potassium iodide**

What are the adverse effects of iodides?

Anaphylactoid reaction—angioedema and swelling of the larynx
Chronic iodide intoxication (iodism)
Brassy taste and burning in the mouth
Soreness of the teeth and gums
Swelling of the eyelids
Coryza and sneezing simulating a cold
Respiratory problems
Enlarged parotid and submaxillary glands

IONIC INHIBITORS

Give two examples of ionic inhibitors.

Perchlorate (ClO_4^-) and **thiocyanate**

What is their mechanism of action?

They competitively inhibit the concentration of iodide by blocking the iodide transport mechanism.

What are the clinical uses of the ionic inhibitors?

Ionic inhibitors have been used in the past to treat Graves' disease and **amiodarone**-induced thyrotoxicosis. However, their use has diminished in favor of other options.

RADIOACTIVE IODINE

Why use radioactive iodine (I_{131})?

Because the thyroid gland very avidly takes up iodine, a dose of radioactive iodine can ablate thyroid tissue, which results in *permanent* reduction of thyroid activity.

In whom do you use it?

In adults over the age of 21 who have hyperthyroidism. It is also the best form of treatment when Graves' disease has been refractory to antithyroid drugs or has persisted after subtotal thyroidectomy.

Is there any evidence that iodine causes cancer?

No

What are the adverse effects?

A high incidence of delayed hypothyroidism

What are the contraindications?

Radioactive iodine should not be used in pregnant women or nursing mothers.

THYROID STORM

What is it?

A life-threatening medical emergency characterized by extreme effects of hyperthyroidism.

What causes it?

Illness, surgery, or other stress in a patient who is already thyrotoxic

How do you a manage a patient who has thyroid storm?

Supportive therapy (oxygen, fluids)
β-Adrenergic blockers to manage hypertension and tachycardia
Propylthiouracil or **methimazole**
Intravenous sodium iodine
Glucocorticoids to inhibit peripheral conversion of T_4 to T_3

31

Sex Steroids and Reproductive Drugs

What are the three major categories of sex steroids?

1. Estrogens
2. Progestins
3. Androgens

How do natural estrogens, progestins, and androgens work?

In general, because all of these agents are steroids, the compounds will enter the cell and bind to a cytosolic receptor. The Steroid-receptor complex will then travel to the nucleus of the cell and activate gene transcription. This results in the synthesis of proteins that regulate physiologic functions.

ESTROGENS

What are estrogens?

The estrogens are compounds involved in normal female development and regulation of the menstrual cycle (Figure 31–1).

What are the three main estrogens produced by the female body?

1. Estradiol
2. Estrone
3. Estriol

Which of these estrogens is the principal secretory product of the ovary?

Estradiol. It is the most potent.

What are the precursors to estrogen synthesis?

Androstenedione and testosterone (Figure 31–2)

What are estrogen's most important physiological effects?

Regulates growth and maturation of the reproductive organs
Stimulates endometrial growth
Reduces bone resorption and maintains normal structure of the skin and blood vessels
Increases levels of thyroxine-binding globulin

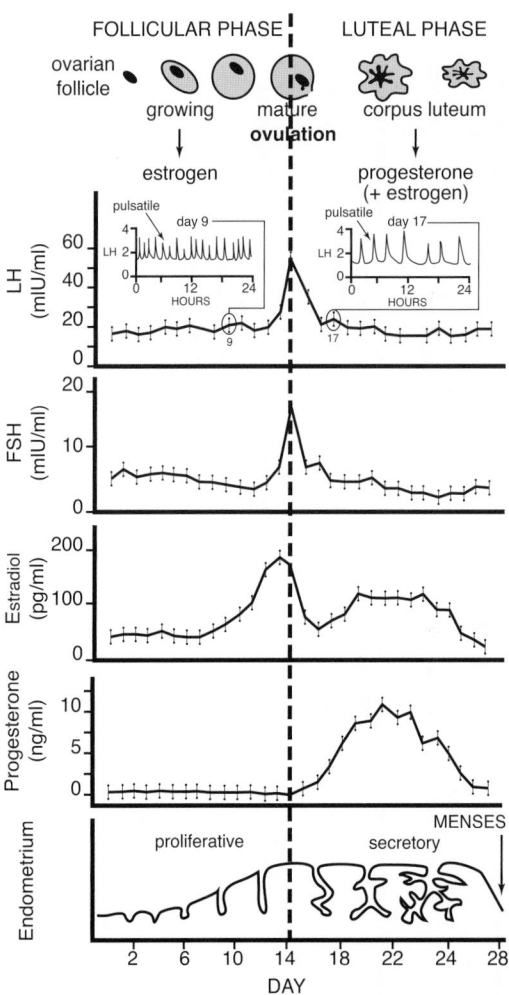

Figure 31–1. Hormonal relationships of the human menstrual cycle. Average daily values of LH, FSH, estradiol (E$_2$), and progesterone in plasma samples from women exhibiting normal 28-day menstrual cycles. Changes in the ovarian follicle (top) and endometrium (bottom) also are illustrated schematically. Frequent plasma sampling reveals pulsatile patterns of gonadotropin release. Characteristic profiles are illustrated schematically for the follicular phase (day 9, inset on left) and luteal phase (day 17, inset on right). Both the frequency (number of pulses per hour) and amplitude (extent of change of hormone release) of pulses vary throughout the cycle. (From Brunton LL, Lazo JS, Parker KL [eds.]. *Goodman & Gilman's The Pharmacological Basis of Therapeutics*, 11th ed. New York: McGraw-Hill, 2006, p. 1546. Redrawn with permission from Thorneycroft et al., 1971.)

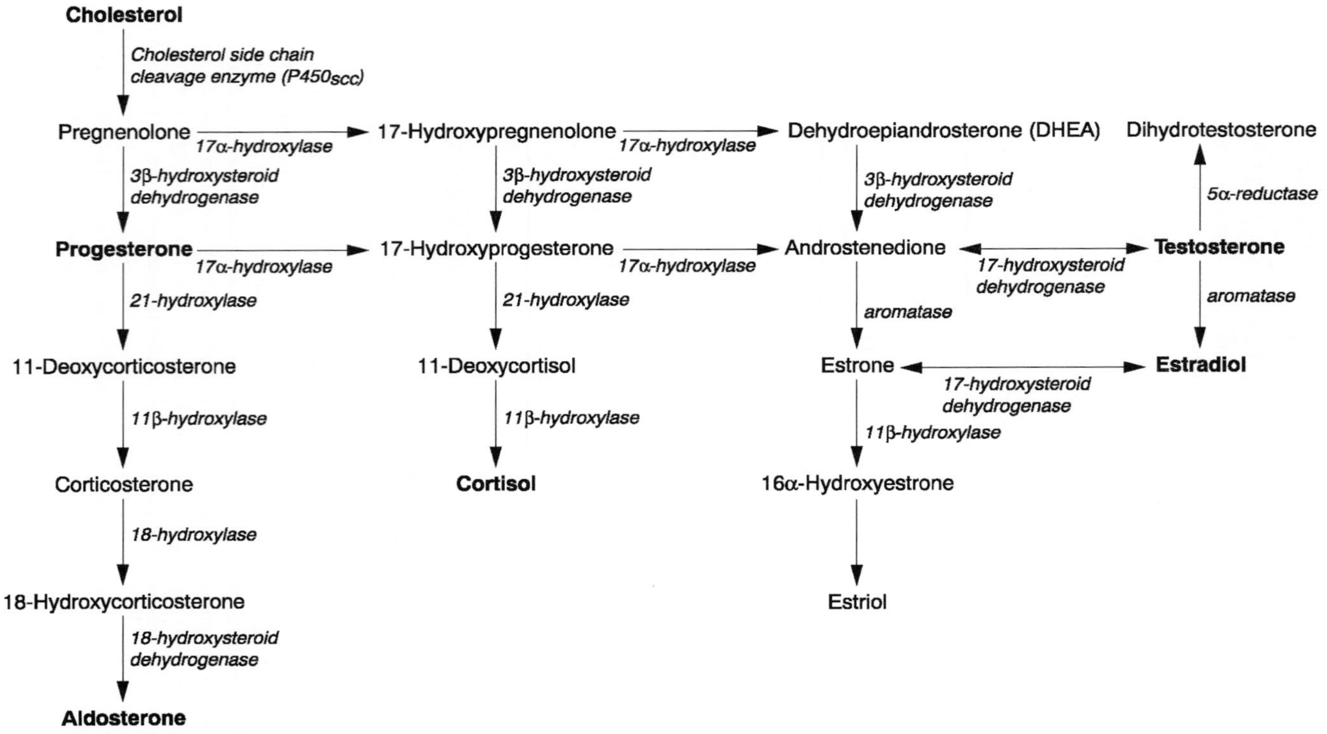

Figure 31-2. Steroid hormone synthesis. (Redrawn with permission from Gallia G, Hann CL, Hewson WH. *The Pharmacology Companion*. La Jolla, CA: Alert & Oriented Publishing Company, 1997, Fig 7.2.)

Increases HDL and triglyceride levels and decreases LDL levels

Promotes coagulation of the blood

Give examples of estrogens that are currently used clinically.

Estradiol
Estrone
Ethinyl estradiol
Quinestrol
Mestranol

What are the clinical uses of estrogens?

An important therapeutic use of estrogens is treatment of primary hypogonadism in young girls.

Estrogens are used in oral contraceptives in combination with progestins. They suppress FSH secretion and therefore inhibit ovulation.

Estrogens are used in postmenopausal hormone replacement therapy. They help reduce the risk of cardiovascular disease, osteoporosis, hot flashes, and vaginitis.

What is the route of administration?

Estrogens are effective when given transdermally and intramuscularly. Estrogens can also be given orally, although there is a large first-pass hepatic metabolism.

What are the potential toxic effects of estrogen replacement?

Postmenopausal bleeding

Endometrial hyperplasia

Breast tenderness

Cholestasis

Over long periods there is an increased risk of endometrial cancer, thromboembolism, hypertriglyceridemia, hypertension, MI, and hepatic adenoma.

Name four *absolute* contraindications to estrogen replacement therapy.

1. Breast cancer
2. Pregnancy
3. Liver disease
4. History of thrombophlebitis

SELECTIVE ESTROGEN RECEPTOR MODULATORS

TAMOXIFEN (NOLVADEX)

What is tamoxifen?

A nonsteroidal drug that acts as a competitive inhibitor of estradiol in breast tissue and an agonist on endometrial tissue

When is it used?

In the treatment of breast cancer in postmenopausal women

Are there adverse effects?

Yes—hot flashes, nausea and vomiting, endometrial cancer, venous thrombosis, and menstrual irregularities

RALOXIFENE (EVISTA)

What is it?

Raloxifene and actually **tamoxifen** as well belong to a class of drugs known as selective estrogen receptor modulators (SERMs). This means that they act as estrogen agonists at some receptors and antagonists at other receptors. **Tamoxifen** is a first-generation SERM, while raloxifene is a second-generation SERM.

What is it used for?

Preventive treatment of osteoporosis in postmenopausal women. **Raloxifene** acts as an estrogen agonist on bone and has antagonistic effects on breast tissue; thus, like tamoxifen, it reduces the risk of breast cancer.

What is the route of administration?

PO

What are the adverse effects?	Thromboembolic events, hot flashes **Raloxifene** does not stimulate endometrial tissue as **tamoxifen** does and thus does not increase the risk of endometrial cancer
What are the contraindications to this drug?	Pregnancy

CLOMIPHENE (CLOMID)

Describe this drug.	**Clomiphene** is a partial agonist at estrogen receptors in the pituitary gland. This drug prevents normal feedback inhibition of estrogens on the hypothalamus and pituitary and increases release of LH and FSH from the pituitary. This subsequently stimulates ovulation.
How is clomiphene used therapeutically?	To treat infertility in anovulatory women
What are the adverse effects?	Hot flashes Ovarian enlargement Multiple simultaneous births Visual disturbances

PROGESTINS

Name the most important progestin of the human body.	Progesterone is the prototypical progestin. It is synthesized in the ovary, testis, and adrenal gland from circulating cholesterol. Luteinizing hormone stimulates its synthesis (see Figure 31–2).
What are the physiological effects of progesterone?	Stimulates lipoprotein lipase activity and increases fat deposition Increases insulin response to glucose Promotes glycogen storage in the liver Increases body temperature Regulates maturation of the endometrium Increases development of breast secretory glands
Give some examples of synthetic progestins.	**Medroxyprogesterone acetate** **Norethindrone** **Norethindrone acetate** **Norgestrel**
What are the therapeutic uses of progestins?	**Contraception**—used either alone or with estradiol **Hormone replacement therapy** in combination with **estrogen** to reduce the risk of endometrial cancer associated with **estrogen** therapy alone. Also used when **ovarian suppression** is necessary, for example, in the treatment of dysmenorrhea and endometriosis. **Diagnosis of estrogen secretion**—If menstruation occurs after administration of **progesterone** in amenorrheic patients, it can be concluded that the uterus has been stimulated by estrogen.

How can progestins be administered?	PO or IM
Describe the adverse effects.	Weight gain, depression, acne, hypertension, edema, and thrombophlebitis.

PROGESTIN INHIBITORS—MIFEPRISTONE (RU 486)

Describe mifepristone.	It is a competitive inhibitor of progestins at progesterone receptors.
When do you use it?	This controversial "morning after" drug is used as an abortifacient. It is usually given concomitantly with prostaglandin E or prostaglandin F to increase myometrial contractions.
Are there adverse effects?	Yes—heavy uterine bleeding, GI effects (nausea, vomiting, anorexia), and abdominal pain

DANAZOL (DANOCRINE)

Describe danazol.	**Danazol** is a drug that acts as a partial agonist at progesterone, androgen, and glucocorticoid receptors.
When is it used?	The drug is used to treat endometriosis.
What are the adverse effects?	Weight gain Edema Acne Reduced HDL cholesterol levels

ANDROGENS

What are androgens?

Androgens are a group of 19-carbon steroids derived from cholesterol.

Name four androgens produced by the testes.

1. Testosterone
2. Dihydrotestosterone
3. Dehydroepiandrosterone
4. Androstenedione

Which is the principal androgen?

Testosterone

Where is testosterone produced?

In the testis, the adrenal gland, and (to a small degree) the ovary

What is testosterone produced from?

Progesterone and dehydroepiandrosterone (Figure 31–2)

What are the physiological effects of the androgens?

The androgens' effects can be broken down into two categories:
1. Anabolic—increase in overall body growth, muscle mass, and red blood cell production
2. Androgenic—growth of the larynx and skeleton, development of facial hair, darkening of the skin

Give some examples of synthetic androgens.

Testosterone cypionate—injectable
Oxandrolone (Oxandrin)
Stanozolol (Winstrol)
Fluoxymesterone (Halotestin)

How are the synthetic analogues administered?

Because of significant first-pass metabolism, androgens are best injected or given transdermally. Some synthetic analogues, like those listed above, can be given orally but are more hepatotoxic and less effective that way.

What is the primary clinical use of synthetic androgens?

Replacement therapy in male hypogonadism. On occasion it is used to promote growth in prepubertal boys.

Describe the toxicities of synthetic androgen treatment.	1. Behavioral effects including excessive rage or hostility
	2. Increased LDL/HDL ratio
	3. Stunted growth due to premature closure of the epiphyseal plates
	4. In women: hirsutism, depression of menses, acne, and clitoral enlargement
	5. In males: decreased spermatogenesis, gynecomastia, acne, testicular atrophy, prostatic hypertrophy

Name a contraindication to androgen use.	Pregnancy

ANDROGEN ANTAGONISTS

Name the four categories of androgen antagonists and give examples of each.	1. Gonadotropin-releasing analogues—**gonadorelin** or **leuprolide**
	2. Receptor inhibitors—**flutamide** and **cyproterone**
	3. Steroid synthesis inhibitors—**ketoconazole** and **spironolactone**
	4. 5α-reductase inhibitors—**finasteride**
	See Figure 31–3.

GONADORELIN (FACTREL)

What is it?	This drug is a synthetic GnRH analogue.

In what clinical situations is this drug used?	For stimulation of gonadotropins (when given in pulsatile form) or suppression of gonadotropins when given in continuous form. Suppression therapy is used in the treatment of endometriosis, prostate cancer, and central precocious puberty. Stimulation therapy is mainly for hypogonadotrophic hypogonadism. Leuprolide, goserelin, and nafarelin are also synthetic GnRH analogues.

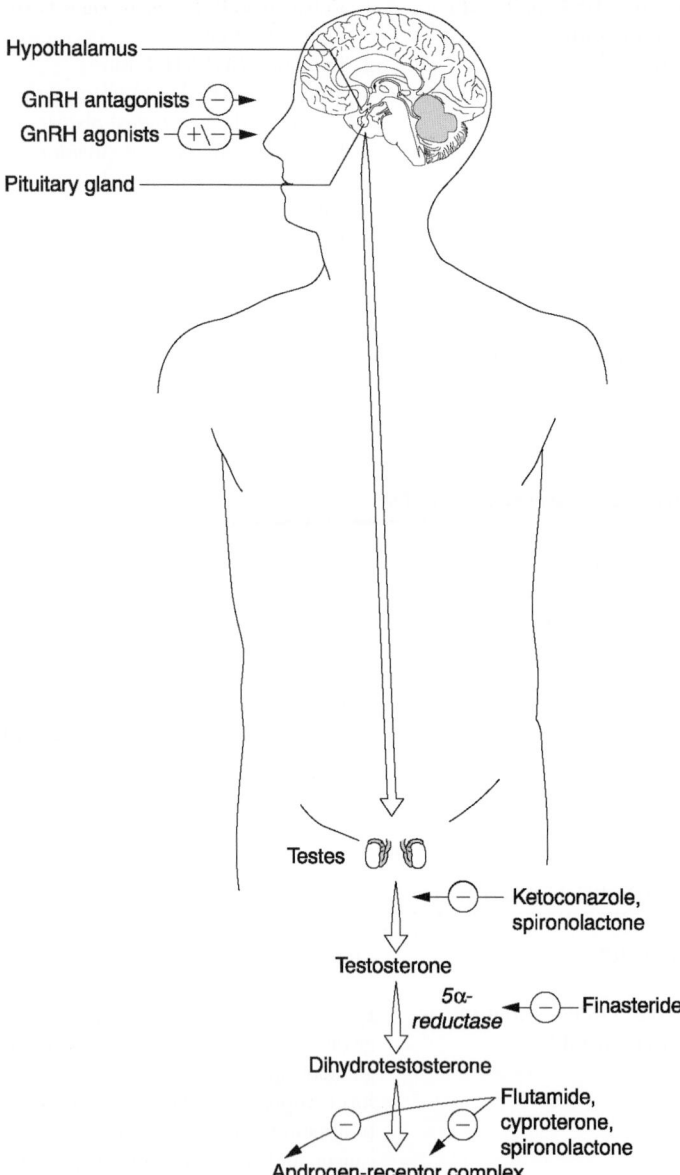

Figure 31–3. Sites of action of some antiandrogen drugs.

FLUTAMIDE (EULEXIN) AND **BICALUTAMIDE** (CASODEX)

How do these drugs work?	They are nonsteroidal drugs that act as competitive antagonists at the androgen receptors.
When are they used?	In combination with a GnRH analogue to treat patients with advanced **prostate cancer**
What are the side effects?	Hepatitis and gynecomastia

CYPROTERONE

What is cyproterone?	It is a steroid that is also a competitive antagonist at androgen receptors. It is used in the treatment of women with hirsutism.

KETOCONAZOLE

Why does an antifungal work as an antiandrogen?	**Ketoconazole** inhibits several of the cytochrome P-450 enzymes involved in steroid synthesis. See *Chapter 47—Antifungal Drugs,* for more information on this drug.

FINASTERIDE (PROSCAR, PROPECIA)

How does it work?	5α-Reductase is an enzyme responsible for the conversion of testosterone to dihydrotestosterone (DHT). Cells of the prostate are stimulated to grow by DHT. **Finasteride** inhibits this enzyme and thus reduces cell proliferation in the prostate.
When is it used?	Benign prostatic hyperplasia (BPH) **Propecia** is used to treat hair loss.
What are the side effects?	Loss of libido, erectile dysfunction

FEMALE CONTRACEPTION

What are the three different kinds of oral contraceptives currently available?

1. Combination estrogen-progestin tablets that are taken in constant doses throughout the menstrual cycle
2. Combination estrogen-progestin tablets in which the progestin concentration slowly increases to mimic the natural cycle
3. Progestin-only preparations

What kinds of implantable or injectable contraception are currently available?

These are primarily progestin-only agents. Examples include **norgestrel** (Norplant) and Progestasert, a intrauterine device that releases low amounts of progesterone over the course of a few years.

How do oral contraceptives work?

They work primarily by preventing ovulation. In addition, they change the properties of cervical mucus and impair implantation of fertilized ova.

What are the adverse effects of combination oral contraceptives?

Formation of blood clots—major toxic effect
Increased risk of breast cancer—The evidence for this is *questionable*. However, *convincing evidence* exists that combination oral contraceptives *reduce* the incidence of both endometrial and ovarian cancer.
Minor toxicities include:
Breast tenderness
Headache
Gallbladder disease
Acne
Weight gain

What is the most common side effect of progestin-only contraceptives?

Irregular, unpredictable breakthrough bleeding. The incidence decreases over time, and amenorrhea is typical after 1 year of use.

What are the absolute contraindications for combination oral contraceptives?

Pregnancy
History of thromboembolic disease
Myocardial infarction
Coronary artery disease
Cerebrovascular disease
Congenital hyperlipidemia
Breast or endometrial cancer

ERECTILE DYSFUNCTION

What drugs are used to treat erectile dysfunction?

Sildenafil (Viagra)
Vardenafil (Levitra)
Tadalafil (Cialis)

How do they work?

These drugs inhibit phosphodiesterase (PDE) V. This, in turn, results in an increase in cGMP, which relaxes the smooth muscle of the corpora cavernosa and facilitates blood flow to the penis.

Which of the three medications has the longest half life?

Sildenafil and **vardenafil** have half lives of 4 hrs, while **tadalafil** has a half life of 18 hrs.

Are there any toxic effects?

Yes. Headache and flushing are most common. Alterations in color vision (bluish-green hue to objects) have been reported with **sildenafil**. Priapism can occur with all three medications.

When are these drugs contraindicated?

In patients who are concurrently taking organic nitrates, because the combination can cause severe hypotension

32

Corticosteroids and Inhibitors

What are the two major groups of corticosteroids?	Mineralocorticoids and glucocorticoids
Where are corticosteroids produced?	In the adrenal cortex—specifically in the zona glomerulosa (mineralocorticoids) and the zona fasciculata (glucocorticoids)
Describe the functions of the two major pharmacological groups of corticosteroids.	1. **Glucocorticoids**—primarily affect metabolism, inflammation, and immune responses 2. **Mineralocorticoids**—affect fluid and electrolyte balance The biological activity of the synthetic corticosteroids discussed here ranges from strict glucocorticoid to strict mineralocorticoid activity (Figure 32–1).
How are corticosteroids administered?	They can be given orally, topically, IV, aerosolized, or via IM injection.

GLUCOCORTICOIDS

How do glucocorticoids work?	Both glucocorticoids and mineralocorticoids enter the cell and bind to a cytosolic receptor. The steroid receptor complex then enters the nucleus and alters gene expression by binding to specific DNA receptors.
What are the major physiological effects of glucocorticoids?	**Anti-inflammatory effects**— Glucocorticoids inhibit the number and function of lymphocytes, eosinophils, basophils, and monocytes; increase neutrophils at the site of injury; and decrease the release of arachidonic acid, the major precursor

Short-Acting Glucocorticoids (8 – 12 hr)

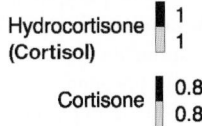

Hydrocortisone (Cortisol) — 1 / 1

Cortisone — 0.8 / 0.8

Intermediate-Acting Glucocorticoids (18 – 36 hr)

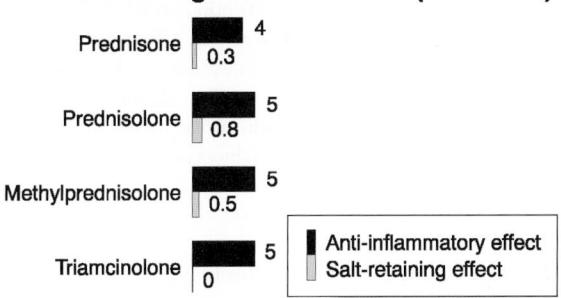

Prednisone — 4 / 0.3

Prednisolone — 5 / 0.8

Methylprednisolone — 5 / 0.5

Triamcinolone — 5 / 0

■ Anti-inflammatory effect
▨ Salt-retaining effect

Long-Acting Glucocorticoids (1 – 3 days)

Betamethasone — 35 / 0

Dexamethasone — 30 / 0

Paramethasone — 10 / 0

Mineralocorticoids

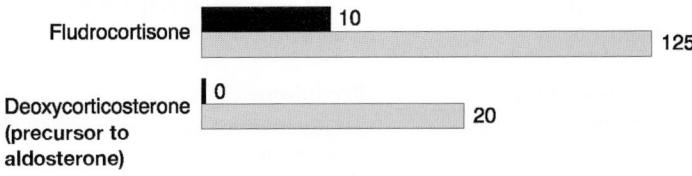

Fludrocortisone — 10 / 125

Deoxycorticosterone (precursor to aldosterone) — 0 / 20

Figure 32–1. Pharmacological properties of some commonly used natural and synthetic corticosteroids. Activities are all relative to hydrocortisone = 1. Time refers to duration of action. (Redrawn with permission from Mycek MJ, Harvey RA, Champe PC [Harvey RA, Champe PC, eds.]. *Lippincott's Illustrated Reviews: Pharmacology,* 2nd ed. Philadelphia: Lippincott-Raven Publishers, 1997, p. 255.)

to prostaglandins, by blocking the enzyme phospholipase A_2.

Metabolic effects—Glucocorticoids stimulate gluconeogenesis, lipolysis, and lipogenesis, resulting in an increase in plasma glucose levels that provides energy for the body to fight infection, trauma, debilitating disease, or other stresses.

Catabolic effects—Glucocorticoids can cause muscle, bone, lymphoid, skin, and fat catabolism.

Immunosuppressive effects—Glucocorticoids inhibit the function of lymphocytes, monocytes, and eosinophils

Name the major natural glucocorticoid of the human body.

Cortisol (hydrocortisone)

What hormone normally controls cortisol secretion?

Adrenocorticotropic hormone (ACTH)

How is cortisol transported in the blood?

Ninety percent of cortisol is bound to plasma proteins.

How is cortisol metabolized?

Primarily in the liver

Does cortisol have any mineralocorticoid properties?

Yes! This is an important reason for the hypertension associated with Cushing's syndrome.

Name a few of the synthetically produced glucocorticoids.

Prednisone (Deltasone)
Triamcinolone (Aristocort)—often used topically
Dexamethasone (Decadron)
Beclomethasone (Beclovent)
Betamethasone (Celestone)
There are many more. Their names usually end in "one," which will help you recognize them.

How do the synthetically produced glucocorticoids

They differ with respect to the route of administration, half-life, and ratio of

differ from one another and from naturally occurring glucocorticoids?

glucocorticoid-to-mineralocorticoid activity. In general, the synthetic agents are longer-acting (Figure 32–1) and have better absorption through lipid barriers.

What are the therapeutic uses of synthetic glucocorticoids?

The list of inflammatory or immunological conditions that respond to glucocorticoid therapy is extremely lengthy. It includes but is not limited to:

Adrenal insufficiency (Addison's disease)—in conjunction with a mineralocorticoid

Congenital adrenal hyperplasia

Asthma (beclomethasone)

Collagen vascular diseases

Ocular disease—uveitis, exophthalmos, optic neuritis

Lung maturation in a fetus (betamethasone)—helps increase production of surfactant

Skin disease—contact dermatitis, urticaria

Chemotherapy—prednisone for Hodgkin's disease

Diagnosis of Cushing's syndrome— dexamethasone suppression test

Cerebral edema—dexamethasone

Inflammation reduction in general— rheumatoid arthritis and osteoarthritis, inflammatory bowel disease

What are the adverse effects of glucocorticoids?

Long-term use of glucocorticoids can cause a large number of side effects. The most important include:

Adrenal suppression—Sudden termination of glucocorticoid therapy is not recommended because it will not allow time for the normal hypothalamic-pituitary-adrenal axis to regain control.

Metabolic disorders including diabetes, muscle wasting, and osteoporosis

Increased risk of infections

CNS effects such as a psychosis or euphoria
Stimulation of peptic ulcers
Iatrogenic Cushing's syndrome—weight gain, moon face, acne, increased growth of body hair
To avoid these effects, it is important to *use as low a dose as possible, choose local over systemic therapy when possible,* and *taper the steroids* after achieving a therapeutic response.

MINERALOCORTICOIDS

What is the major mineralocorticoid in the body?

Aldosterone

What controls the secretion of aldosterone?

ACTH and the renin-angiotensin system

Describe the function of aldosterone.

Aldosterone acts on the renal tubule cells to increase reabsorption of sodium, bicarbonate, and water in exchange for the excretion of potassium.

Name some synthetic mineralocorticoids.

Fludrocortisone (Florinef)
Desoxycorticosterone

What are mineralocorticoids responsible for?

Fluid and electrolyte balance, especially of sodium and potassium

What is fludrocortisone used for?

Replacement therapy after adrenalectomy or for primary and secondary adrenocortical insufficiency

What side effects can be seen with fludrocortisone therapy?

Hypokalemia
Congestive heart failure due to volume overload

ADRENOCORTICOSTEROID ANTAGONISTS

Do adrenocorticosteroid antagonists inhibit both glucocorticoid and mineralocorticoid activity?

Yes

AMINOGLUTETHIMIDE (Cytadren)

How does aminoglutethimide work?

It inhibits cytochrome P-450, which catalyzes the rate-limiting step of conversion of cholesterol to pregnenolone. This reduces the biosynthesis of all physiological steroids.

How is it used?

To decrease hypersecretion of cortisol in patients who have Cushing's syndrome

To reduce estrogen production in the treatment of breast cancer (largely replaced by tamoxifen)

Are there adverse effects?

Yes. Gastrointestinal and neurological side effects are seen, along with a transient maculopapular rash.

METYRAPONE (Metopirone)

What is the action of this drug?

It reduces corticosteroid biosynthesis by inhibiting the final step in the pathway (11- hydroxylation). This occurs in the cytochrome P-450 system.

What are the clinical uses?

Testing adrenal function, decreasing hypercorticism due to adrenal tumor

What are the side effects of metyrapone?

Hirsutism
Salt and water retention
Dizziness

KETOCONAZOLE (Nizoral)

What is the role of ketoconazole?

Although **ketoconazole** is mainly used as an antifungal agent, at higher doses it also inhibits steroid synthesis, so it has been used to treat hirsutism, adrenal cancer, and Cushing's syndrome.
See *Chapter 47—Antifungal Drugs,* for further details.

MIFEPRISTONE AND SPIRONOLACTONE

How do these drugs work?

They are both antagonists at receptor sites. **Mifepristone** is a glucocorticoid antagonist while **spironolactone** antagonizes the mineralocorticoid receptor.

When are they used?

Mifepristone (RU-486) is used to treat Cushing's disease and has also been used as an antiprogestogen to terminate early pregnancy.

Spironolactone, a diuretic, can also be used to treat hirsutism in women and hyperaldosteronism.

33

Insulins and Oral Hypoglycemic Drugs

TREATMENT STRATEGIES FOR DIABETES

What is the general treatment strategy for insulin-dependent diabetes (type 1)?

Patients with this disease have an absolute deficiency of insulin because of enormous β-cell destruction. Treatment includes:
Dietary and exercise instruction
Parenteral insulin (usually a mix of different classes to match physiological outputs)

What is the general treatment strategy for non–insulin-dependent diabetes (type 2)?

This disease is frequently associated with low-to-normal insulin levels and target-organ insulin resistance. Treatment includes:
Dietary modification
Weight reduction
Oral hypoglycemic agents: monotherapy or in combinations
Insulin for cases that are not well controlled with all of the above.

INSULIN

What is the structure of insulin?

It is a 51–amino acid protein consisting of two polypeptide chains connected by disulfide bonds.

Where does insulin work?

Insulin binds to proteins in the circulation and cell membrane receptors. Insulin does **not** enter the cell nucleus.

What type of receptor does insulin bind to?

Tyrosine kinase

What are the effects of insulin?

Insulin affects almost every tissue in the body, but the most important target organs are:

Liver—promotes glucose storage as glycogen; increases triglyceride synthesis

Muscle—facilitates protein and glycogen synthesis as well as potassium uptake

Adipose tissue—improves triglyceride storage by activating plasma lipoprotein lipase; reduces circulating free fatty acids

What are the types of insulin preparations used clinically?

There are three main classes of insulin:

1. **Short-acting**—**insulin lispro** (Humalog), **insulin aspart**, **insulin glulisine**, and **regular insulin** (Humulin)
2. **Intermediate-acting**—**isophane insulin suspension** (**neutral protamine Hagedorn** [NPH]) and **insulin zinc suspension** (lente)
3. **Long-acting**—**insulin zinc suspension extended** (ultralente), **insulin glargine**

Different classes of insulins are often combined for maximim efficacy.

Which types of insulin are used for management of hyperglycemic emergencies?

Lispro and regular, because they can be given intravenously and work rapidly

What are the sources of insulin?

Animal insulin preparations made from beef and pork have largely been replaced by human insulin, which can be made through bacterial DNA recombinant technology.

Table 33–1. Pharmacokinetics and Compatibility of Various Insulins

	Insulin preparations	Onset	Peak	Duration	Compatible mixed with
Rapid-Acting	Insulin Injection (Regular)	0.5 to 1		8 to 12	All
	Lispro Insulin Solution	0.25	0.5 to 1.5	6 to 8	Ultralente, NPH
Intermediate-Acting	Isophane Insulin Suspension (NPH)	1 to 1.5	4 to 12	24	Regular
	Insulin Zinc Suspension (Lente)	1 to 2.5	7 to 15	24	Regular, semilente
Long-Acting	Extended Insulin Zinc Suspension (Ultralente)	4 to 8	10 to 30	> 36	Regular, semilente

(©1999 by Facts and Comparisons. Table adapted with permission from Drug Facts and Comparisons, p. 616, 1999, bound edition. St. Louis, MO: Facts and Comparisons, a Wolters Kluwer Company.)

What determines the onset, peak, and duration of action of a particular type of insulin preparation?

The mixture ratio of **zinc protamine** and other substances to **insulin** determines the rate of release (Table 33–1).

What is the standard route for the administration of insulin?

Subcutaneous injection

What are adverse effects of insulin use?

Symptoms of hypoglycemia—diaphoresis, vertigo, tachycardia

Insulin allergy—an IgE-mediated reaction

Insulin antibodies—IgG-mediated, most commonly seen with animal insulin preparations

Lipodystrophy—a change in the fatty tissue surrounding the injection site

ORAL HYPOGLYCEMIC AGENTS

What are five major classes of oral hypoglycemic agents?

1. Sulfonylureas
2. Meglitinides
3. Biguanides
4. α-glucosidase inhibitors
5. Thiazolidinediones (glitazones)

Can these classes be used in combination to achieve glycemic control?

Yes. For example, a sulfonylurea may be used with a biguanide.

SULFONYLUREAS

Give examples of sulfonylureas.

Chlorpropamide (Diabinese)—first generation; has the longest duration of action

Tolbutamide (Orinase)—first generation

Autohexamide (Dymelor)—first generation

Glyburide (Micronase)—second generation; *high potency*

Glipizide (Glucotrol)—second generation; *high potency*

Glimepiride (Amaryl)—second generation

How do sulfonylureas work?

They are known as secretagogues because their primary action is to stimulate the release of endogenous insulin from β cells of the pancreas. Other actions include reducing serum glucagon levels and increasing binding of insulin to target receptors.

How do sulfonylureas work at the cellular level?

By closing K^+ channels on β-cell membranes. This causes cell depolarization and triggers insulin release.

What are the adverse effects of sulfonylureas?

Hypoglycemia due to an overdose or liver/kidney failure—most important

Gastrointestinal distress

Pruritus

Hyperinsulinemia

Agranulocytosis and aplastic anemia (rare)

Chlorpropamide in particular has a tendency to cause a **disulfiram**-like reaction if taken with **ethanol**

What are the pharmacokinetics of the sulfonylureas?

These agents are metabolized in the liver and excreted by the kidneys. **Glyburide** is also eliminated through feces.)

What are contraindications to the use of sulfonylureas?

Liver or renal insufficiency and pregnancy

What drugs potentiate the effects of sulfonylureas?

Aspirin
Monoamine oxidase inhibitors
Ethanol
Phenylbutazone
Probenecid
Allopurinol
Chloramphenicol
Dicumarol
Sulfonamides

What drugs _reduce_ the effects of sulfonylureas?

Phenobarbital
β-adrenergic blockers
Rifampin
Cholestyramine
Loop and thiazide diuretics

MEGLITINIDES

Name the drugs that belong to this class	**Repaglinide** (Prandin) **Nateglinide** (Starlix)
Which group of drugs are repaglinide and nateglinide similar to?	They are very similar to the sulfonylureas in terms of their mechanism of action. These medications work by stimulating the release of insulin; their onset of action, however, is quicker. Therefore, they are most commonly taken just prior to meals.
Where are these drugs metabolized?	In the liver. They are excreted through the bile.
What are its adverse affects?	Again very similar to those of the sulfonylureas Hypoglycemia (The reported incidence is lower than sulfonylureas, however.) **Repaglinide** can cause severe hypoglycemia in patients taking **gemfibrozil**.

BIGUANIDES

Name two biguanides.	1. **Metformin** (Glucophage) 2. **Phenformin**—withdrawn owing to an association with severe lactic acidosis
What is their mechanism of action?	They increase glucose uptake and utilization by the muscles and adipose tissue of the body. Their exact mechanism is not known for certain. However, studies indicate that **metformin** works primarily through a reduction in hepatic gluconeogenesis. Unlike sulfonylureas, their effects are not dependent on functional islet cells.

Does metformin cause a hypoglycemia?

No. Because they do not stimulate insulin release, the incidence of hypoglycemia is very low.

Does metformin improve lipid profiles?

Yes. It reduces LDL and raises HDL. It is the only hypoglycemic agent proven to reduce mortality in type 2 diabetics.

What are the contraindications to the use of metformin?

Renal or liver disease
Cardiac failure requiring medication
Chronic hypoxic lung disease
It is also recommended that **metformin** be withheld prior to a radiologic procedure using an IV iodinated contrast medium because of the potential for acute renal failure induced by the contrast medium.

How is metformin metabolized?

It is excreted unchanged in the urine and does not undergo hepatic metabolism. Tubular secretion is the major route of elimination.

What are the adverse effects?

Lactic acidosis, especially in patients with liver/renal failure, heart failure medications, or alcoholism
Gastrointestinal reactions are most common (diarrhea, nausea, upset stomach)
Decreased absorption of vitamin B_{12} and folate may occur with long-term therapy.

α-GLUCOSIDASE INHIBITORS

Name two drugs that are within this class.

Acarbose (Precose)
Miglitol (Glyset)

How do acarbose and miglitol work?

Both of these drugs inhibit **α glucosidase**, an enzyme in the intestinal brush border. This delays the absorption of complex starches from the gastrointestinal tract.

What are their advantages over other oral hypoglycemic agents?

They do not cause a reactive hypoglycemia since they do not stimulate insulin release or increase the actions of insulin on target tissues.

How are they metabolized?

Acarbose and **miglitol** are metabolized exclusively within the GI tract, mostly by intestinal bacteria but also by digestive enzymes.

What are the adverse effects?

Gastrointestinal symptoms (flatulence, bloating, diarrhea)

THIAZOLIDINEDIONES (Glitazones)

Give three example of this class.

Troglitazone (Rezulin)—withdrawn from the U.S. market
Rosiglitazone (Avandia)
Pioglitazone (Actos)

How do these drugs work?

They both lower blood glucose levels by improving the target-cell (liver and skeletal muscle) response to insulin. They are dependent on the presence of insulin for their activity. Other actions include a decrease of hepatic glucose output, which is commonly seen in NIDDM.

Where in the cell do they act?

The mechanism is thought to involve binding to nuclear receptors called peroxisome proliferator-activated receptor γ that regulate the transcription of a number of insulin-responsive genes.

Do thiazolidinediones cause hypoglycemia?

No. When used alone they do not predispose to hypoglycemia.

What are the adverse effects?

Troglitazone was removed from the market because of severe hepatotoxicity.
Rosiglitazone and **pioglitazone** can also cause hepatotoxicity, but to a much lesser degree.
Other adverse affects from this class of drugs include anemia, weight gain, and headache.

34

Drugs That Affect Calcium Homeostasis and Bone Metabolism

Where in the body is the major storage reservoir of calcium and phosphorus?	The skeleton contains 99% of total body calcium and phosphorus.
Name the principal regulators of plasma Ca^{2+} within the body.	Parathyroid hormone (PTH) 1,25 Dihydroxyvitamin D (calcitriol) Calcitonin

HYPOCALCEMIA

What are the most common presenting signs of hypocalcemia?	Muscular excitability—tetany Paresthesias Laryngospasm Seizures Chvostek's and Trousseau's signs
What is Chvostek's sign?	Facial muscle spasm that occurs when the facial nerve is tapped anterior to the ear.
What is Trousseau's sign?	Carpal spasm after occlusion of blood flow in the forearm with a blood pressure cuff
What are the most common causes of hypocalcemia?	Chronic renal failure Hypoparathyroidism Vitamin D deficiency Malabsorption
What are the pharmacological treatment options for hypocalcemia?	1. Calcium salt preparations 2. Vitamin D preparations

CALCIUM SALT PREPARATIONS

Name four of the more common calcium salt preparations.	1. **Calcium chloride** (Tums) 2. **Calcium gluceptate** 3. **Calcium gluconate** 4. **Calcium carbonate**
What are the adverse effects of calcium supplementation?	Calcium supplements may cause peripheral vasodilation or transient tingling. Also, rapid infusion of calcium can cause cardiac arrhythmias.

VITAMIN D AGENTS

Name three of the more common vitamin D agents currently available.	1. **Calcitriol** (Calcijex)—the vitamin D metabolite of choice for quickly raising serum calcium levels 2. **Ergocalciferol** (Drisdol) 3. **Calciferol**
How does vitamin D work?	It stimulates absorption of calcium and phosphate from the intestine and also decreases the renal excretion of calcium.
What are the common clinical indications for the use of vitamin D supplements?	Osteoporosis, chronic renal failure, nutritional rickets (caused by inadequate dietary intake of vitamin D), metabolic rickets (caused by tissue resistance to vitamin D), osteomalacia, hypoparathyroidism
What are the side effects of these agents?	Vascular calcification, nephrocalcinosis, and soft-tissue calcification

HYPERCALCEMIA

What are the most common symptoms of hypercalcemia?	Hypercalcemia can be a life-threatening condition. Patients may demonstrate dehydration, renal stones, constipation, abdominal pain, weakness, confusion, and delirium—"Groans, bones, and psychiatric overtones."

What conditions or diseases will cause hypercalcemia?

CHIMPANZEES:
Calcium supplementation
Hyperparathyroidism
Iatrogenic (caused by thiazide diuretics)
Malignancy/Milk alkali syndrome
Paget's disease
Addison's disease
Neoplasm
Zollinger-Ellison syndrome
Excess vitamin D
Excess vitamin A
Sarcoid

List the pharmacological treatment options for the treatment of hypercalcemia.

1. Bisphosphonates
2. Calcitonin
3. Plicamycin
4. Glucocorticoids
5. Loop diuretics.

BISPHOSPHONATES

Give four examples of drugs in this category.

Etidronate (Didronel)
Pamidronate (Aredia)
Alendronate (Fosamax)
Risedronate (Actonel)

What is the difference between the first- and second-generation bisphosphonates?

First-generation drugs such as **etidronate** are associated with osteomalacia (bone demineralization) and therefore are currently used very rarely. The second-generation bisphosphonates such as **pamidronate** and **alendronate** are more potent and less toxic.

How do these drugs work?

They *inhibit osteoclastic activity*—more specifically, they reduce both the resorption and formation of hydroxyapatite crystals.

What is their route of administration?

Pamidronate—IV only
Etidronate—oral or IV
Alendronate and **risedronate**—oral

For what conditions are bisphosphonates used?

Malignancy-associated hypercalcemia (breast and prostate cancer)

Paget's disease of the bone
Postmenopausal osteoporosis

What are the adverse effects?	Bone pain in patients who have Paget's disease, usually around the pagetic lesion Osteomalacia (etidronate) Esophagitis Nausea and diarrhea

CALCITONIN (CALCIMAR)

What is it?	A 32–amino-acid peptide synthesized and secreted by the parafollicular C cells of the thyroid gland
What are the physiological actions of calcitonin?	It decreases osteoclastic bone resorption as well as calcium and phosphate reabsorption from the kidney. **Calcitonin** essentially opposes the actions of parathyroid hormone.
For what conditions is calcitonin used?	Paget's disease and osteoporosis
What type of calcitonin is used?	Although **human calcitonin** is available, **salmon calcitonin** is often used because it is more potent and has a longer half-life. Tolerance occurs after chronic use.
What are the adverse effects?	Allergic reaction and nausea; flushing, redness, or tingling of the face

PLICAMYCIN (MITHRACIN)

What is plicamycin?	A cytotoxic antibiotic that also lowers serum calcium concentration
How does it work?	**Plicamycin** is thought to lower serum calcium levels by blocking bone resorption.
For what conditions is it used?	Because of its high systemic toxicity, it is reserved for the short-term treatment of malignancy-associated hypercalcemia and Paget's disease of the bone.

What are the adverse effects?

Sudden thrombocytopenia followed by hemorrhage
Hepatic and renal toxicity

GLUCOCORTICOIDS

How do glucocorticoids decrease plasma calcium levels?

They reduce plasma calcium concentration by decreasing the intestinal absorption of calcium and increasing its renal excretion.

What conditions respond best to glucocorticoid (prednisone) therapy?

Hypercalcemic states secondary to sarcoidosis and lymphoma. See *Chapter 32—Corticosteroids and Inhibitors*, for a more detailed discussion of glucocorticoids.

OTHER AGENTS

What is the role of thiazide diuretics in the treatment of hypercalcemia?

Thiazides increase serum calcium levels and therefore are *never* used in the treatment of hypercalcemia. See *Chapter 23—Diuretics*, for further information.

What is the role of loop diuretics in hypercalcemia?

These agents, along with aggressive saline hydration, are often used to reduce serum calcium levels in acute hypercalcemia.

Section VII

Musculoskeletal
System

35

Anti-inflammatory Drugs and Acetaminophen

What is inflammation?

The reaction of vascularized living tissue to injury

How is inflammation mediated by the body?

Inflammation is initiated and sustained through chemical mediators such as prostaglandins, prostacyclins, bradykinin, histamine, interleukin-1, and leukotrienes.

What exactly are prostaglandins?

Prostaglandins are local mediators (they do not circulate in the blood) that have a variety of physiological actions. They are a member of a group of compounds known as eicosanoids.

What is an eicosanoid?

An eicosanoid is any biologically active compound derived from arachidonic acid, including prostaglandins, leukotrienes, prostacyclin, and thromboxane.

What is arachidonic acid?

Arachidonic acid is a 20-carbon fatty acid that serves as the precursor for prostaglandin and structurally similar compounds. Arachidonic acid is found in the phospholipids of cell membranes and is liberated by phospholipase A_2.

What are the two major enzymes that use arachidonic acid as a substrate?

Cyclooxygenase and lipoxygenase. Cyclooxygenase has two isoforms: cyclooxygenase 1 (COX-1) and cyclooxygenase 2 (COX-2) (Figure 35–1).

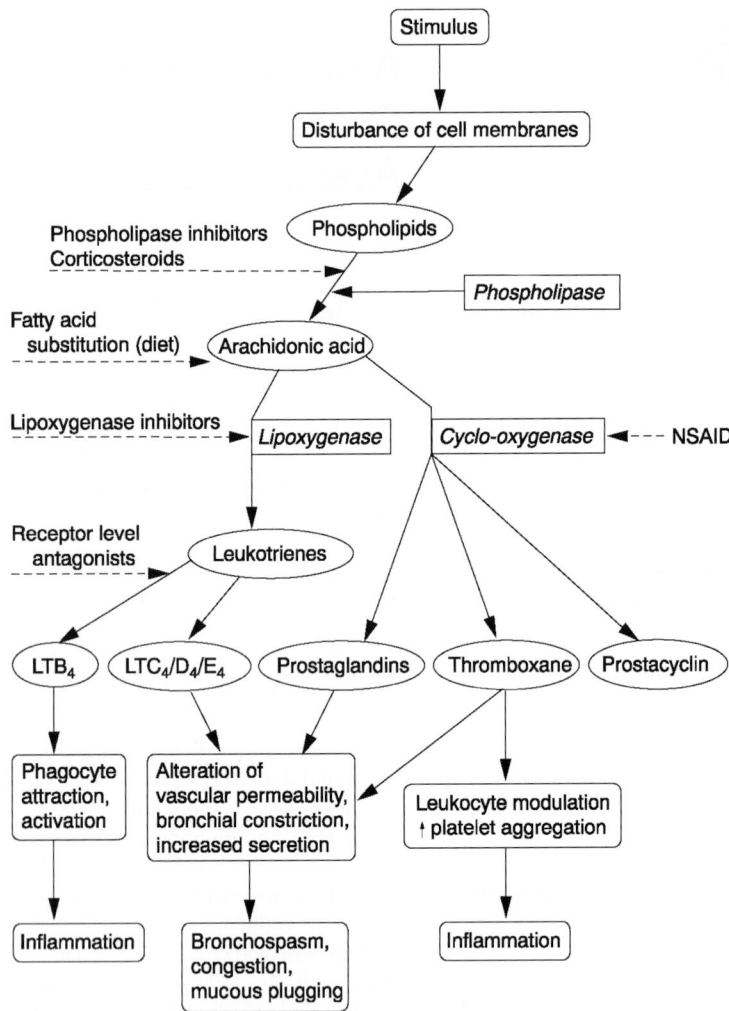

Figure 35–1. Scheme for mediators derived from arachidonic acid and sites of drug action (*dashed arrows*). (Redrawn with permission from Katzung BG. *Basic & Clinical Pharmacology,* 9th ed. New York: McGraw-Hill, 2004, p. 581.)

Give some examples of prostaglandins and leukotrienes and state their role in inflammation.	Prostaglandin E_2 (PGE_2)—erythema Prostaglandin I_2 (PGI_2)—vasodilation Leukotriene C_4—edema Leukotriene D_4—vasodilation PGE_2, PGI_2, leukotriene B_4—pain/tenderness

NONSTEROIDAL ANTI-INFLAMMATORY DRUGS (NSAIDS)

What are NSAIDs?

These drugs are a class of chemically dissimilar agents that act by reversibly inhibiting the synthesis of cyclooxygenase and, subsequently, that of prostaglandin and thromboxane.

Name several groups of NSAIDs and give examples of each, including any unique traits they may have.

NSAIDs can be divided into groups based on chemical structure:

Salicylates:
Acetylsalicylic acid (aspirin)
Diflunisal (Dolobid)—poor antipyretic properties

Pyrazolones:
Phenylbutazone—very toxic; can cause agranulocytosis and aplastic anemia. Currently not used.

Indoleacetic Acids:
Indomethacin —used in acute gouty arthritis, ankylosing spondylitis, and to close a patent ductus arteriosus (PDA) that remains open because of prostaglandin involvement.
Sulindac (Clinoril)
Etodolac (Lodine)
Diclofenac (Voltaren)
Ketorolac (Toradol)—excellent analgesic properties; commonly used as an alternative to opioids
Tolmetin (Tolectin)
Nabumetone (Relafen)

Propionic Acids:
Naproxen (Naprosyn)
Ketoprofen (Orudis)
Ibuprofen (Motrin, Advil)
Flurbiprofen (Ansaid)
Oxaprozin (Daypro)

Oxicams:
Piroxicam (Feldene)—long half-life permits once-daily dosing
Meloxicam (Mobic)

Fenamates:
Mefenamic acid
Meclofenamic acid.
This group is rarely used today because of side effects.
COX-2 Selective Inhibitors:
Celecoxib (Celebrex)
Rofecoxib (Vioxx)
Valdecoxib (Bextra)

How does COX-1 differ from COX-2?

The two isoforms of cyclooxygenase are remarkably similar yet have some important differences. Recent studies indicated that COX-2 was more involved in producing inflammatory mediators, while COX-1 was predominantly responsible for the production of cytoprotective prostaglandins formed by the gastric mucosa. Thus selective inhibition of COX-2 was postulated to produce anti-inflammatory effects without the unwanted GI side effects.

How does aspirin differ in its action from the other NSAIDs?

Aspirin is unique among NSAIDs by acetylating cyclooxygenase **irreversibly.** All the other NSAIDs inhibit cyclooxygenase in a reversible manner.

What are the four main therapeutic uses of NSAIDs?

1. **Anti-inflammatory**—frequently used for osteoarthritis, gout, rheumatoid arthritis, ankylosing spondylitis, and dysmenorrhea
2. **Analgesia**—alleviate mild to moderate pain
3. **Antipyretic effect**
4. **Antiplatelet activity**—due to the irreversible decreased production of thromboxane

Aspirin's antiplatelet activity lasts 7 to 10 days (life span of the platelet); it is often used in the treatment of myocardial ischemia, transient ischemic attacks, and stroke. COX-2 inhibitors do not have any antiplatelet actions.

How do NSAIDs decrease a patient's fever or pain?

The antipyretic and anti-inflammatory effects of NSAIDs are due to inhibition of prostaglandin synthesis at thermoregulatory centers in the hypothalamus.

How are the NSAIDs metabolized?

They are converted to water-soluble conjugates in the liver and cleared by the kidney. If the hepatic system is overwhelmed, the half-life of the drug will increase dramatically.

Describe the adverse effects of NSAIDs.

Epigastric distress, nausea, and vomiting—the most common side effects. These effects occur because most NSAIDs inhibit prostaglandins that normally stimulate production of the protective mucus of the stomach and small intestine.

Cardiovascular disorders—Because fatal stroke and myocardial infarction were reported with the COX-2 inhibitors rofecoxib and valdecoxib, they have been withdrawn from the market. Celecoxib is still available but only under strict physician supervision. Other newer COX-2 inhibitors are undergoing trials.

Coagulation disorders—Aspirin should be stopped at least 1 week before surgery.

Renal toxicity can be induced by sustained large dosages of NSAIDs.

Hypersensitivity—Approximately 15% of patients will experience urticaria or bronchoconstriction.

Reye's syndrome risk—When given to children who have a fever secondary to a viral infection, **aspirin** has been associated with an increased incidence of Reye's syndrome, which is characterized by cerebral edema and hepatitis.

The newer NSAIDs have a lower incidence of gastric disturbances but a higher incidence of renal damage.

What is salicylism?

When plasma levels of NSAIDs go beyond the maximum therapeutic range, patients develop salicylate toxicity, or salicylism. The features of salicylism can vary with plasma levels:

Mild:
Tinnitus
Vertigo
Respiratory stimulation

Severe:
Coma
Metabolic acidosis

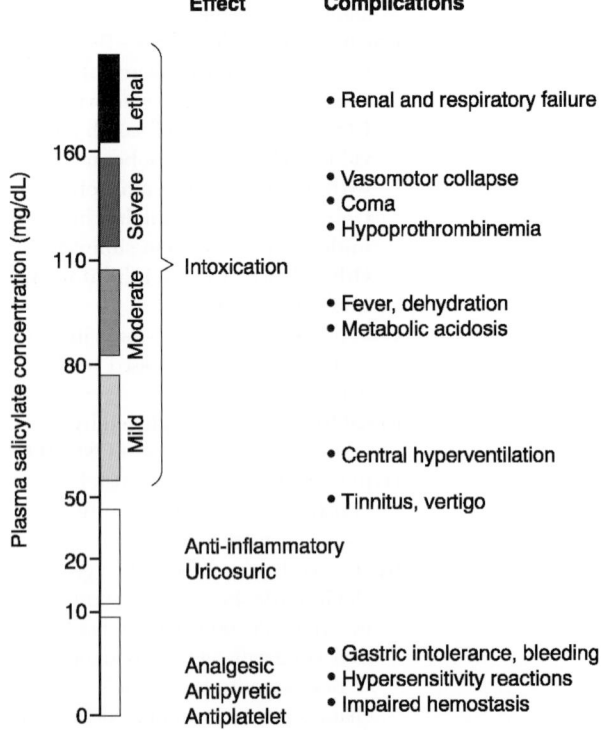

Figure 35–2. Approximate relationships of plasma salicylate levels to pharmacodynamics, also associated complications. (Modified and reproduced with permission from Hollander J, McCarty D Jr. *Arthritis and Allied Conditions.* Philadelphia: Lea & Febiger, 1972.)

Delirium
Hallucinations
Respiratory and renal depression
Figure 35–2.

What is the treatment for salicylate toxicity?

Maintaining respiration and circulation, minimizing drug absorption (via gastric lavage), and maximizing elimination (alkalinizing the urine enhances elimination)
Correct any metabolic acidosis or respiratory alkalosis that may occur.

What other agents are used to treat inflammation?

Corticosteroids, such as **prednisone**. These agents are discussed further in *Chapter 32—Corticosteroids and Inhibitors.*

ANTIRHEUMATIC DRUGS

What are the major classes of drugs used in the therapy of rheumatoid arthritis (RA)?

Disease Modifying Antirheumatic Drugs (DMARDs)
NSAIDS and COX-2 Inhibitors
Glucocorticoids
Analgesic drugs

Why are some antirheumatic drugs known as disease modifying drugs or slow acting agents?

Unlike NSAIDS, continuous therapy with some of these agents can actually delay or even prevent the progression of joint disease. They often take months to become effective. The use of one or more of these agents has become the standard of care

What are some of the key DMARDs ?

1. **Methotrexate**
2. **Leflunoamide**
3. **Etanercept**
4. **Infliximab**
5. **Anakinra**
6. **Adalimumab**
7. **Penicillamine**
8. **Gold Salts**
9. **Hydroxychloroquine**
10. **Sulfasalazine**

METHOTREXATE (RHEUMATREX)

What is it?

Methotrexate is a folate antagonist that has been used in a variety of clinical settings such as cancer, psoriasis, or graft vs. host disease

How does this drug work in rheumatoid arthritis?

It suppresses the immune system by inhibiting proliferation of lymphocytic cells. This helps slow the appearance of new erosions in joints.

When is this drug used?

After a failed trial of NSAIDs, **methotrexate** either alone or in combination with another DMARD has become the cornerstone in the treatment of RA.

What are the toxicities of this drug?

When used for RA, the doses required are much less than when it is used as an antineoplastic agent. The most common adverse effects are nausea and mucosal ulcers. Cirrhosis of the liver and decreased white blood cell count can also occur. See Chapter 39 for further information on **methotrexate**.

LEFLUNOMIDE (ARAVA)

How does this drug work?

By blocking the enzyme **dihydroorotate dehydrogenase** (DHODH) it causes a block in the creation of uridine monophosphate, a key component of the pyrimidines needed for RNA synthesis.

What are the clinical indications for leuflonamide?

Can be used alone or in combination with methotrexate for RA.

What are the adverse effects?

Headache, diarrhea, nausea, and liver toxicity. Do not use in pregnancy.

ETANERCEPT (ENBREL)

What is the mechanism of action for this drug?	Tumor necrosis factor alpha (TNF-α) is a proinflammatory cytokine involved in RA. **Etanercept** binds two molecules of TNF-α together and prevents them from activating cellular receptors.
When is this drug used?	The combination of **methotrexate** and **etanercept** has shown to reduce symptoms in RA more effectively than either one alone.
What are its toxicities?	In general, well tolerated. Injection site reactions may occur.

INFLIXIMAB (REMICADE)

What is it?	An IgG monoclonal antibody
How does it work?	Binds directly to TNF-α and inactivates it
When is this drug used clinically?	For RA, it is often used in conjunction with **methotrexate**. It is often used to treat Crohn's disease as well.
How is this drug administered?	IV
What are its potential hazards?	Infusion reactions such as fever/chills Development of anti-**infliximab** antibodies Predisposition to infections

ADALIMUMAB (HUMIRA)

How does this drug work?	Similar to **etanercept** and **infliximab**, **adalimumab** also works to decrease TNF activity. Adalimumab, however, works by directly binding TNF-α receptor sites.

When is this drug used?	Usually in combination with **methotrexate** after other drugs have failed.
What is the route of administration for this drug?	Subcutaneous injection only.
What are its toxicities?	Headache, nausea, or rash at the injection site

ANAKINRA (KINERET)

How does this drug work?	Blocks interleukin IL-1receptors.
How is this drug used?	Usually in combination with **methotrexate** after failing one or more of the other DMARDs
What are the adverse effects?	Predispose to infections. Neutropenia especially if used in combination with a TNF blocker.

PENICILLAMINE AND GOLD SALTS

When are these agents used for rheumatoid arthritis?	These drugs have fallen out of favor and are being chosen less often because they are not as effective as the newer agents and are more toxic.
How do they work?	**Penicillamine**: an analog of the amino acid cysteine interferes with the production of immunoglobulin **Gold Salts**: suppresses phagocytosis and lysosomal enzyme activity
What are the potential toxic effects?	**Penicillamine**: nephritis, aplastic anemia **Gold Salts**: dermatitis, GI disturbances, aplastic anemia

HYDROXYCHLOROQUINE

How does this drug work?	Exact mechanism of immunosuppression is unclear but it may interfere with the activity of T lymphocytes as well as inhibit DNA/RNA synthesis
Whats its role in RA?	Usually used in conjunction with an NSAID or **methotrexate**
What are its toxic effects?	Rash, retinal damage, bone marrow depression

SULFASALAZINE

What is the mechanism of action?	Exact mechanism still under investigation. It may cause immunosuppression through inhibition of IL-1, TNF-α, and other proinflammatory mediators.
How is it used in RA?	In the U.S. after a patient fails monotherapy with NSAIDs, **methotrexate** is commonly used. In Europe, **sulfasalazine** is preferred.
What are its adverse effects?	Allergic reactions including rash, fever, Stevens–Johnson syndrome, hepatitis, and bone marrow suppression
	In men, it decreases number and motility of sperm.

ACETAMINOPHEN (TYLENOL)

What is acetaminophen?

Acetaminophen is an over-the-counter antipyretic and analgesic medication that is routinely administered.

How does acetaminophen work?

This drug acts by inhibiting cyclooxygenase and thus prostaglandin synthesis in the CNS. It has much less of an effect on cyclooxygenase in peripheral tissues, which accounts for its **weak anti-inflammatory effects**.

What are the general clinical indications for acetaminophen?

Fever and mild-to-moderate pain

What are other, more specific clinical uses for this drug?

Patients who have peptic ulcer disease or hemophilia tolerate **acetaminophen** better than NSAIDs. **Acetaminophen** is also indicated for children who have viral infections, because **aspirin** increases the risk of Reye's syndrome.

How does acetaminophen affect platelets?

Acetaminophen does not affect platelet function, nor does it have any effect on blood clotting time.

Can acetaminophen be administered to gout patients who are taking probenecid?

Yes. Unlike **aspirin**, **acetaminophen** does not antagonize the uricosuric agent **probenecid**.

What is the metabolism of this drug?

Acetaminophen is metabolized in the liver by the cytochrome P-450 system.

What are the important side effects of acetaminophen?

Acetaminophen has a negligible side-effect profile except for hepatotoxicity, which is the main concern when overdoses occur.

Why does acetaminophen cause hepatotoxicity?

Toxic doses of **acetaminophen** surpass the liver's supply of glutathione, a compound that normally binds to and inactivates dangerous metabolites of **acetaminophen** such as N-acetyl-p-benzoquinone. Without glutathione, these metabolites will bind to hepatic proteins and cause necrosis.

What can be given to counteract the adverse effects of acetaminophen?

N-acetylcysteine (Mucomyst) can be administered. It has a sulfhydryl group similar to glutathione and therefore acts as a temporary substitute to bind any free toxic metabolites.

36

Drugs Used to Treat Gout

What is gout?

Gout is a familial metabolic disease associated with high blood levels of uric acid (hyperuricemia). The disease is characterized by attacks of arthritis and urinary calculi, which are caused by deposits of sodium urate crystals in joints, cartilage, and the kidneys (Figure 36–1).

What are the common clinical signs and symptoms of gout?

During the initial attacks, the usual presentation is sudden pain in a single joint, most often the metatarsophalangeal joint of a great toe.

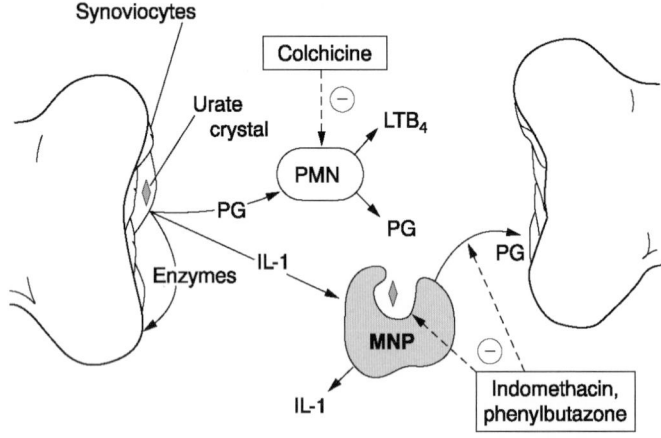

Figure 36–1. Pathophysiological events in a gouty joint. Synoviocytes phagocytose urate crystals and then secrete inflammatory mediators, which attract and activate polymorphonuclear leukocytes (PMNs) and mononuclear phagocytes (MNPs, or macrophages). Drugs active in gout inhibit crystal phagocytosis and the release of inflammatory mediators by PMNs and MNPs. PG = prostaglandin; IL-1 = interleukin-1; LTB$_4$ = leukotriene B$_4$. (Redrawn with permission from Katzung BG. *Basic and Clinical Pharmacology,* 7th ed. Stamford, CT: Appleton & Lange, 1998, p. 596.)

Whom does gout usually affect?

Men. Onset is usually in the 40s.

What is uric acid?

Uric acid is the end product of **purine metabolism** and is excreted mainly via the kidney (Figure 36–2).

What is the definition of hyperuricemia?

Hyperuricemia is usually defined as a serum concentration of uric acid greater than 7 mg/dL. It is important to note that hyperuricemia is not always associated with gout; however, gout is always preceded by hyperuricemia.

What are the causes of hyperuricemia?

Idiopathic enzyme defects in purine metabolism—90% of cases (This is known as *primary gout.*)

Disease states associated with the rapid production and destruction of cells—myeloproliferative disorders and malignancies, especially those treated with chemotherapy or radiation (This is known as *secondary gout.*)

Weakly acidic drugs such as clofibrate, thiazides, and salicylates can cause decreased renal excretion of uric acid.

Other causes include excessive alcohol intake, kidney disease, high-purine diets, starvation, and obesity.

How is gout treated?

It depends on whether the patient is suffering from an acute attack or chronic gout. In general the treatment strategy is as follows:

Reduce inflammation (via NSAIDs).

Facilitate the excretion of uric acid (via uricosuric agents).

Decrease the production of purines (via allopurinol).

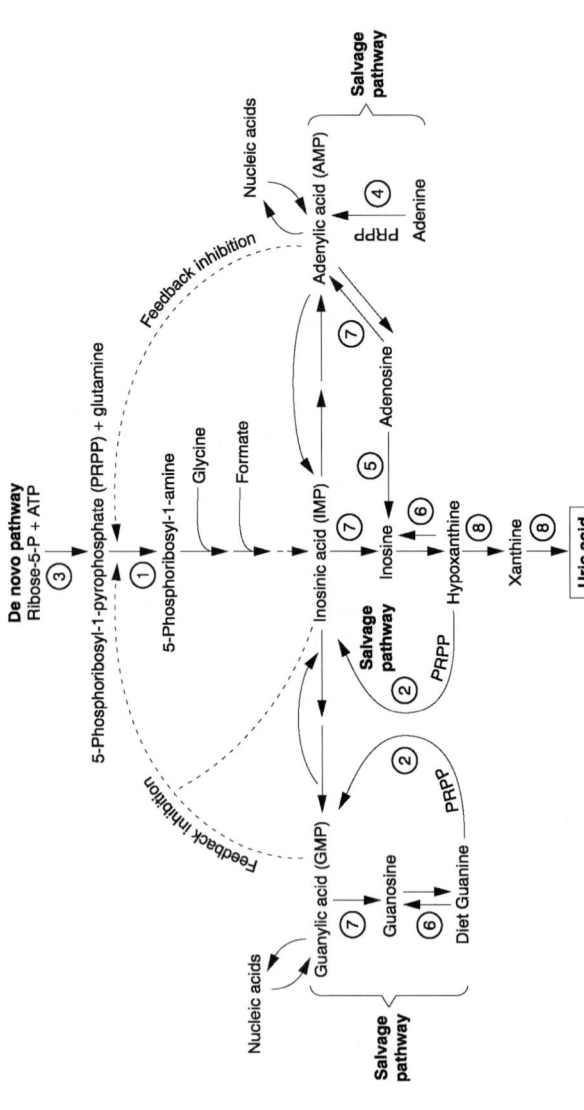

Figure 36–2. Outline of purine metabolism. ① Amidophosphoribosyltransferase. ② Hypoxanthine guanine phosphoribosyltransferase. ③ PP-ribose-P synthetase. ④Adenine phosphoribosyltransferase. ⑤Adenosine deaminase. ⑥ Purine nucleoside phosphorylase. ⑦ 5′-nucleotidase. ⑧ Xanthine oxidase. (Modified and redrawn with permission from Kelley WN, Wyngaarden JB. Clinical syndromes associated with hypoxanthine-guanine phosphoribosyl transferase deficiency. In Stanbury JB et al [eds]. *Metabolic Basis of Inherited Disease.* New York: McGraw-Hill, 1982, p. 1115.)

ACUTE GOUT

What pharmacological agents are available for treating an acute attack of gout?	**Indomethacin** **Phenylbutazone** **Colchicine**
Aspirin is an NSAID—can it be used in the treatment of gout?	No! **Aspirin**, because it is a salicylate, inhibits uric acid secretion into the renal tubules and therefore is contraindicated in the treatment of gout.

INDOMETHACIN (INDOCIN)

What is its therapeutic use?	It is the drug of choice to treat **acute attacks** of gout.
What is this drug's mechanism of action?	It reversibly inhibits cyclooxygenase. Consequently the production of prostaglandins and thromboxane, which are responsible for inflammation, is reduced.
State indomethacin's adverse effects.	Headache, vertigo Abdominal distress Renal toxicity Hypersensitivity reactions See *Chapter 35—Anti-inflammatory Drugs and Acetaminophen*, for a more detailed discussion of NSAIDs.

PHENYLBUTAZONE (AZOLID)

What is the classification of this drug?	**Phenylbutazone**, like **indomethacin**, is an NSAID.
What is the mechanism of action?	The same as that of **indomethacin**
What is phenylbutazone's therapeutic use?	**Phenylbutazone** was used more often in the past for treating acute cases of gout. However, because it has a high incidence of side effects, it is not often used today.

State the adverse effects of this drug.	Vomiting Skin rash Aplastic anemia and agranulocytosis

COLCHICINE

What is the mechanism of action?	**Colchicine** reduces the inflammatory response by binding to microtubular protein, thus inhibiting neutrophil migration and phagocytic activity. (Neutrophils are largely responsible for the inflammation and pain associated with gout.) **Colchicine** also decreases the formation of leukotriene B_4.
Does colchicine affect the production or excretion of uric acid?	No
What is this drug's route of administration?	PO or IV
State colchicine's therapeutic use.	*Colchicine is primarily used to prevent recurrent attacks of acute gout.* It can also be used in the treatment of chronic gout.
What are the adverse effects of colchicine?	Most common effects—GI distress (vomiting, diarrhea, abdominal pain) Acute poisoning after large doses can lead to nephrotoxicity, bloody diarrhea, and shock. With chronic use—possible agranulocytosis, alopecia, and aplastic anemia Myopathy has been reported (rare).
What are the relative contraindications to colchicine use?	**Colchicine** is contraindicated in patients who have GI disease, hepatitis, or renal disease.

CHRONIC GOUT

What pharmacological options are available for chronic gout?	Colchicine (*see above*) Uricosuric agents—**probenecid** and **sulfinpyrazone** **Allopurinol**

URICOSURIC AGENTS

What are they?	Weak organic acids that interfere with the renal processing of uric acid
Give two examples.	1. **Probenecid** (Benemid) 2. **Sulfinpyrazone** (Anturane)
What is the mechanism of action of these drugs?	The actions of uricosuric agents are dependent upon their serum concentrations: **At low concentrations** they reduce the renal excretion of uric acid by inhibiting uric acid secretion into the renal tubules. **At therapeutic concentrations** they increase uric acid excretion by inhibiting uric acid reabsorption in the proximal tubule. It is important to remember that low doses of uricosuric agents and salicylates such as **aspirin** actually *increase* serum uric acid concentration.
What is the route of administration for these drugs?	PO. It is completely absorbed and lasts for approximately 12 hours.
What is their therapeutic use?	The treatment of chronic gout (to avoid attacks) and severe hyperuricemia. These drugs are *not* indicated in the treatment of acute attacks of gout.
What are the adverse effects of probenecid and sulfinpyrazone?	They can precipitate an acute attack of gouty arthritis in the early stages of treatment. Gastrointestinal distress Allergic dermatitis

ALLOPURINOL (LOPURIN)

What is it?	**Allopurinol** is an isomer of hypoxanthine.
What is xanthine oxidase?	Xanthine oxidase is the enzyme that catalyzes the terminal steps of uric acid synthesis. It converts hypoxanthine to xanthine and xanthine to uric acid (see Figure 36–2).
How does allopurinol work?	**Allopurinol** and its metabolite **alloxanthine** competitively inhibit the enzyme xanthine oxidase.
What are the therapeutic uses of allopurinol?	Treatment of chronic gout Treatment of the hyperuricemia associated with Lesch-Nyhan syndrome, hematological disorders (polycythemia vera, myeloid metaplasia), or for the prevention of renal calculi by antineoplastic therapy
State the route of administration for allopurinol.	PO
Can you combine allopurinol with other antigout drugs?	Yes. Because urate-lowering drugs can initially precipitate an acute gout attack, **colchicine** is often given concurrently with **allopurinol** or the uricosuric agents.
What are this drug's adverse effects?	**Allopurinol** is usually well tolerated but can cause hypersensitivity reactions (allergic dermatitis, fever) and GI distress (diarrhea, abdominal pain). Attacks of acute gout may occur during the initial months of therapy. Therefore it is important to concomitantly use NSAIDs or **colchicine**.
Are allopurinol, probenecid, and sulfinpyrazone indicated in the treatment of acute attacks?	No. These drugs are usually begun once the acute attack is under control. Remember to use **indomethacin** and **colchicine** for acute attacks.

37

Autacoids and Autacoid Antagonists

What is an autacoid?

This word is derived from the Greek words *autos* (self) and *akos* (medicinal agent or remedy)—hence, **self agent.** Autacoids can be thought of as locally acting hormones because they are formed by the tissues on which they act.

Name two of the principal autacoids within the body.

1. Serotonin
2. Histamine

Although ergot alkaloids are not truly autacoids, they are discussed in this chapter because of their important actions on smooth muscle.

Are these the only autacoids of the body?

No. Several other compounds, such as bradykinins and prostaglandins, are included in this group, but histamine and serotonin are the most likely to be tested on the USMLE Step 1 exam ✎.

SEROTONIN AND SEROTONIN ANTAGONISTS

What is serotonin?

Serotonin (5-hydroxytryptamine, or 5-HT) is an indole ethylamine found in both plant and animal tissues.

What is serotonin derived from?

The amino acid L-tryptophan

Where is most of the serotonin in the body found?

The enterochromaffin cells of the GI tract contain approximately 90%, the CNS contains most of the remaining 10%.

How does serotonin exert its actions?

Through several major 5-HT cell membrane receptor subtypes

What enzyme is responsible for the metabolism of serotonin?	Monoamine oxidase
What are this agent's physiological actions?	Neurotransmission Vasoconstriction (except for skeletal muscle and heart, where it causes vasodilation) Contraction of GI smooth muscle Stimulation of pain receptors
Name six serotonin agonists.	**Sumatriptan** (Imitrex)—prototypical agonist at the 5-HT$_1$ receptor **Naratriptan** (Amerge) **Rizatriptan** (Maxalt) **Eletriptan** (Relpax) **Almotriptan** (Axert) **Zolmitriptan** (Zolmig)
What are these agents used for?	To treat acute migraine headaches. They are not intended for prophylaxis.
How are they administered?	Sumatriptan can be administered IV, PO, or through a nasal spray. The other agents are taken orally.
What are the adverse effects of these agents?	Coronary artery vasospasm, myocardial infarction, and arrhythmias are important to remember but fortunately are very rare. More commonly patients may experience paresthesias, fatigue, or drowsiness.
When should sumatriptan not be administered?	Avoid in patients concurrently taking an MAO inhibitor because it will potentiate the effects of the medicine. Also avoid in patients who have a history of cardiovascular disease or uncontrolled hypertension.

Name two serotonin inhibitors and describe their clinical uses.

Ondansetron (Zofran)—treatment of nausea and vomiting associated with surgery and chemotherapy

Cyproheptadine (Periactin)—treatment of allergic rhinitis and occasionally GI hypermotility in carcinoid tumor

Are these drugs selective serotonin inhibitors?

No. They block 5-HT receptors, but they also inhibit H_1 and α receptors. This accounts for the multiple clinical effects of these drugs.

What are the adverse effects of these drugs?

Ondansetron—diarrhea, and headache
Cyproheptadine—sedation, dizziness

HISTAMINE AND HISTAMINE BLOCKERS

What is the mechanism of action?

Histamine formed from the amino acid histidine exerts its effects primarily by binding to H_1 and H_2 receptors, which are located on cell surfaces and mediate a variety of physiological responses.

Where is histamine found within the body?

Within granules of mast cells and basophils. Histamine is especially concentrated in the skin, GI system, and lung.

What is its physiological role?

Histamine, when released from mast cells and basophils, constricts bronchioles (H_1 receptors)

Constricts intestinal smooth muscle (H_1 receptor)

Stimulates sensory nerve endings mediating pain and itching (H_1 receptors)

Lowers blood pressure (H_1 and H_2 receptors)

Stimulates gastric HCL secretion (H_2 receptors)

Increases permeability of skin capillaries (H_1 receptors)

What are the clinical uses of histamine?

Histamine itself is of no use clinically. However, histamine blockers are very important.

Name some first-generation H₁-receptor blockers and their clinical uses.

Diphenhydramine (Benadryl)—allergic reactions, motion sickness, insomnia
Hydroxyzine (Atarax)—allergic reactions
Promethazine (Phenergan)—motion sickness
Clemastine (Tavist)—allergic reactions
Chlorpheniramine (Aller–Chlor)—allergic reactions
There are more, but these are some of the more common.

Do H₁ blockers selectively block H₁ receptors?

No. In fact, they block muscarinic, alpha-adrenergic, and serotonin receptors.

Name four second-generation H₁ blockers.

Fexofenadine (Allegra)
Loratadine (Claritin)
Cetirizine (Zyrtec)
Desloratadine (Clarinex)

What is the main advantage of second-generation H₁ blockers over their first-generation counterparts?

These drugs are much less lipid-soluble and therefore have little CNS-sedating effect. They are also more selective for the H₁ receptor than first-generation drugs.

When are they used clinically?

They are very beneficial for treating seasonal allergic rhinitis.

What are the adverse effects of H₁ blockers?

First-generation H₁ blockers are known to cause sedation, dry mouth, and urinary retention (cholinergic blockade). They can also cause orthostatic hypotension (alpha blockade). Second-generation blockers overall are very safe, although sedation can occur at very high doses.

Name a few H₂-receptor blockers.

Cimetidine, ranitidine, famotidine, nizatidine
These drugs are discussed further in *Chapter 38—Drugs Used to Treat Gastrointestinal Disorders.*

ERGOT ALKALOIDS

What are ergot alkaloids?	A group of compounds produced by the fungus *Claviceps purpurea*
What is their mechanism of action?	The ergot alkaloids interact with adrenoreceptors, 5-HT receptors, and dopamine receptors.
What are their physiological actions?	Vasoconstriction of small vessels Stimulation of uterine muscle
Give some examples of ergot alkaloids.	**Bromocriptine** **Ergonovine** **Ergotamine**
What are these agents' clinical uses?	Acute Migraine—**ergotamine**, through actions on serotonin receptors, diminishes cerebrovascular pulsations. Hyperprolactinemia—**bromocriptine** Postpartum hemorrhage—**ergonovine** has been used after the delivery of the placenta in order to control bleeding. Contraindicated during pregnancy.
What are the adverse effects?	Prolonged vasoconstriction—may result in gangrene (**Nitroprusside** can be administered to treat ergotamine-induced vasoconstriction.) Diarrhea, nausea, vomiting Unwanted uterine contractions CNS psychosis

Section VIII

Gastrointestinal System

38

Drugs Used to Treat Gastrointestinal Disorders

DRUGS USED TO TREAT ACID-PEPTIC DISEASE

What is acid-peptic disease?

Acid-peptic disease includes peptic ulcer (gastric and duodenal), gastroesophageal reflux, and pathological hypersecretory states such as Zollinger-Ellison syndrome.

What is the pathogenesis of peptic ulcer disease?

Factors that play an important role include:
Gastric acid and pepsin secretion
Decreased mucosal resistance to acid
Helicobacter pylori infection

What are the therapeutic options for treating peptic ulcer disease?

Antacids—neutralize gastric acid
H_2-receptor blockers and proton pump inhibitors—reduce gastric acid secretion
Mucosal protective agents—enhance mucosal surface
Antimicrobial therapy—to treat *H. pylori;* current regimens include triple therapy with bismuth, metronidazole, and tetracycline

ANTACIDS

What are gastric antacids?

Gastric antacids are weak bases that react with gastric hydrochloric acid to form a salt and water. The net result is increased gastric pH.

Name the active ingredients of antacids.

Calcium carbonate (Tums)
Aluminum hydroxide
Magnesium hydroxide (Milk of Magnesia)

List the major side effects of
each.

Calcium carbonate's side effects
include **nephrolithiasis** and **fecal
compaction.**

Aluminum hydroxide reacts with
hydrochloric acid to form aluminum
chloride, which is insoluble and
causes **constipation.**

Magnesium hydroxide produces
magnesium salts, which, because they
are poorly absorbed, cause the
diarrhea commonly associated with
this compound.

H$_2$-RECEPTOR BLOCKERS

**What factors increase gastric
acid secretion?**

Three principal agonists control gastric
acid secretion: histamine, acetylcholine,
and gastrin.

**What biochemical
mechanism do these three
factors share?**

The final common pathway of these
compounds is through activation of the
H^+/K^+- ATPase proton pump (Figure
38–1).

**How effective are H$_2$-
receptor blockers in
reducing gastric acid?**

H$_2$-receptor blockers are capable of
reducing more than 90% of basal
secretions of gastric acid after a single
dose.

**Do these agents have
additional therapeutic
value?**

They have been shown to be effective in
promoting the healing of duodenal and
gastric ulcers as well as relieving
esophageal reflux disease.

**Name four H$_2$-receptor
blockers.**

1. **Cimetidine** (Tagamet) —prototype
2. **Ranitidine** (Zantac)
3. **Famotidine** (Pepcid)
4. **Nizatidine** (Axid)

**How can H$_2$ blockers be
given?**

IV or PO

**What are the side effects of
H$_2$-receptor blockers?**

In general they are well tolerated. The
longest clinical experience is with
cimetidine, but the other drugs

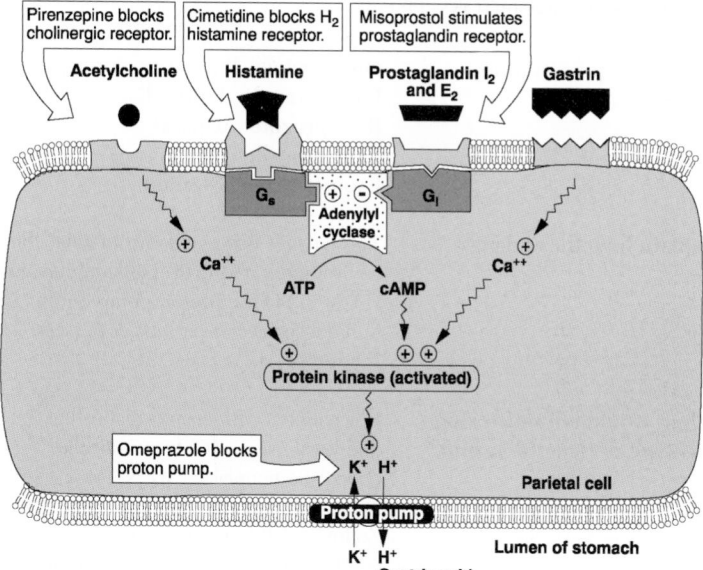

Figure 38–1. Effects of acetylcholine, histamine, prostaglandin I_2 and E_2, and gastrin on gastric acid secretion by the parietal cells of the stomach. G_s and G_i are membrane proteins that mediate the stimulatory or inhibitory effect of receptor coupling to adenylyl cyclase. (Redrawn with permission from Howland RD, Mycek MJ [Harvey RA, Champe PC, eds.]. *Lippincott's Illustrated Reviews: Pharmacology*, 3rd ed. Baltimore: Lippincott Williams & Wilkins, 2006, p. 325.)

associated with this class are similar. Most common side effects include nausea, headache, dizziness.

Cimetidine is known to create unwanted endocrinological effects such as gynecomastia and elevated serum prolactin levels (resulting in galactorrhea). Confusional states in the elderly may be seen.

Are there any important drug-drug interactions associated with H₂ blockers?

Yes. Cimetidine is a strong inhibitor of the cytochrome P-450 system and therefore can slow the metabolism of drugs normally broken down through this system. Examples include **warfarin, quinidine, benzodiazepines, procainamide**, and **phenytoin**.

PROTON PUMP INHIBITORS (PPIs)

Name five proton pump inhibitors.	**Omeprazole** (Prilosec)—prototype **Lansoprazole** (Prevacid) **Rabeprazole** (Aciphex) **Pantoprazole** (Protonix) **Esomeprazole** (Nexium)
Explain how these drugs work.	These drugs become active in an acidic environment and irreversibly inhibit the H^+/K^+- ATPase proton pump on the luminal surface of parietal cells (see Figure 38–1).
When would administering this type of drug be useful?	For patients with esophageal reflux, duodenal or gastric ulcer, multiple endocrine neoplasia (MEN), or a hypersecretory condition such as Zollinger-Ellison syndrome. Also used in combination with antibiotics to eradicate *H. pylori*
How effective are proton pump inhibitors?	They can essentially inhibit 100% of gastric acid secretion with a single daily dose.
How are they administered?	PO or IV
What are the potential side effects?	Most commonly these drugs are well tolerated, but they can cause nausea or diarrhea. In animal (*not human*) studies, long-term administration of large doses of omeprazole has caused development of gastric carcinoid tumors.

MUCOSAL PROTECTIVE AGENTS

Name the drugs belonging to this class.	**Sucralfate** (Carafate) **Bismuth** **Misoprostol** (Cytotec)

Sucralfate (Carafate)

What is sucralfate?	Sucralfate is a sulfated disaccharide developed for use in treating peptic ulcer disease.

What is its major mechanism of action?	Polymerization and selective binding to necrotic ulcer tissue, where it acts as a barrier to acid, pepsin, and bile.
What other actions are possible?	**Sucralfate** may also directly adsorb bile salts and may stimulate endogenous prostaglandin synthesis.
Can sucralfate be taken with H_2-receptor blockers or proton pump inhibitors?	No. **Sucralfate** requires an acid pH to be activated and should not be administered simultaneously with either H_2-receptor blockers or proton pump inhibitors.

Bismuth

How does bismuth work?	Like sucralfate, bismuth compounds appear to work by selectively binding to an ulcer, coating it and protecting it from acid and pepsin.
What other therapeutic actions are possible?	Bismuth compounds may have some antimicrobial activity against *H. pylori*. When bismuth compounds are combined with antimicrobials (**metronidazole** and **tetracycline**), ulcer healing rates of up to 98% have been reported.

Misoprostol

How does this drug work?	**Misoprostol** is a prostaglandin E_1 analogue that decreases gastric acid secretion and stimulates production of mucin and bicarbonate.
What are the clinical indications for administering misoprostol?	Currently it is seldom used because of its adverse effects and minimal benefits. In the past it was used for peptic and duodenal ulcers induced by long-term NSAID therapy.
What are its major side effects?	Diarrhea in up to 30% of patients who take the drug, unwanted uterine contractions (contraindicated in pregnancy), and exacerbations of inflammatory bowel disease.

PROKINETIC AGENTS

What conditions can be treated with prokinetic agents?	Gastroesophageal reflux and gastroparesis

Name two drugs in this class.	1. **Cisapride** (Propulsid) 2. **Metoclopramide** (Reglan)

Cisapride

How does cisapride work?	It stimulates the release of acetylcholine at the myenteric plexus, which results in increased esophageal sphincter tone and therefore decreased reflux.

What are its toxicities?	Prolonged QT interval and cardiac arrhythmias—generally no longer available in the United States because of these severe adverse effects. Can only be used by patients who have failed all other treatments and have undergone an ECG.

Metoclopramide

Which receptors does metoclopramide stimulate?	5-HT_3 and D_2 receptors in gastric smooth muscle, which results in acceleration of GI emptying. It is a first-line agent. Works primarily on the small intestine.

Other than gastroparesis, what else is metoclopramide used for?	The drug is beneficial in reducing the nausea and vomiting associated with chemotherapeutic agents.

What types of adverse effects can be seen with this drug?	Extrapyramidal side effects are the most important (parkinsonism and tardive dyskinesia) Diarrhea Drowsiness

ANTIEMETIC DRUGS

State the major categories of antiemetics and give an example of each.	H_1 antihistamines—**diphenhydramine** Phenothiazines—**prochlorperazine** (Compazine)

Marijuana—**dronabinol** (Marinol)
$5-HT_3$ inhibitors—**ondansetron** (Zofran)
Corticosteroids—**dexamethasone**
Benzamides—**metoclopramide**

What are the clinical indications for these drugs?	Any condition that is inducing moderate to severe emesis, such as chemotherapy or GI infection.
	Each of the antiemetic drugs is discussed in greater detail in other chapters (see index).
Can these drugs be used in combination?	Yes. Corticosteroids, for example, can be combined with **ondansetron** to provide an even greater anti-emetic effect.

INFLAMMATORY BOWEL DISEASE (IBD) THERAPIES

Into what two major subtypes is IBD usually divided?	Ulcerative colitis Crohn's disease
What are the pharmacological options for treating these diseases?	**Sulfasalazine**, antibiotics (**metronidazole**, **ciprofloxacin**), glucocorticoids, immunosuppressive agents such as azathioprine, **methotrexate**, and **cyclosporine**, and immunomodulators such as **infliximab**. Glucocorticoids, antibiotics, and immunosuppressive agents are discussed in greater detail elsewhere in the text but are mentioned here for completeness.

Sulfasalazine (Azulfidine)

How does it work?	**Sulfasalazine** suppresses proinflammatory mediators such as IL-1 and TNF-α. Its exact mechanism of action is still under investigation.
What conditions is it used to treat?	It works much better against the symptoms of ulcerative colitis than Crohn's disease, since Crohn's often involves the small bowel, where the drug is not active.

What are its side effects?	Vomiting diarrhea, nausea
When should sulfasalazine not be prescribed?	Because **sulfasalazine** also has a sulfonamide component, it should be avoided in patients with sulfa allergies.

Infliximab

What is it?	It is a monoclonal antibody targeted to tumor necrosis factor alpha (TNF-α), one of the principal mediators of inflammation in Crohn's disease
When is it used?	To treat IBD, particularly moderate to severe Crohn's disease. It is particularly good for closing fistulas associated with Crohn's disease and acute flares of this condition. Also used for rheumatoid arthritis.
What are its toxicities?	Respiratory infection and hypotension. Since **infliximab** is given IV, acute reactions such as fever, chills, and urticaria may occur after infusion. Also, antibodies to **infliximab** may develop.

ANTIDIARRHEAL AGENTS

Name two agents widely used for this purpose.	**Loperamide** (Imodium) **Diphenoxylate** (Lomotil)
How do they work?	**Loperamide** and **diphenoxylate** are derivatives of **meperidine**, an opiate, which slows gastrointestinal motility through actions of peripheral μ-opioid receptors. These drugs have very few if any CNS effects. (See Chapter 19 for further details on opiates.)

LAXATIVES

How are laxatives classified?	These drugs are generally classified by simplified mechanism of action, that is, as stimulants, osmotic agents, bulking agents, and stool softeners.

STIMULANTS

Give some examples of stimulant laxatives.	**Castor oil** **Senna** (Senokot) **Phenolphthalein** (Ex-Lax) **Bisacodyl** (Dulcolax)
What are the side effects of stimulant laxatives?	Chronic stimulation of the colon can lead to chronic colonic distention and thus perpetuation of the perceived need for laxatives.

BULKING AGENTS

Name some members of this group.	These agents, which are usually insoluble during the digestive process, include: Hydrophilic colloids (from indigestible parts of fruits and vegetables) Agar Methylcellulose Bran
How do these agents work?	They are nonabsorbable agents that increase water retention and stool bulk. This distends the bowel and stimulates peristalsis.

OSMOTIC AGENTS

Name two agents in this group.	Saline cathartics (**magnesium citrate** and **magnesium hydroxide**) Nondigestible sugars such as **lactulose** and **sorbitol**
How do they work?	They osmotically draw water into the lumen of the digestive tract, which then stimulates motility.

STOOL SOFTENERS

How do these agents work?	By emulsifying stool, these agents soften it and make its passage easier.
Name some stool softeners.	Examples include **mineral oil** and **docusate sodium** (Colace).

Section IX

Immune System

39   Antineoplastic Drugs

What is the definition of a neoplasm?

The word "neoplasm" simply refers to a collection of abnormally proliferating cells. *Benign neoplasms* do not invade surrounding tissue. *Malignant neoplasms* can invade and metastasize to all parts of the body and are usually fatal.

Name the five stages of the cell cycle.

1. G_1—synthesis of components needed for DNA synthesis
2. S—DNA synthesis
3. G_2—growth and replication of cytoplasmic constituents
4. M—mitosis
5. G_0.—resting phase

What is the significance of a cell cycle–specific (CCS) antineoplastic agent?

"Cell cycle–specific" means that the drug will primarily affect the cells that are actively replicating or cycling through G_1 to M (see Figure 39–1). Cell cycle–specific drugs include:
Antimetabolites
Mitotic inhibitors
Bleomycin
Etoposide
Steroid hormones

What are cell cycle–nonspecific (CCNS) drugs?

CCNS drugs kill cells whether they are cycling or resting (G_0). They are more toxic but are more effective for slow-growing tumors. Cell cycle–nonspecific agents include alkylating agents, **cisplatin**, nitrosoureas, and antibiotics.

What are the options for treating cancer in addition to chemotherapy?

Surgery, immunotherapy, and radiotherapy are often used initially to reduce the neoplastic cell burden (debulking); this is often followed by chemotherapy

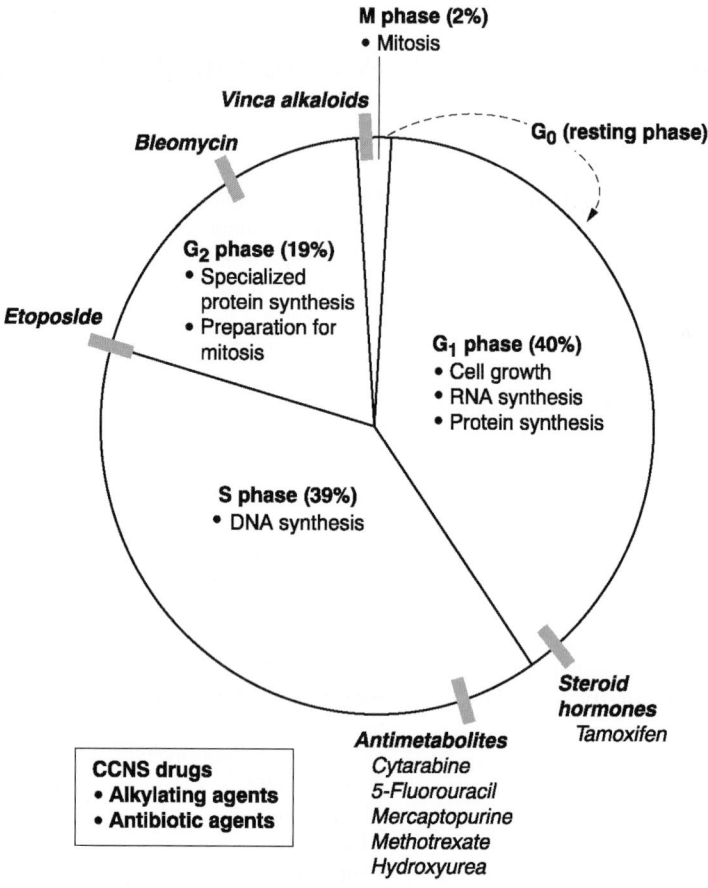

Figure 39–1. Cell cycle–specific antineoplastic drugs. The percentages indicate the approximate percentage of time spent in each phase by a typical malignant cell. The duration of the G_1 phase, however, can vary markedly.

State six classes of antineoplastic agents and give examples of each.

1. **Alkylating agents—mechlorethamine, cyclophosphamide, melphalan, lomustine, streptozocin, cisplatin, busulfan, dacarbazine, procarbazine**

2. **Antibiotics—dactinomycin, doxorubicin, daunorubicin, bleomycin**

3. **Antimetabolites—methotrexate, 6-mercaptopurine, cytarabine, 5-fluorouracil, hydroxyurea**

4. **Hormones and related agents— flutamide, tamoxifen, leuprolide,** glucocorticoids
5. **Mitotic inhibitors—vinblastine, vincristine, etoposide,** paclitaxel (Figure 39–2)
6. **Monoclonal antibodies— rituximab, trastuzumab, gemtuzumab**

How does resistance to chemotherapeutic drugs develop?	Neoplastic cells can defend themselves in several ways including: Increased DNA repair Changes in target enzymes Drug inactivation Decreased drug accumulation Alternative metabolic pathways
Can antineoplastic drugs be used in combination?	Yes. Many cancer treatment protocols involve more than one drug simultaneously.

ALKYLATING AGENTS

What are alkylating agents?	A group of cell cycle–nonspecific compounds that transfer an alkyl group, usually to the N^7 nitrogen atom of guanine residues in one or both strands of DNA. This prevents further replication of tumor cells. All alkylating agents are carcinogenic and thus can lead to secondary cancer.
What are two major classes of alkylating agents?	Nitrogen mustards (Mechlorethamine, Cyclophosphamide, Infosfamide, Melphalan, Chlorambucil) and nitrosoureas (carmustine, lomustine, streptozocin)

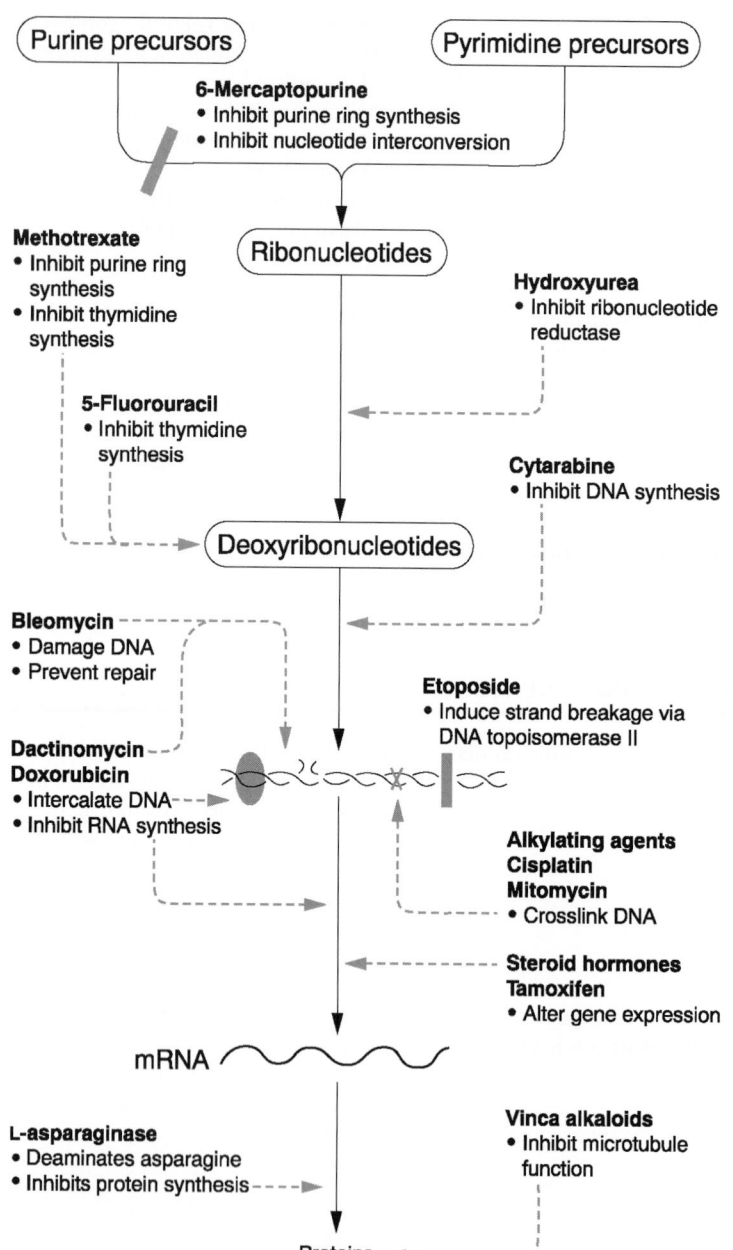

Figure 39–2. Cancer chemotherapeutics and their sites of action. (Adapted and redrawn with permission from Stanbury J et al. *Metabolic Basis of Inherited Disease,* 4th ed. New York: McGraw-Hill, 1989, Fig. 27-45.)

NITROGEN MUSTARDS

Mechlorethamine (Mustargen)

What is its mechanism of action?	**Mechlorethamine** binds with the N^7 nitrogen of guanine in DNA. This, in turn, results in cross-linking between guanine residues, strand breaks, and miscoding mutations.
How is this drug used clinically?	Formerly used as a component of MOPP (**mechlorethamine**, Oncovin [**vincristine**], **procarbazine**, and **prednisone**) therapy in Hodgkin's disease. It has been largely replaced by cyclophosphamide melphan, and more stable agents.
How does resistance to this drug occur?	Decreased permeability of the drug or increased DNA repair.
What is its route of administration?	IV only
Are there adverse effects?	Yes—severe bone marrow suppression, severe nausea and vomiting, and lacrimation. Extravasation can cause serious harm and requires rapid infiltration with sodium thiosulfate, which deactivates the drug.

Cyclophosphamide (Cytoxan)/Ifosfamide (Ifen)

What is their mechanism of action?	**Cyclophosphamide** and **ifosfamide** are activated in the cytochrome P-450 system. The metabolite of these drugs, called phosphoramide mustard, cross-links DNA and RNA strands.
How is cyclophosphamide used clinically?	For treating ovarian and breast carcinoma, Hodgkin's and non-Hodgkin's lymphoma, and all of the leukemias. It is also used as an immunosuppressive agent in transplantation.
When is ifosfamide used clinically?	To treat testicular carcinoma and sarcoma.

What is the preferred route of administration?	PO for both drugs, but they can be given IV.
Both drugs have similar toxic effects. What are they?	Hemorrhagic cystitis: can be minimized with the injection of MESNA (sodium -2- mercaptoethane sulfonate) GI effects (nausea and vomiting) Bone marrow suppression Neurotoxicity with **ifosfamide** Severe alopecia Gonadal suppression

Melphalan (Alkeran)

Explain melphalan's mechanism of action.	This drug is a phenylalanine derivative of nitrogen mustard that cross-links strands of DNA and RNA.
How is melphalan used clinically?	For treating multiple myeloma in combination with other agents
What are the adverse effects?	Bone marrow suppression, leukopenia, and thrombocytopenia. Can also cause pulmonary infiltrates and fibrosis.

Chlorambucil (Leukeran)

What is it?	A nitrogen mustard that has a mechanism of action and toxicity profile very similar to **melphalan**.
What is it used for?	It is a standard agent for patients with CLL. May also be used for folicular lymphoma.
What are its toxicities?	Moderate bone marrow suppression GI distress

NITROSOUREAS

Lomustine (CeeNu) and Carmustine (BiCNU)

How do these drugs work?	**Lomustine** and **carmustine** alkylate DNA, which results in strand breakage and inhibition of protein synthesis.
Describe the solubility of these agents.	Lomustine and **carmustine** are very lipophilic molecules, which partially accounts for their CNS activity.

What are the clinical uses?	Treatment of brain tumors
State the adverse effects.	Both drugs cause delayed bone marrow depression (usually 4 to weeks after onset of use), GI effects (nausea and vomiting), and flushing of the skin and conjunctiva. High doses can cause pulmonary fibrosis and renal failure.

Streptozocin (Zanosar)

State the mechanism of action.	**Streptozocin** is an alkylating agent that inhibits DNA synthesis by cross-linking strands of DNA.
What is the clinical use?	Treatment of pancreatic islet cell carcinoma and malignant carcinoid tumors. It is given IV.
Describe the adverse effects.	GI effects (nausea and vomiting) and renal failure

OTHER ALKYLATING AGENTS

Cisplatin (Platinol)

How does it work?	**Cisplatin** is a member of the platinum coordination complex along with **carboplatin** and **oxaliplatin**. They all attach to mucleophilic sites on DNA and form both intrastrand and interstrand crosslinks. This leads to inhibition of DNA replication and transcription.
When do you use cisplatin?	For treating testicular, bladder, lung, and ovarian carcinomas. It is used in combination with other agents.
How are cisplatin, carboplatin, and oxaliplatin administered?	Usually IV, but they can be given intraperitoneally for ovarian cancer.
What are the adverse effects?	Nephrotoxicity—the number one toxicity, which can be limited with aggressive hydration and mannitol Ototoxicity Paresthesias Severe vomiting

Carboplatin (Paraplatin)

What is its clinical use?	Treatment of ovarian carcinomas
Are there adverse effects?	Yes—bone marrow suppression and anemia but not kidney, CNS, or ototoxicity like cisplatin

Oxaliplatin (Eloxatin)

What is its clinical indication?	Colorectal cancer
What are its adverse effects?	Anaphylactic reactions, leukopenia, nausea, and vomiting

Busulfan (Myleran)

State the mechanism of action.	This drug cross-links strands of DNA.
How is it used clinically?	**Busulfan** is effective for treating chronic myelocytic leukemia (CML).
What are the adverse effects?	Pulmonary fibrosis, hyperpigmentation Bone marrow suppression

Dacarbazine (DTIC)

Describe the mechanism of action.	This drug becomes activated in the liver and subsequently inhibits DNA and RNA synthesis via formation of toxic methyl carbonium ions.
What is the clinical use?	Treatment of Hodgkin's lymphoma (part of the ABVD regimen) and melanoma ABVD = Adriamycin, bleomycin, vinblastine, dacarbazine
How is it administered?	IV
State the adverse effects.	GI effects (nausea and vomiting), hepatotoxicity, and bone marrow suppression

Temozolomide (Temodar)

What is it?	An analogue of **dacarbazine**.
When should it be used?	**Temozolomide** is specifically indicated for glioblastoma multiforme.

What is its mechanism of action?	Same as that of **dacarbazine**.
How is it administered?	Orally
What are its adverse effects?	Nausea and vomiting

Procarbazine (Matulane)

How does this drug work?	**Procarbazine** forms hydrogen peroxide, which in turn creates free radicals that cause DNA strand lysis. It also inhibits RNA synthesis.
What is the clinical use?	Treatment of Hodgkin's disease (part of the MOPP regimen) MOPP = mechlorethamine, vincristine (**Oncovin**), procarbazine, prednisone
Does it have any significant drug reactions?	Yes. Since procarbazine mildly inhibits MAD, patients should avoid eating foods high in tyramine. Also it can cause a disulfiram-type reaction with alcohol.
List the adverse effects.	Myelosuppression and GI irritation. Also, **procarbazine** like most alkylating agents, is leukemogenic and teratogenic. Behaviorial disturbances such as hallucinations have been reported.

ANTIBIOTICS

| **Where do these antineoplastic antibiotics originate?** | From various strains of the soil fungus *Streptomyces* |

DACTINOMYCIN (COSMEGEN)

| **How does it work?** | **Dactinomycin** binds to the double helix of DNA and forms a dactinomycin-DNA complex, which in turn inhibits the actions of DNA-dependent RNA polymerase. The drug may also cause DNA single-strand breaks. |
| **When do you use dactinomycin?** | In combination with **vincristine** to treat Wilms' tumor and rhabdomyosarcoma in children. It is also used with **methotrexate** for choriocarcinoma. Ewing's tumor and Kaposi's sarcoma also show response to the drug. |

What is the route of administration?	IV. Extravasation can cause serious damage.
How does resistance to this drug occur?	Through increased efflux of the medication from the cell
List the adverse effects.	Bone marrow depression and GI distress are usually the dose-limiting toxicities. Skin abnormalities associated with prior radiation therapy may occur.

DOXORUBICIN (ADRIAMYCIN) AND DAUNORUBICIN (CERUBIDINE)

How do these two drugs work?	They are anthracycline antibiotics whose antitumor activity may result from several mechanisms: They bind to adjacent base pairs along the sugar-phosphate backbone of DNA, thus blocking DNA and RNA synthesis. They disrupt cell membranes. They generate oxygen radicals, which cause single-strand breaks in DNA.
What are the clinical indications?	**Doxorubicin** is used to treat acute leukemias, multiple myeloma, and cancers of the breast, endometrium, ovary, thyroid, and lung. **Daunorubicin** is used for treating acute leukemias (acute myelogenous leukemia [AML] and acute lymphocytic leukemia [ALL]).
How are these two drugs administered?	Both must be administered intravenously because they are inactivated in the stomach. Extravasation can lead to extensive tissue damage.
Describe the pharmacokinetics of these drugs.	They are distributed to almost all of the tissues except the CNS. Both drugs are extensively metabolized in the liver and excreted primarily through the bile.
How does resistance to these drugs occur?	Increased efflux out of the cell DNA repair

Are there adverse effects?

Yes. Irreversible cardiotoxicity is the most important (✎ common board question); this effect may be a result of the oxygen-free radical production. These drugs can also cause bone marrow depression, alopecia, GI distress, and stomatitis. Patients may also complain of a reddish color to their urine.

What are idarubicin, epirubicin, and valrubicin?

They are newer structural analogs of the naturally occurring anthracycaline antibiotics daunorubicin and doxorubicin

What are they used for?

Idarubicin is predominantly used for acute leukemia while **eprubicin** is used for solid tumors such as breast cancer. **Valrubicin** is used for urinary bladder carcinoma.

What are the advantages of using these drugs?

Less cardiotoxicity then seen with the older antibiotics.

BLEOMYCIN (BLENOXANE)

How does it work?

Bleomycin combines with Fe^{2+} to form a complex that reacts with oxygen to produce free radicals, which cause strand scission and DNA fragmentation.

What are the clinical uses?

Bleomycin is a component of the regimen for testicular carcinoma. It is usually used in combination with **vinblastine, etoposide** or **cisplatin.** In Hodgkin's disease, it is part of the ABVD regimen.

How is bleomycin administered?

It can be given by intramuscular, intravenous, subcutaneous, or intracavitary routes.

Describe the adverse effects.

Pulmonary toxicity (✎ **board question**)
Fever and chills
Mucocutaneous toxicity including ulcers, hyperpigmentation, erythema
Hypersensitivity reactions (anaphylaxis)
Unique in that it causes very little myelosuppression

MITOMYCIN (MUTAMYCIN)

Describe the mechanism of action.

Mitomycin is metabolically reduced to an alkylating agent, which inhibits DNA synthesis.

When is mitomycin used clinically?

Carcinoma of the cervix, lung, bladder, and colon

What are the adverse effects?

GI effects (nausea, vomiting, loss of appetite) and severe bone marrow suppression

ANTIMETABOLITES

How can antimetabolites be further subdivided?

Into folate analogs (**methotrexate**), purine analogs (**6-mercaptopurine, 6-thioguanine, fludarabine, cladrabine**), and pyrimidine analogs (**cytarabine, 5-FU, capecitabine, gemcitabine**)

METHOTREXATE (FOLEX)

How does it work?

Methotrexate is a folic acid antagonist that prevents the conversion of dihydrofolate to tetrahydrofolate by inhibiting the action of **dihydrofolate reductase.** This results in decreased synthesis of thymidylate, amino acids, and purine nucleotides, which make up DNA and RNA.

Describe methotrexate's clinical uses.

Methotrexate is used in treating the following conditions:
Choriocarcinoma, head and neck cancers
Lung cancer
 ALL
Non-Hodgkin's lymphoma
Breast cancer
Methotrexate has a number of other clinical uses, including the treatment of psoriasis and rheumatoid arthritis.

How does resistance to methotrexate occur?

Decreased absorption of the drug
Increased levels or mutated form of dihydrofolate reductase

How can methotrexate be given and where is it metabolized?

Through several different routes: IM, IV, orally, or intrathecally. MTX is metabolized in the liver.

What are the adverse effects of methotrexate?

Bone marrow suppression, stomatitis, erythema, rash
GI hemorrhagic enteritis
Neurotoxicity (seizures, encephalopathy)
Hepatotoxicity
Nephrotoxicity with high dosages.
Alkalinization of the urine and hydration help to limit this toxicity.

What is the "leucovorin rescue"?

Toxic effects upon normal cells can be minimized with the administration of **leucovorin** (folinic acid), which is preferentially absorbed by normal cells but not by neoplastic cells. **Leucovorin** essentially bypasses the enzyme blocked by **methotrexate** (Figure 39–3).

6-MERCAPTOPURINE (PURINETHOL)

Describe how this drug works.

6-Mercaptopurine (6-MP) is a purine analogue that enters target cells and then is converted to 6-thioinosinic acid by hypoxanthine guanine phosphoribosyl transferase (HGPRT). This active compound then inhibits a number of enzymes in purine interconversion. Dysfunctional DNA and RNA is formed and thus cell replication is terminated.

State the clinical uses.

Treatment of ALL and AML

What is the mode of administration?

PO

How does resistance to 6-mercaptopurine occur?

Decreased levels of HGPRT leads to an inability to convert the drug into its active form.
Increased metabolism of the drug to thiouric acid.

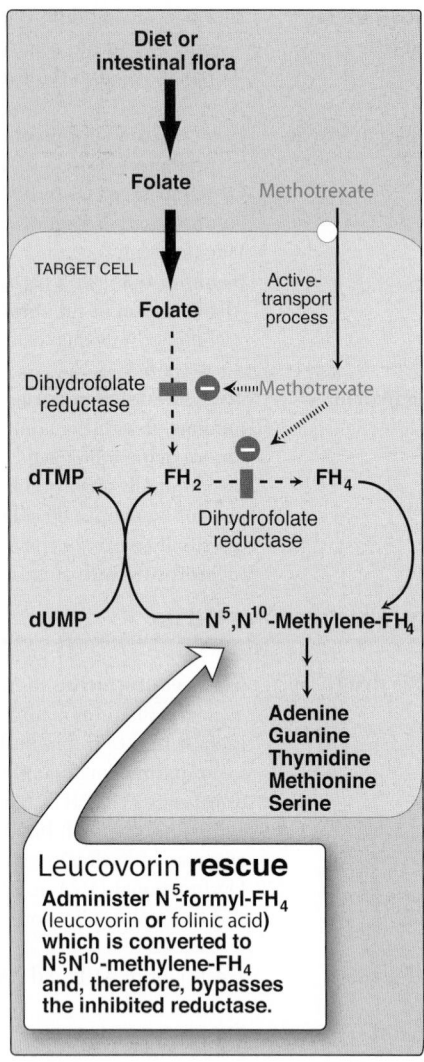

Figure 39–3. Mechanism of action of methotrexate and the effect of administration of leucovorin. FH_2 = dihydrofolate; FH_4 = tetrahydrofolate; dTMP = deoxythymidine monophosphate; dUMP = deoxyuridine monophosphate. (With permission from Howland RD, Mycek MJ [Harvey RA, Champe PC, eds.]. *Lippincott's Illustrated Reviews: Pharmacology,* 3rd ed. Baltimore: Lippincott Williams & Wilkins, 2006, p. 458.)

Are there any important drug interactions to keep in mind?	Yes. Patients who are also taking **allopurinol** must be given a reduced dosage of **mercaptopurine** because **allopurinol** inhibits xanthine oxidase, the same enzyme responsible for the metabolism of **mercaptopurine**. Toxic levels are achieved quickly if the dosage is not decreased.
Describe the adverse effects.	Bone marrow suppression and hepatotoxicity

6-THIOGUANINE

How does it work?	Similar to 6-MP. It must first be converted to a nucleotide form which then inhibits the creation of the purine ring.
When is this drug used?	Acute nonlymphocytic leukemia in combination with daunorubicin and cytarabine
What are its toxicities?	Very similar to 6-MP

CLADRIBINE (LEUSTATIN)

How does it work?	After being converted to cladribine triphosphate, it incorporates into the 3'-terminus of DNA and prevents chain elongation. It also is a potent inhibitor of ribonuceotide reductase.
What is it used for?	Hairy cell leukemia-first line agent, CLL, and non-Hodgkin's lymphoma. It has largely replaced the drug pentostatin.
What are its adverse effects?	Bone marrow suppression, peripheral neuropathy, and fever

FLUDARABINE (FLUDARA)

What is its mechanism of action?	Fludarabine, like cladribine, is a prodrug that must be activated to a nucleotide to become cytotoxic. It effectively terminates chain elongation when incorporated into DNA. This drug also inhibits DNA polymerase, primase, and ligase as well as RNA functioning.

How is administered?	IV. Toxic when given orally.
When is it used clinically?	CLL and low grade lymphoma
What are its adverse effects?	Bone marrow suppression GI distress (nausea, vomiting, diarrhea) Neurologic toxicity can also occur.

CYTARABINE (CYTOSAR-U)

How does this drug function?	**Cytarabine** is a pyrimidine analogue that enters cells and is then activated by phosphorylation. The triphosphate form (ARA-CTP) then prevents DNA synthesis by blocking chain elongation.
What is its clinical use?	**Cytarabine** is very much limited to the treatment of AML.
What is the route of administration?	IV
Describe the adverse effects.	Severe bone marrow suppression Stomatitis Gastrointestinal distress

5-FLUOROURACIL (ADRUCIL)

How does this drug work?	Like **cytarabine**, 5-fluorouracil acts as a pyrimidine analog. It enters cells and is converted to 5FdUMP, which then inhibits the enzyme **thymidylate synthetase**. The result is inhibition of DNA synthesis through lack of thymine nucleotides. 5FdUMP also inhibits RNA synthesis. Leucovorin is administered with 5-FU because it increases the binding of 5-FU to thymidylate synthetase thereby potentiating the antitumor effect of 5-FU.
State the clinical use.	Treatment of breast carcinoma and GI (gastric, pancreatic, and colorectal) carcinomas Topically for solar keratosis and basal cell carcinoma.

How is this drug administered?	Because of its severe toxicity to the GI tract, 5-fluorouracil is given intravenously.
Describe the adverse effects.	Myelosuppression, stomatitis, and oral and GI mucosa ulcers. Sometimes after prolonged infusions, an erythematous desquamation of the palms and soles can occur. This is known as "hand-foot syndrome."

GEMCITABINE (GEMZAR)

What is it?	An analog of the nucleoside deoxycytidine
How does it work?	It is first activated through triphosphorylation and then becomes incorporated into DNA in places which would normally contain cytosine. This prevents further replication. Also inhibits ribonucleotide reductase.
What is it used for?	Primarily for metastatic adenocarcinoma of the pancreas. Also used for non-small cell lung cancer, ovarian, bladder, esophageal, and head and neck cancer.
How is it administered?	IV
What toxicities should be monitored?	Myelosuppression Elevated LFTs Hemolytic uremic syndrome—rare

CAPECITABINE (XELODA)

How does it work?	Similar to 5-FU. It actually is converted to 5-FU within cells.
What is its advantage over 5-FU?	It is well absorbed orally.
What is it used for?	Metastatic breast and colorectal cancer.
What are its adverse effects?	Similar to 5-FU. GI distress. Watch for toxicity in patients with hepatic or renal impairment.

HORMONES AND RELATED AGENTS

FLUTAMIDE (EULEXIN), NILUTAMIDE (NILANDRON), AND BICALUTAMIDE (CASODEX) (SEE ALSO CHAPTER 31)

How do these drugs work?

They are nonsteroidal antiandrogens that inhibit ligand binding and subsequent translocation of the androgen receptor to the nucleus.

What are the clinical uses?

These drugs are used in combination with a GnRH such as **leuprolide** for the treatment of advanced prostate cancer.

State the adverse effects.

Flushing, mastodynia, and variable degrees of decreased libido.
Hot flashes and back pain can also occur
Visual problems: **nilutamide**
Gynecomastia
Reversible hepatotoxicity

TAMOXIFEN (NOLVADEX)

What is it?

A nonsteroidal antiestrogen that competitively inhibits estradiol at estrogen receptors

How is tamoxifen used clinically?

It is a first-line agent for women with estrogen receptor–positive breast cancer and is most effective in postmenopausal women.

State the route of administration.

PO

What are the adverse effects?

Hot flashes, GI effects (nausea and vomiting), and menstrual bleeding. Long-term effects include thromboembolic disease and possibly increased risk of endometrial cancer.

What is toremifene (Fareston)?

An agent very similar to **tamoxifen**. Also used in breast cancer treatment, with a similar toxicity profile.

What is raloxifene (Evista)?

Like **tamoxifen** and **toremifene**, **raloxifene** is a drug that acts as a partial agonist at estrogen receptors. It is used primarily for the prevention and treatment of osteoporosis.

| **How does raloxifene differ from tamoxifen?** | **Raloxifene** does not appear to stimulate endometrial growth and is not associated with increased risk of endometrial cancer. |

AROMATASE INHIBITORS

| **What are aromatase inhibitors (AI) ?** | They are drugs that inhibit the enzyme aromatase, which is responsible for the conversion of androstenedione and testosterone to estrogen. |

| **Give some examples of aromatase inhibitors** | **Aminoglutethimide**—1st generation
Formestane—2nd generation
Anastroloze and **letrozole**—3rd generation
Exemestane—3rd generation |

Aminoglutethimide

| **When is this drug used?** | It was the first AI developed. Rarely used now because of toxicities.
Mentioned for historical purposes only.
Similarly, **formestane** is rarely used today |

Anastrozole (Arimidex)/Letrozole (Femara)

| **What are they used for?** | Both of these drugs are nonsteroidal agents that are used for postmenopausal women with early-stage or advanced hormone-receptor positive breast cancer. |

| **What are their adverse effects?** | Asthenia, nausea, diarrhea. **Letrozole** can cause bone pain, hot flashes, GI upset |

Exemestane (Aromasin)

| **What is it?** | It is a **steroidal irreversible** inhibitor of aromatase. |

| **What are its indications?** | Advanced breast cancer in postmenopausal women that has progressed after tamoxifen therapy |

| **What are its adverse effects?** | Nausea, fatigue, and hot flashes |

LEUPROLIDE (LUPRON) AND GOSERELIN (ZOLADEX)

How do these drugs work?	**Leuprolide** and **Goserelin** are long-acting synthetic gonadotropin-releasing hormone analogues that, when administered in a continuous fashion, are used to inhibit the release of FSH and LH from the anterior pituitary. Thus the synthesis of estrogen and androgen is reduced.
What are their clinical uses?	The treatment of prostate cancer and endometriosis
How are they administered?	**Leuprolide** is injected subcutaneously, while **Goserelin** is generally implanted intramuscularly.
Are there adverse effects?	Yes—hot flashes and impotence

GLUCOCORTICOIDS

Give two examples of glucocorticoids used as antineoplastic agents.	1. **Prednisone** 2. **Hydrocortisone**
What are their clinical uses?	Treatment of Hodgkin's lymphoma, non-Hodgkin's lymphoma, ALL, and myeloma
List the adverse effects.	Increased incidence of infection Hyperglycemia Osteoporosis Gastric and duodenal ulcers See *Chapter 32—Corticosteroids and Inhibitors*, for more information on glucocorticoids.

MITOTIC INHIBITORS

VINBLASTINE (VELBAN) AND VINCRISTINE (ONCOVIN)

Describe the mechanism of action.	Both of these drugs, also known as vinca alkaloids, bind tubulin and prevent the assembly of microtubules. This inhibits formation of the mitotic spindle and arrests the cell at metaphase.

What are their clinical uses?

Vinblastine—component of a protocol for Hodgkin's disease, Kaposi's sarcoma, and the VBC (vinblastine, bleomycin, cisplatin) regimen for testicular carcinoma

Vincristine—component of MOPP for Hodgkin's lymphoma and regimens used to treat childhood lymphatic leukemias, Wilms' tumor, choriocarcinoma, and Ewing's sarcoma

How are these two drugs administered?

IV

Does resistance occur?

Yes. Resistant tumor cells are often found to have increased levels of P-glycoprotein, a membrane transport pump that causes the efflux of **vinblastine** and **vincristine**.

Are there adverse effects?

Vinblastine produces more bone marrow suppression than does **vincristine**. Vin*B*lastine— *B*one marrow suppression

Vincristine induces a peripheral neuropathy, paralytic ileus, and areflexia

Both drugs can cause GI irritation, phlebitis, or cellulitis

PACLITAXEL (TAXOL)/DOCETAXEL (TAXOTERE)

How do paclitaxel and docetaxel work?

These drugs bind the β-tubulin subunit, **promoting** the formation of microtubules and preventing their disassembly. The result is that bundles of malformed microtubules are created, which arrests the cell in mitosis.

What is the clinical use?

Paclitaxel and **docetaxel** are used for treating ovarian, lung, and breast carcinoma. **Docetaxel** is more potent because of its chemical structure.

Which route of administration is used for these drugs?

IV

List the adverse effects.

Bone marrow suppression (neutropenia, thrombocytopenia): treatment with a granulocyte colony-stimulating factor (filgrastim) can help.

Hypersensitivity reactions such as urticaria or dyspnea. Pretreatment with steroids and histamine blockers will help prevent these unwanted effects.

GI effects (nausea and vomiting)

Peripheral edema: greater with **docetaxel**

Peripheral neuropathy

MONOCLONAL ANTIBODIES

TRASTUZUMAB / RITUXIMAB

How do they work?

Trastuzumab binds to and inactivates breast cancer cells that express a surface protein called human epidermal growth factor 2 (HER2)

Rituximab binds to the CD20 antigen found on B lymphocytes. CD20 plays a part in cell cycle initiation and differentiation.

What are they used for?

Some 25% to 30% of patients with breast cancer will express the HER2 surface protein on their tumor cells.

Trastuzumab is used specifically for this population subset. **Rituximab** is used in the treatment of low-grade lymphoma.

What are the adverse effects?

Trastuzumab: The most important one to remember is congestive heart failure. Others include the usual nausea, vomiting, and abdominal pain seen with so many antineoplastic drugs.

Rituximab: infusion reactions can occur which may be fatal. Pretreatment with histamine blockers and bronchodilators will help alleviate the hypotension, angioedema, and bronchospasm that may occur. Neutropenia has occasionally been reported.

Name four other monoclonal antibodies.

Bevacizumab, cetuximab, gemtuzumab, alemtuzumab

What are they used for?

Bevacizumab is an antivacular endothelial growth factor (VEGF) used for metastatic colon cancer in combination with 5-FU.

Cetuximab is an antiepidermal growth factor (EGF) also used for metastatic colon cancer.

Gemtuzumab is an antibody directed against the CD33 surface protein which is expressed on myeloid cells used for refractory cases of AML.

Alemtuzumab is an anti-CD52 antibody for CLL.

What are their adverse effects?

Bevacizumab: diarrhea, hypertension, stomatitis, bowel perforation, and stroke are serious but fortunately rare

Cetuximab: initial treatment can cause hypotension and difficulty breathing

Gemtuzumab: bone marrow suppression and hepatic toxicity

Alemtuzumab: acute infusion reactions, and the depletion of hematopoietic cells and T cells
Opportunistic infection

MISCELLANEOUS ANTINEOPLASTIC AGENTS

HYDROXYUREA (HYDREA)

What is it?	**Hydroxyurea** is a urea analogue that prevents DNA synthesis by inhibiting the enzyme **ribonucleotide reductase**.
How is this drug used clinically?	For treating CML, polycythemia vera, sickle cell disease, and melanoma
What are the adverse effects?	Bone marrow suppression Nausea and vomiting Diarrhea

ETOPOSIDE (VEPESID) AND TENIPOSIDE (VUMON)

What is the mechanism of action of etoposide and teniposide?	They inhibit the function of the **DNA topoisomerase II**–DNA complex, which causes double-stranded DNA breaks during DNA replication.
How are etoposide and teniposide used clinically?	**Etoposide** is used for small cell carcinoma of the lung, and testicular carcinoma. **Teniposide** is used as a second-line agent for ALL, gliomas, and neuroblastomas.
How are they administered?	**Etoposide** can be given IV or orally, whereas **teniposide** is given IV only.
How does resistance to these drugs occur?	Through increased efflux of drug or a decrease in DNA topoisomerase II expression
State the adverse effects.	Nausea and vomiting Alopecia Bone marrow suppression (leukopenia, thrombocytopenia) is the dose limiting toxicity.

ASPARAGINASE

What type of drug is this?	It is actually an enzyme that hydrolyzes serum asparagines to aspartic acid and ammonia. Some tumor cells need an external source of asparagines to grow. Without them they are not capable of synthesizing proteins to replicate.
When is it used clinically?	To treat pediatric ALL in combination with **vincristine** and **prednisone.**
What are the adverse effects?	Severe hypersensitivity reactions Pancreatitis Seizures and coma

IMATINIB

What is it?	A selective tyrosine kinase inhibitor. Tyrosine kinase is a critical signal transduction protein. Without it cells are not able to proliferate.
What is used for?	CML in a blast crisis and gastrointestinal stromal tumor.
How is it given?	Orally
What are the adverse effects?	Fluid retention, edema hepatotoxicity, thrombocytopenia, or neutropenia.

GEFINITIB

What is its mechanism of action?	Blocks epidermal growth factor receptor
How is it used?	Nonsmall cell lung cancer that has failed to respond to other therapy.
How is it administered?	Orally
What are its toxic effects?	Intersitial lung disease—rare Diarrhea, nausea, and skin rashes most common.

IRONOTECAP/TOPETECAN

What are they?	They are derivatives of an earlier drug called **camptothecin.**
How do they work?	These drugs work in the S phase of the cell cycle. They bind to and inhibit the enzyme topoisomerase 1. Subsequently, DNA cannot repair itself.
What are the clinical indications?	**Ironotecan:** used for colon or rectal carcinoma in conjunction with 5-FU. **Topetecan:** previously treated patients with ovarian and small cell lung cancer.
Does resistance develop?	Yes. Similar to all neoplastic drugs, resistance can occur through mutation in the binding site of topoisomerase 1 or increased efflux of the drug out of the cell.
How are they administered and excreted?	IV infusion. Eliminated through the kidneys
What are the adverse effects?	Bone marrow suppression particularly with **topetecan** **Irinotecan** causes a severe, delayed diarrhea.

40

Immunomodulators

What are the two major branches of the immune system?

Cell-mediated immunity, which is largely composed of T cells, and **humoral immunity,** which consists of B cells, plasma cells, and antibodies

What is an immunomodulator?

A substance that either suppresses or stimulates the immune system

Name and give an example of five major classes of immuno*suppressants*

1. Antibiotics (**cyclosporine, tacrolimus, sirolimus**)
2. Cytotoxic drugs (**azathioprine, cyclophosphamide**)
3. Enzyme Inhibitors (**mycophenolate mofetil**)
4. Corticosteroids (**prednisone**)
5. Antibody reagents

See Figure 40–1 for sites of action.

Give two examples of an immuno*stimulant*.

Aldesleukin
Interferon

ANTIBIOTICS

CYCLOSPORINE (SANDIMMUNE)

Where does this drug come from?

It was originally isolated from a soil fungus.

How does this drug work?

It inhibits production of interleukin-2 (IL-2), which is critical for T cell–mediated immunity.

Specifically how does it block IL-2 production?

The drug binds to a cytoplasmic receptor protein called cyclophilin. This cyclophilin-cyclosporine complex then inhibits a protein called **calcineurin,** which is required to dephosphorylate NFAT (nuclear factor of activated T

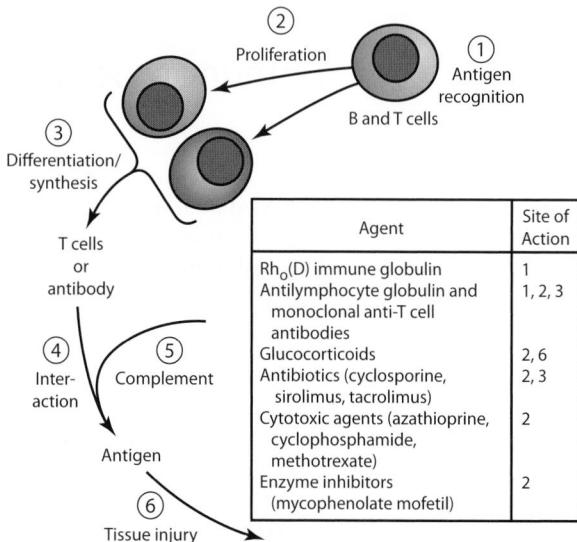

Figure 40–1. The sites of action of immunosuppressive agents on the immune response. (With permission from Katzung BG [ed.]. *Basic & Clinical Pharmacology*, 9th ed. New York: McGraw-Hill, 2004, p. 940.)

cells). NFAT is critical for the transcription of IL-2. Without it, production is effectively blocked.

Does it also affect humoral immunity?

Cyclosporine is highly selective for the suppression of cell-mediated immunity.

When is this drug used?

In the transplantation of solid organs
To treat graft-versus-host disease in bone marrow transplant recipients and rheumatoid arthritis. It is also used topically to treat psoriasis.

How is this drug metabolized?

By the hepatic P-450 system. Therefore drugs that either induce or suppress this system can affect plasma levels of cyclosporine.

What are potential side effects?

Renal dysfunction is the dose-limiting toxicity. Also watch for neurotoxicity (limb paresthesias, tremor, and seizures can occur), hyperkalemia, hypertension, hirsutism, and gingival hyperplasia.

TACROLIMUS (FK506)

How does this drug work, and is it similar to cyclosporine?	It is. **Tacrolimus**, like **cyclosporine**, inhibits IL-2 by blocking calcineurin. However it binds to a different cellular receptor (FKBP-12) rather than cyclophilin. The selectivity for T-cell suppression is also analogous to **cyclosporine**.
How does this drug compare to cyclosporine?	**Tacrolimus** is a newer drug and is approximately 100 times more potent.
Where is it metabolized?	It is metabolized extensively in the liver and has similar drug interactions as **cyclosporine**.
When is this drug used clinically?	In organ transplantation. It is often used in combination with glucocorticoids.
What are its potential hazards?	Similar to those of cyclosporine. **Nephrotoxicity** is the major problem, which can be exacerbated with coadministration of cyclosporine or other nephrotoxic drugs. Hypertension, hyperkalemia, and diabetes can also occur. Neurotoxicity is **more** common than with cyclosporine. Hirsutism and gingival hyperplasia, however, **do not** occur.

SIROLIMUS (RAPAMUNE)

What is it?	A macrolide produced by a soil mold. It was previously called **rapamycin**.
How does it work ?	**Sirolimus** works differently than **cyclosporine** or **tacrolimus**. It acts by inhibiting mammalian target of rapamycin (mTOR) protein kinases, which in turn prevents cell cycle progression and blocks the ability of T cells to proliferate in response to IL-2 stimulus.

How is it administered and metabolized?

Orally. High fat diets reduce absorption. It is metabolized extensively in the hepatic cytochrome P450 system. Therefore, other drugs, such as **allopurinol**, which inhibit the P450 system, can increase plasma levels.

What are its clinical uses?

As adjunctive therapy in combination with cyclosporine or tacrolimus and glucocorticoids for renal transplantation

What are the adverse effects of sirolimus?

Hyperlipidemia, that may require treatment. Patients treated with **sirolimus** and **cyclosporine** do experience interactions. **Sirolimus** aggravates **cyclosporine**-induced renal dysfunction, while **cyclosporine** increases **sirolimus**-induced hyperlipidemia.
Other adverse effects of **sirolimus** include leukopenia, thrombocytopenia, and infection.

CYTOTOXIC DRUGS

CYCLOPHOSPHAMIDE (CYTOXAN)

See *Chapter 39—Antineoplastic Drugs*

How does this drug work?

Cyclophosphamide is also used as an antineoplastic agent. As stated in Chapter 39, it is a prodrug that is activated to a cytotoxic alkylating agent by the cytochrome P-450 system. Although it affects both B and T lymphocytes, B cells are affected to a much greater degree because they have a slower rate of recovery.

When is this drug used?

For the treatment of autoimmune diseases including hemolytic anemia, systemic lupus erythematosus (SLE), rheumatoid arthritis (RA), and Wegener's granulomatosis
Organ transplantation

What are potential side effects?

Hemorrhagic cystitis alopecia, GI distress, sterility, and pancytopenia

AZATHIOPRINE (IMURAN)

How does this drug work?	**Azathioprine** is also a prodrug that becomes active only after it is modified by various enzymes into 6 mercaptopurine (6-MP) and subsequently into 6-thioIMP. These products block the de novo purine synthesis pathway. Both B and T lymphocytes are suppressed after the administration of **azathioprine**.
When is this drug used?	**Azathioprine** is largely used in kidney transplantation and the treatment of autoimmune disorders such as hemolytic anemia.
Give an example of an important drug interaction with azathioprine.	**Azathioprine** is metabolized by xanthine oxidase. **Allopurinol** blocks the breakdown of **azathioprine** because it inhibits xanthine oxidase. Consequently, patients taking **allopurinol** along with **azathioprine** have an increased risk of toxicity.
What are the potential toxic effects?	Bone marrow suppression Increased risk of cancer GI irritation

MYCOPHENOLATE MOFETIL (CELLCEPT)

How does mycophenolate mofetil work ?	This drug is converted into mycophenolic acid, which inhibits the enzyme inosine monophosphate dehydrogenase (IMP). IMP is used in the de novo pathway of purine (specifically guanine) synthesis.
What similarity does it share with azathioprine?	They both block the purine synthesis pathway.
When is it used?	Organ transplantation It can be used in combination with cyclosporine and glucocorticoids. It has largely replaced **azathioprine** because of a better safety profile.

What are the main adverse effects to monitor?	GI side effects, drug-induced fever, leukopenia
Does it affect B- and T-cell lines equally?	Yes. The inhibition of IMP causes both a B- and T-cell suppression.

ADRENOCORTICAL STEROIDS

See *Chapter 32—Corticosteroids and Inhibitors*

Name the synthetically produced glucocorticoids used for their systemic immunosuppressive effects.	**Prednisone** **Methylprednisone** **Betamethasone** **Dexamethasone**
How do they work?	Corticosteroids **inhibit phospholipase A2**. This leads to inhibition of the biosynthesis of arachidonic acid and subsequently the production of leukotrienes, cytokines, and prostaglandins. Recent studies suggest they also **interfere with transcription factors** required to activate **T-cell genes** and immune complexes.
What are the toxicities?	Immune suppression requires long-term use of steroids. This is associated with a wide variety of side effects including infections, ulcers, weight gain. (see Chapter 32).

ANTIBODIES

What are Mabs?	"Mabs" is the acronym for monoclonal antibodies. Two of the monoclonal antibodies currently in use include **muromonab-CD3** and **daclizumab**.
How does muromonab-CD3 (okt3) work?	It binds to the CD3 antigen on the surface of human thymocytes and mature T lymphocytes. This results in a blockade of T cell function. The non functional circulating T cells are depleted from the blood stream and peripheral lymph node organs such as the spleen. This occurs secondary to complement activated cell death.

In what situation would muromonab-CD3 be used?

Acute organ transplant rejection. Circulating T cellls disappear from the blood within minutes of infusion. When **muromonab** is administered, it transiently stimulates the release of cytokines from T cells. It is, therefore, very important to premedicate the patient with glucocorticoids, which help prevent this release of cytokines.

What are its toxicities?

Cytokine release syndrome can follow the first dose. Symptoms range from mild fever/chills, headache and diarrhea to severe seizures, aseptic meningitis, pulmonary edema and cardiac arrest. Because of these potential problems **muromonab** has fallen out of favor and is being replaced with newer antibodies such as **daclizumab** and **basiliximab**.

DACLIZUMAB (ZENAPAX)/BASILIXIMAB (SIMULECT)

What are daclizumab and basiliximab?

They are synthetic antibodies produced by recombinant DNA technology. Thus, they are less antigenic than **muromonab-CD3**.

State the mechanism of action of these drugs.

Competitively binds to the alpha subunit of the IL-2 receptor expressed on T lymphocytes and therefore blocks T-cell activation

When would daclizumab and basiliximab be beneficial?

In preventing an episode of acute rejection after renal transplantation

What side effects do you have to watch for?

GI irritation, headache, and muscle pain

RH$_O$(D) IMMUNE GLOBULIN (RHOGAM)

What is it?

It's a human IgG preparation that contains antibodies against red cell Rh(D) surface antigens.

| When is it used? | RhoGam is used for prevention of Rh hemolytic disease of the newborn. It is given to an Rh-negative mother whenever fetal red cells have been suspected to enter the mother's circulation (ectopic pregnancy, miscarriage, or transplacental hemorrhage). |

ANTITHYMOCYTE GLOBULIN

What is it?	**Antithymocyte globulin** is usually produced in rabbits by immunization against human thymus cells. **Antithymocyte** globulin binds to T cells and depletes them from circulation through cell death and also causes T cell dysfunction.
What is it used for?	Used in the treatment of acute renal transplant rejection in combination with other immunosuppressants
Name the toxicities associated with the use of lymphocyte immune globulin.	Hypersensitivity reactions including serum sickness and anaphylaxis. Premedication with glucocorticoids can reduce these symptoms. Also watch for thrombocytopenia, leukopenia and viral infections.

IMMUNOSTIMULANTS

ALDESLEUKIN

What is aldesleukin?	It is a synthesized form of interleukin-2 made by recombinant DNA technology.
What does it do?	It stimulates the production of cytotoxic T cells and natural killer cells.
What is it used for?	To treat metastatic renal cell carcinoma and melanoma
What should be monitored during Aldesleukin therapy?	Cardiovascular status. Hypotension and reduced organ perfusion leading to death may occur. Risk of infections is also high.

INTERFERONS

What are interferons?	Interferons are types of cytokines. They can enhance immune activities including increased phagocytosis by macrophages and augmented cytotoxicity by T lymphocytes. There are three major types of interferons—namely, alpha (α), beta (β), and gamma (γ).
What are they used for?	**Alpha**—hairy cell leukemia, malignant melanoma, Kaposi's sarcoma, and hepatitis B **Beta**—multiple sclerosis **Gamma**—increases leukocyte activity in patients with chronic granulomatous disease
What side effects are associated with interferon therapy?	Fever, hypersensitivity reactions

Section X

Antimicrobial Drugs

41

Introduction to Antimicrobial Drugs

What are four critical factors that determine the selection of an antimicrobial drug?

1. **Identity of the organism**—usually identified through Gram's stain or culture
2. **Safety of the drug**
3. **Site of infection**—for example, some drugs cross the blood-brain barrier whereas others do not.
4. **Patient's medical history**—allergies, immune status, renal and hepatic condition, pregnancy, and lactation status

See *Appendix B—Recommended Antimicrobial Agents Against Selected Organisms*.

Name four large classes of antimicrobial agents, give examples of each, and describe their mechanisms of action.

1. **Cell wall synthesis inhibitors**—*Examples:* Penicillins, **cycloserine**, cephalosporins, **vancomycin**. These drugs block the cross-linking of peptidoglycan chains, which is the final step in bacterial cell wall synthesis.
2. **Protein synthesis inhibitors**—*Examples:* **Tetracycline**, aminoglycosides, **erythromycin, clindamycin, chloramphenicol**. These agents bind to bacterial ribosomes.
3. **DNA synthesis inhibitors**—Quinolones and fluoroquinolones block nucleic acid synthesis by inhibiting DNA gyrase. **Rifampin** inhibits DNA-dependent RNA polymerase. The sulfonamides inhibit synthesis of folate, which is a critical component of DNA.
4. **Cell membrane disrupters**—Polyene antimicrobials such as **amphotericin B** bind to components of fungal cell membranes.

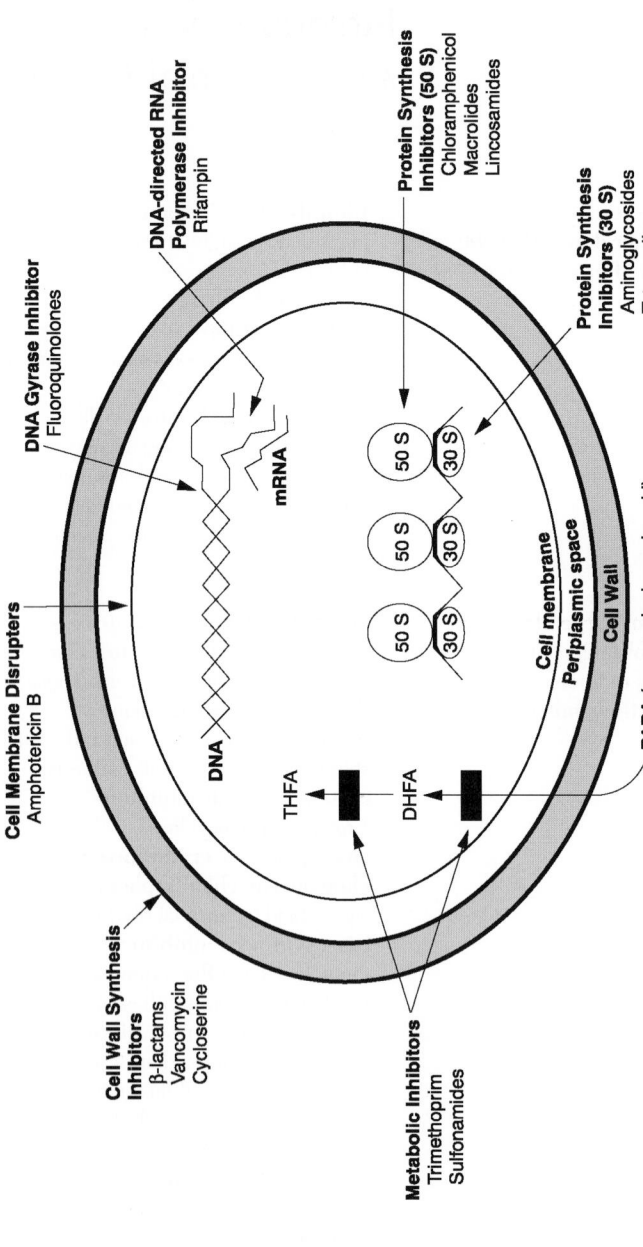

Figure 41–1. Site of action of various antimicrobial agents. (Redrawn with permission from Gallia G, Hann CL, Hewson WH. *The Pharmacology Companion.* La Jolla, CA: Alert & Oriented Publishing Company, 1997, p. 150, Fig. 5.1.)

Figure 41–1.
Each of these groups is discussed in
detail in succeeding chapters.

What do bacteriostatic drugs do?	They arrest the growth and replication of bacteria, thus giving the body's immune system a chance to destroy and remove the pathogens.
What do bactericidal drugs do?	Bactericidal drugs kill bacteria outright.
Which drugs are considered bactericidal?	Aminoglycosides Quinolones **Cycloserine** **Vancomycin** Carbapenems Penicillins Cephalosporins **Trimethoprim-sulfamethoxazole**
Which drugs are considered bacteriostatic?	**Chloramphenicol** **Nitrofurantoin** **Clindamycin** **Tetracycline** **Erythromycin** **Lincomycin**
What is meant by the chemotherapeutic spectrum of an antibiotic?	The term "chemotherapeutic spectrum" refers to the types of microorganisms affected by a given agent. Thus, a broad-spectrum agent affects a wide variety of microorganisms.
Can antibiotics be used in combination?	Yes. Sometimes, for example, in the empiric treatment of pneumonia, combination drug therapy is required. However, whenever possible, it is best to use single-agent therapy to limit the risk of toxicity and resistance.
What is drug resistance?	The term "drug resistance" refers to the ability of a microorganism to withstand a drug that was previously toxic to it.

Name the four basic mechanisms by which microorganisms can become resistant to antibiotics and give an example of each.

1. **Production of drug-inactivating enzymes**—β-lactamase, an enzyme that binds to certain penicillins, is a prime example of an enzyme that counteracts the effects of an antibiotic.
2. **Changes in drug penetration**—The effectiveness of aminoglycosides and tetracycline, for example, depends on their ability to reach high intracellular concentrations. Bacteria may adapt to become impermeable to these antibiotics or increase their ability to excrete these antibiotics.
3. **Changes in receptor structure**—Antibiotics such as **erythromycin** bind to certain receptors. Microorganisms can sometimes cause these receptors to mutate so that they have very little affinity for antibiotics.
4. **Alterations of metabolic pathways**—Bacteria may acquire the ability to use preformed folic acid, thus bypassing the inhibitory actions of sulfonamides.

What is meant by empiric therapy?

Early intervention through the use of an antibiotic before a pathogen is identified

What is the benefit of empiric therapy?

Because early intervention usually helps to improve the outcome of an infection, antibiotics are sometimes used before a Gram's stain or culture of the pathogen is obtained. Physicians use information from the history, physical examination, and any other completed diagnostic tests to determine which antibiotic to use.

What is meant by antimicrobial prophylaxis?

Antimicrobial prophylaxis is the use of antibiotics to *prevent* disease. Examples include prevention of tuberculosis among individuals who are in close contact with infected patients and pretreatment of patients with artificial heart valves who are undergoing dental procedures.

42   Penicillins

To what classification of drug does penicillin belong?

Penicillin is a member of a group of drugs known as β-lactams because of their characteristic four-membered lactam ring (Figure 42–1). They are bactericidal agents.

Define β-lactamase.

β-lactamase is a bacterial enzyme that hydrolyzes the amide bond of the β-lactam ring. It is also known as penicillinase.

What are penicillin-binding proteins (PBPs)?

Penicillin-binding proteins are enzymes that are involved in the synthesis of the cell wall and in the maintenance of the morphological structure of bacteria.

What are transpeptidases?

Transpeptidases are bacterial enzymes responsible for cross-linking peptidoglycan chains, which is the final step in bacterial cell wall synthesis.

What is the major mechanism by which penicillins kill bacteria?

Penicillins bind to PBPs and inhibit the transpeptidase step, which results in bacterial cell lysis.

What additional mechanism is involved?

Penicillins also release autolysins, bacterial degradative enzymes involved in the normal remodeling of the bacterial cell wall.

Which type of organisms are *not* susceptible to penicillins?

Organisms that are not actively growing or do not have a cell wall

Do penicillins enter the CNS?

Normally these drugs do not distribute well into the CNS. However, when the meninges are inflamed, as occurs in meningitis, penicillins easily reach

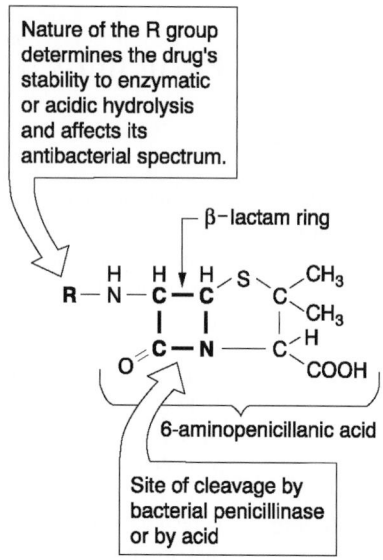

Nature of the R group determines the drug's stability to enzymatic or acidic hydrolysis and affects its antibacterial spectrum.

β−lactam ring

6-aminopenicillanic acid

Site of cleavage by bacterial penicillinase or by acid

Figure 42–1. Structural features of β-lactam antibiotics. (Redrawn with permission from Howland RD, Mycek MJ [Harvey RA, Champe PC, eds.]. *Lippincott's Illustrated Reviews: Pharmacology,* 3rd ed. Baltimore: Lippincott Williams & Wilkins, 2006, p. 354.)

therapeutic concentrations within the CNS.

How are the penicillins classified?

Penicillins, among the most common and important antibiotics, can be classified as follows:
Natural penicillins
Antistaphylococcal penicillins
Antipseudomonal penicillins
Extended-spectrum penicillins

NATURAL PENICILLINS

Give four examples of natural penicillins and their routes of administration.

1. **Penicillin G**, the prototype drug—oral, intravenous, intramuscular
2. **Penicillin V**—oral only
3. **Penicillin G procaine** (Crysticillin AS)—intramuscular only
4. **Penicillin G benzathine** (Bicillin LA)—intramuscular only

How do the various natural penicillins differ from each other?

These drugs all work the same way; they differ in their route of administration and stability to gastric acid.

What can natural penicillin be used for?

Natural penicillin has a large spectrum; however, it affects Gram-positive organisms the most. Clinical indications include infections due to the following:
Streptococci
Meningococci
Clostridium
Listeria
Enterococci
Diphtheria
Anthrax
Syphilis
Spirochetes, such as *Treponema pallidum*
Actinomycosis
Bacteroides species (except *Bacteroides fragilis*)
Anaerobic organisms that do not produce β-lactamase

Describe the absorption of these penicillins.

Absorption depends on their acid stability and protein binding.

Is the absorption of penicillins influenced by food?

Absorption of most penicillins is affected by food; therefore, these drugs (except amoxicillin) should be administered at least 1 to 2 hr before or after a meal.

How are these drugs excreted?

Penicillins are mostly unchanged as they are excreted in the urine (by glomerular filtration and active tubular secretion), although some penicillins, such as nafcillin and ampicillin, undergo hepatic inactivation and are excreted in the bile.

How can the excretion of penicillins be altered?

Excretion by renal tubular secretion can be delayed by coadministration of probenecid, which inhibits the organic acid secretion system.

What are the adverse effects seen with patients who are medicated with penicillin?

Hypersensitivity reactions— anaphylaxis (rare), urticaria, severe pruritus, fever, joint swelling, and bronchospasm—these are the primary toxicities to watch for.

Seizures may occur in patients with poor renal function or in newborns who have immature anion transport systems.

Gastrointestinal disturbances— diarrhea

Hemolytic anemia

Nephritis

Cation toxicity—Because penicillins are combined with sodium or potassium, patients may suffer from excess Na^+ or K^+ (seen only with extremely high doses).

Are these adverse effects seen with all forms of penicillins?

Yes! Remember that these toxicities apply to all forms of penicillins, not just natural penicillins. (Additional or unique toxicities are mentioned later.)

ANTISTAPHYLOCOCCAL PENICILLINS (PENICILLINASE-RESISTANT PENICILLINS)

Give some examples of penicillinase-resistant drugs and indicate their routes of administration.

Methicillin Discontinued in the U.S.
Nafcillin (Unipen)—PO, IV, or IM
Oxacillin (Bactocill)—PO, IV, or IM
Dicloxacillin (Dynapen)—PO, IV, or IM
Cloxacillin (Tegopen)—PO, IV, or IM
Remember—these are the only penicillins that by themselves are resistant to penicillinase.

When do you use penicillinase-resistant penicillins?

These drugs have a very narrow spectrum; they were developed solely for the purpose of killing staphylococci that produce penicillinase.

What should you do if you encounter methicillin-resistant *Staphylococcus aureus*?

Use vancomycin immediately for serious infections.

What is the distinctive toxicity of methicillin?

Although all penicillins have the potential to cause interstitial nephritis, it was most likely with methicillin.

What other toxicity is associated with these drugs?

Methicillin, nafcillin, and some other penicillins occasionally cause granulocytopenia, especially in children.

ANTIPSEUDOMONAL PENICILLINS

Give two examples of antipseudomonal penicillins.

1. **Piperacillin** (Pipracil)
2. **Ticarcillin** (Ticar)
   Mezlocillin, azlocillin, and carbenicillin all belong to this class as well but they have been discontinued in the U.S.

What is the route of administration for piperacillin and ticarcillin?

Both of these drugs are extremely unstable in gastric acid and therefore must be given intravenously or intramuscularly.

Are these drugs inactivated by penicillinase?

Yes. Therefore, they are commonly paired with beta lactamase inhibitors.

What is their antimicrobial spectrum?

Gram-negative bacilli *Enterobactor*, especially *Pseudomonas* species (hence the name).

What toxicity is likely to be seen with ticarcillin?

Platelet dysfunction

EXTENDED-SPECTRUM PENICILLINS

Give some examples of extended-spectrum penicillins and indicate their routes of administration.

Amoxicillin (Amoxil)—PO
Ampicillin (Omnipen)—PO, IV, and IM

Against what organisms can ampicillin and amoxicillin be used?

In general, all of the organisms affected by the natural penicillins plus some Gram-negative organisms such as *Escherichia coli, Proteus mirabilis, Salmonella, Shigella, Haemophilus influenzae,* and *Listeria monocytogenes*

Are these drugs inactivated by β-lactamase?

Yes!

What important toxicities are associated with ampicillin?

In patients with mononucleosis, the incidence of **rash** is extremely high. Ampicillin-induced **pseudomembranous colitis** is another potential side effect.

With what other agents are these two drugs often combined?

β-lactamase inhibitors, which inhibit the enzyme by binding to it and thus protecting the accompanying antibiotic. On their own, β-lactamase inhibitors are not effective in eliminating bacteria.

Give three examples of β-lactamase inhibitors.

1. **Clavulanic acid**
2. **Sulbactam**
3. **Tazobactam**

With which drugs are each of the three β-lactamase inhibitors paired?

Clavulanic acid with **amoxicillin** (Augmentin) or with **ticarcillin** (Timentin)
Sulbactam with **ampicillin** (Unasyn)
Tazobactam with **piperacillin** (Zosyn)

RESISTANCE

Aside from inactivation of the antibiotic by β-lactamase, how else does bacterial resistance develop?

Alteration in target PBPs
Decreased cell permeability, which prevents the antibiotic from penetrating its target

43

Cephalosporins and Other Cell Wall Synthesis Inhibitors

Where did cephalosporins originate?

From the *Cephalosporium acremonium* fungi

How do they work?

They are analogous to penicillins in:
—Binding to specific penicillin-binding proteins
—Inhibition of cell wall synthesis by blocking the transpeptidase step of peptidoglycan synthesis
—Activation of autolytic enzymes

Are cephalosporins bactericidal or bacteriostatic?

Bactericidal

How are cephalosporins subdivided?

Into first, second, third, and fourth generations.
These classifications are based on general features of antimicrobial activity (Figure 43–1).

In general, how do the characteristics of cephalosporins change from first- to fourth-generation agents?

From the first generation to the fourth generation of cephalosporins, there is:
—A decrease in Gram-positive coverage
—An increase in Gram-negative coverage
—An increase in CNS penetration
—An increase in resistance to β-lactamase

FIRST-GENERATION CEPHALOSPORINS

First-generation cephalosporins are active against which organisms?

Gram-positive cocci, including pneumococci, streptococci, and staphylococci
Some **Gram-negative bacilli**, including

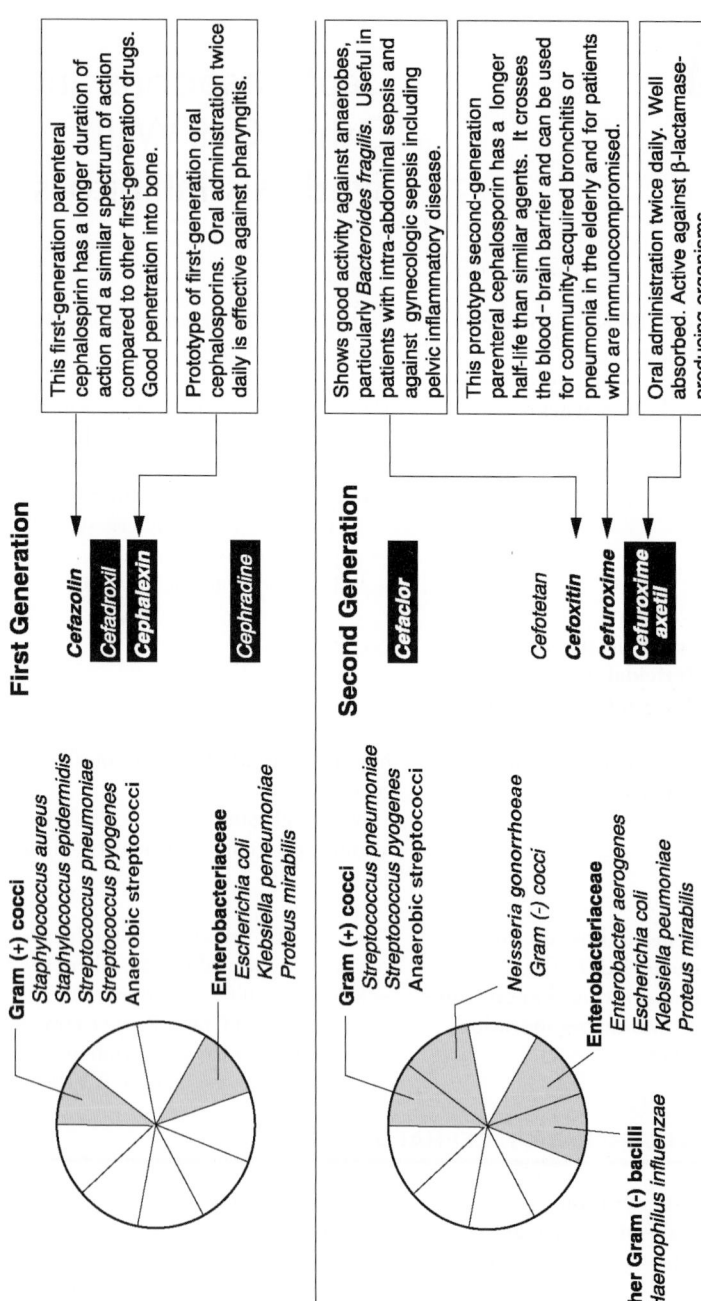

First Generation

This first-generation parenteral cephalosporin has a longer duration of action and a similar spectrum of action compared to other first-generation drugs. Good penetration into bone.

Prototype of first-generation oral cephalosporins. Oral administration twice daily is effective against pharyngitis.

Cefazolin

Cefadroxil

Cephalexin

Cephradine

Gram (+) cocci
Staphylococcus aureus
Staphylococcus epidermidis
Streptococcus pneumoniae
Streptococcus pyogenes
Anaerobic streptococci

Enterobacteriaceae
Escherichia coli
Klebsiella peneumoniae
Proteus mirabilis

Second Generation

Shows good activity against anaerobes, particularly *Bacteroides fragilis*. Useful in patients with intra-abdominal sepsis and against gynecologic sepsis including pelvic inflammatory disease.

This prototype second-generation parenteral cephalosporin has a longer half-life than similar agents. It crosses the blood–brain barrier and can be used for community-acquired bronchitis or pneumonia in the elderly and for patients who are immunocompromised.

Oral administration twice daily. Well absorbed. Active against β-lactamase-producing organisms.

Cefaclor

Cefotetan

Cefoxitin

Cefuroxime

Cefuroxime axetil

Gram (+) cocci
Streptococcus pneumoniae
Streptococcus pyogenes
Anaerobic streptococci

Neisseria gonorrhoeae
Gram (-) cocci

Enterobacteriaceae
Enterobacter aerogenes
Escherichia coli
Klebsiella peumoniae
Proteus mirabilis

Other Gram (-) bacilli
Haemophilus influenzae

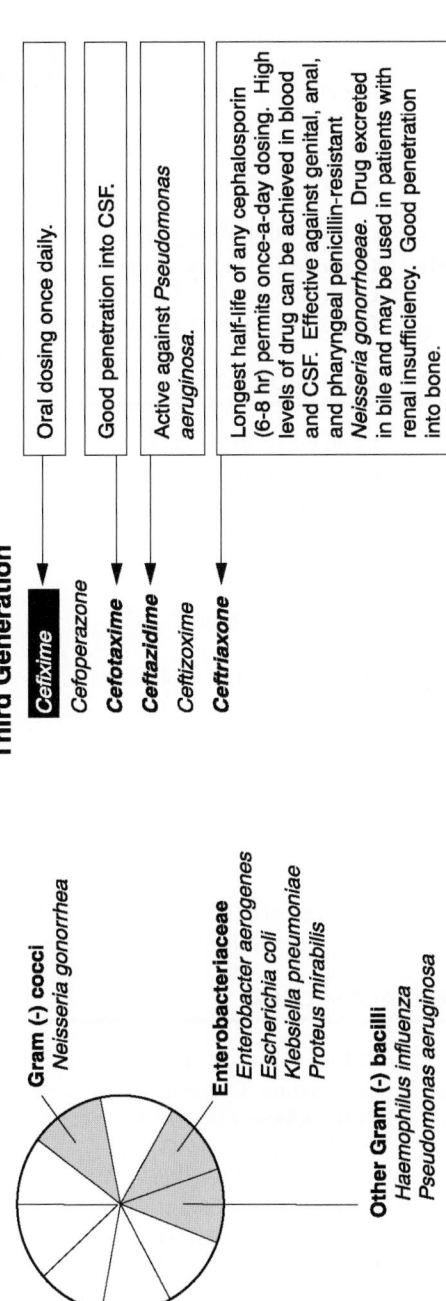

Figure 43–1. Characteristics of some clinically useful cephalosporins. Drugs that can be administered orally are shown in *reverse type*. Drugs with unique traits are shown in *bold*. (Adapted and redrawn with permission from Mycek MJ, Gertner SB, Perper MM [Harvey RA, Champe PC, eds.]. *Lippincott's Illustrated Reviews: Pharmacology*, 2nd ed. Philadelphia: Lippincott-Raven Publishers, 1997, p. 305.)

Proteus mirabilis, Escherichia coli, and *Klebsiella*—**PecK**
Bacteroides fragilis, enterococci, and methicillin-resistant *Staphylococcus aureus* are not covered.

Which drugs are in this group, and what is the route of administration for each?	**Cefadroxil** (Duricef)—oral **Cephalexin** (Keflex)—oral **Cephradine** (Velosef)—oral **Cefazolin** (Ancef)—intravenous

SECOND-GENERATION CEPHALOSPORINS

Name some second-generation cephalosporins and state the route of administration for each.	**Cefaclor** (Ceclor)—PO **Cefuroxime axetil** (Ceftin)—PO **Loracarbef** (Lorabid) —PO **Cefprozil** **Cefotetan** (Cefotan)—IV **Cefoxitin** (Mefoxin)—IV **Cefuroxime** (Zinacef)—IV
What infections can be treated with second-generation cephalosporins?	Second-generation cephalosporins cover the same organisms as first-generation cephalosporins, but they also have somewhat increased activity against Gram-negative organisms including *Haemophilus influenzae, Neisseria,* and *Enterobacter.* Cefoxitin, cefmetazole, and cefotetan can be used to treat anaerobic and aerobic infections, such as those that affect the intra-abdominal area (*B. fragilis*).

THIRD-GENERATION CEPHALOSPORINS

What drugs are in this group, and what is the route of administration for each?	**Cefoperazone** (Cefobid)—IV **Cefotaxime** (Claforan)—IV **Ceftazidime** (Fortaz)—IV **Ceftizoxime** (Cefizox)—IV **Ceftriaxone** (Rocephin)—IV **Cefpodoxime** (Vantin)—PO **Cefdinir** (Omnicef)—PO **Ceftibuten** (Cedax)—PO

Against what organisms do these agents exert action?

Third-generation cephalosporins provide expanded Gram-negative coverage but poor Gram-positive coverage. They are good against *Enterobacter, Citrobacter,* and *Providencia* as well as β-lactamase–producing strains of *Neisseria* and *Haemophilus. Pseudomonas* infection can be treated with ceftazidime and cefoperazone.

FOURTH-GENERATION CEPHALOSPORINS

Name the only fourth-generation cephalosporin currently available in the U.S. and how it is administered.

Cefepine (Maxipine)—IV only

What is the spectrum of fourth generation of cephalosporins?

An expanded range of Gram-positive and Gram-negative organisms over third generation. In particular, it has a better *Pseudomonas* coverage. It is also much more stable against β-lactamase. It is not, however, active against MRSA, enterococci, *B. fragilis,* or *L. monocytogenes.*

GENERAL FEATURES OF THE CEPHALOSPORINS

What are these agents inactive against?

All cephalosporins are inactive against enterococci, methicillin-resistant staphylococci, *Listeria monocytogenes,* and *Clostridium difficile.*

How are the cephalosporins primarily excreted?

Through glomerular filtration. Cefoperazone and ceftriaxone are exceptions; they are excreted in bile.

Are cephalosporins metabolized extensively?

They are excreted largely unchanged.

How does resistance occur?

Through the same mechanisms as pencillins.

In general, what are the adverse effects of the cephalosporins?	**Hypersensitivity reactions** similar to those induced by penicillins. About 10% of patients with penicillin allergy will cross react with cephalosporins (bronchospasm, urticaria).
	Nephrotoxicity
	Intolerance to alcohol (a disulfiram-type reaction) with cefotetan and cefoperazone
	A **positive Coombs' test result,** but rarely associated with hemolytic anemia
	Hypothrombinemia with cefoperazone, due to vitamin K inhibition

OTHER CELL WALL SYNTHESIS INHIBITORS

MONOBACTAMS—**AZTREONAM** (Azactam)

Describe the mechanism of action of the monobactams.	Monobactams disrupt bacterial cell wall synthesis by binding to penicillin-binding proteins and inhibiting peptidoglycan synthesis.
Describe the pharmacokinetics of aztreonam.	Aztreonam is administered via IV or IM routes and is excreted in the urine.
What are the clinical indications for aztreonam?	Primarily aerobic Gram-negative rods (*Pseudomonas, Klebsiella, Serratia*)
What are the adverse effects of aztreonam?	Skin rash Elevated liver function enzymes Gastrointestinal distress (nausea, vomiting)

CARBAPENEMS

What are they?	Carbapenems are synthetic β-lactam antibiotics that are structurally related to the penicillins. They are, however, resistant to β-lactamase.

Give two examples of carbapenems.	**Imipenem** (Primaxin), prototype **Meropenem** (Merrem)
How are they administered?	IV
What is the antibacterial spectrum of this drug?	**Imipenem** is a bactericidal agent active against virtually all Gram-positive, Gram-negative, and anaerobic organisms. **Methicillin**-resistant *Staphylococcus*, **vancomycin**-resistant enterococci (VRE), and *Clostridium difficile* are important exceptions.
What is imipenem usually combined with, and why?	**Imipenem** is usually combined with **cilastatin**. **Imipenem** is inactivated by the enzyme dehydropeptidase, which is found in the brush border of the proximal tubules. **Cilastatin** prevents this inactivation and allows **imipenem** to be used for the treatment of urinary tract infections.
Describe imipenem's adverse effects.	Seizures—provoked by high levels of imipenem GI effects—nausea, vomiting, diarrhea Eosinophilia and neutropenia

VANCOMYCIN (VANCOCIN)

What is vancomycin's mechanism of action?	**Vancomycin** binds to the D-alanyl-D-alanine portion of cell wall precursors and inhibits peptidoglycan polymerization.
Describe this agent's antibacterial spectrum.	**Vancomycin** is a bactericidal agent effective against all Gram-positive organisms. At present it is reserved for treating severe infections caused by methicillin-resistant staphylococci or serious Gram-positive infection in penicillin-allergic patients. It is also used to treat *C. difficile*–induced pseudomembranous colitis and for prophylaxis in patients with prosthetic

heart valves who are undergoing genitourinary or gastrointestinal surgery and are allergic to ampicillin.

How does resistance to vancomycin develop?

Primarily through plasmid-mediated changes in permeability to the drug and decreased binding of **vancomycin** to receptor molecules. Treat vancomycin-resistant organisms with **linezolid** or **quinupristin/dalfoprintin**.

What is vancomycin's usual route of administration?

IV except in treating pseudomembranous colitis, when it is given orally

How is it excreted?

Ninety percent is excreted through glomerular filtration.

What are the adverse effects?

Fever and chills
Shock—a result of rapid administration
Dose-related ototoxicity and
    nephrotoxicity—rare with today's
    preparations
"Red man's syndrome"—facial flushing
    and hypotension due to a rapid
    infusion of the agent, thought to be
    caused by histamine release

BACITRACIN

Describe this agent's antimicrobial spectrum.

Bacitracin is used against Gram-positive organisms.

How does bacitracin work?

It inhibits cell wall synthesis by blocking the transfer of peptidoglycan subunits to a growing cell wall.

What is the usual route of administration?

The use of **bacitracin** is restricted to topical application because of its potential for nephrotoxicity if given systemically.

Are there adverse reactions?

Yes—nausea/vomiting and skin rash

CYCLOSERINE

How does cycloserine work?	**Cycloserine** is a structural analog of D-alanine and therefore blocks the incorporation of D-alanine into peptidoglycans.
When is this drug used?	**Cycloserine** is effective against many Gram-positive and Gram-negative organisms, but it is almost always used to treat tuberculosis caused by strains of *Mycobacterium tuberculosis* that are resistant to first-line drugs.
What are its toxicities?	CNS toxicity—tremors, seizures, confusion, headaches, psychosis

44

Protein Synthesis Inhibitors

How do protein synthesis inhibitors work?	By targeting bacterial ribosomes
Why don't protein synthesis inhibitors work on eukaryotic cells?	Eukaryotic cells have 80S ribosomes composed of 60S and 40S subunits, whereas bacterial cells have 70S ribosomes composed of 50S and 30S subunits. This structural difference allows for selective toxicity. (°S stands for Svedburg unit of sedimentation coefficient.)
Can high doses of drugs such as chloramphenicol and tetracycline result in adverse effects on eukaryotic cells?	Yes, because the eukaryotic mitochondrial ribosome somewhat resembles the bacterial ribosome
Which antibiotics work on the bacterial 30S ribosomal subunit?	Aminoglycosides Tetracyclines **Spectinomycin**

Which antibiotics work on the bacterial 50S ribosomal subunit?	**Chloramphenicol**
	Macrolides—**erythromycin** (E-Mycin),
	    clarithromycin (Biaxin),
	    azithromycin (Zithromax)
	Lincosamides—**clindamycin**
	Telithromycin (Protek)
	Quinupristin/Dalfopristin (Synercid)
	Linezolid (Zyvox)

AMINOGLYCOSIDES

Give some examples of aminoglycosides.	**Amikacin** (Amikin) **Netilmicin** (Netromycin) **Neomycin** (Mycifradin)

Tobramycin (Nebcin)
Gentamycin (Garamycin)
Streptomycin

What is the mechanism of action?

Aminoglycosides cross the outer membrane and enter the periplasmic space through aqueous channels formed by porin proteins. These drugs are then actively transported through the cell membrane by an oxygen-dependent process. They then irreversibly bind to the 30S ribosomal subunit and inhibit protein synthesis by blocking the formation of the **initiation complex** and the **translocation step** (Figure 44–1). They also induce misreading of the mRNA code and promote polysome instability.

Are they bacteriostatic?

No! Aminoglycosides are powerful bactericidal drugs.

What are the pharmacokinetics of the aminoglycosides?

The aminoglycosides penetrate most body fluids well **except for the CSF**. High concentrations of these drugs tend to accumulate in the renal cortex and endolymph of the inner ear, which could account for their nephrotoxicity and ototoxicity.

How are these drugs administered?

Aminoglycosides are usually given IV because they are poorly absorbed after oral administration.

Describe the metabolism of the aminoglycosides.

These drugs are excreted unchanged by the kidneys.

What is the therapeutic use?

Aminoglycosides are used primarily against aerobic Gram-negative enteric bacteria such as *Escherichia coli,*

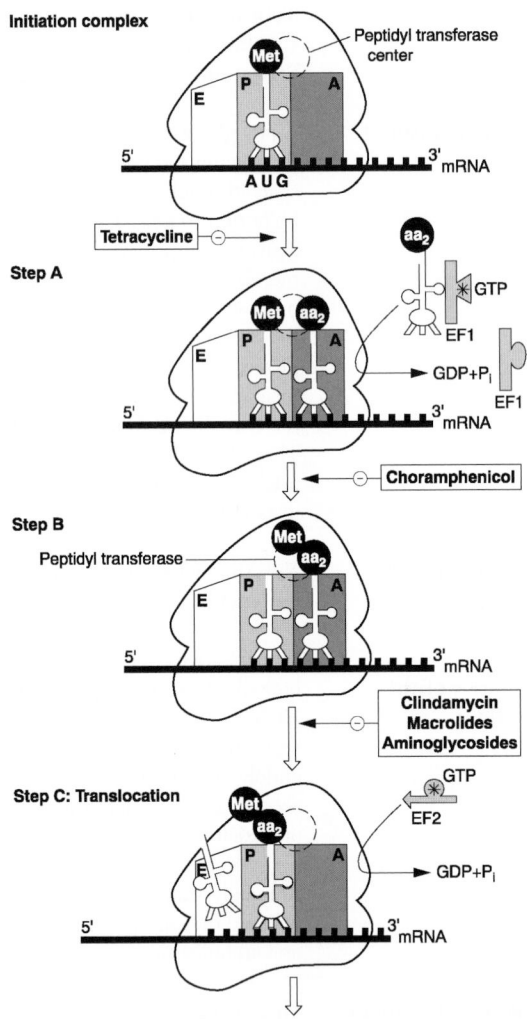

Figure 44–1. Elongation steps in protein synthesis. The first and second cycles of elongation are shown. In *Step A*, aminoacyl-tRNA is placed in the ribosomal A site, beside the P site methionyl-tRNA of the completed initiation complex. In *Step B* the first peptide bond is formed, and in *Step C* the mRNA-peptidyl tRNA complex is translocated to the P site while the deacylated initiator tRNA is moved to the E site. Binding of the next aminoacyl-tRNA (*Step D*) may cause release of deacylated tRNA from the E site, or it may remain in place during peptide bond formation (*Step E*) and then be displaced during translocation (*Step F*). Additional amino acids are added by successive repetition of Steps D-F. *EF* = elongation factors. (Redrawn with permission from Devlin T: *Textbook of Biochemistry with Clinical Correlations.* New York: Wiley-Liss, 1992, p. 740. Adapted with permission of Wiley-Liss, Inc., a division of John Wiley & Sons, Inc.)

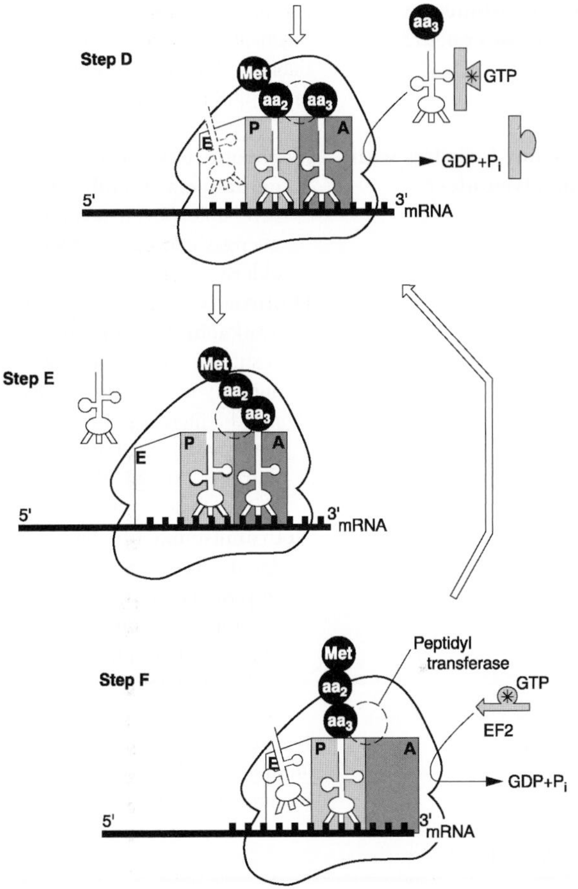

Figure 44–1. *(continued)*

Enterobacter, and *Klebsiella.* They can also be used against *Pseudomonas aeruginosa.* The **aminoglycosides do not cover anaerobes** because oxidative metabolism is required for uptake of these drugs. Frequently, aminoglycosides are coadministered with β-lactams to extend the spectrum and take advantage of the synergism between these two classes of drugs.

How does resistance to aminoglycosides occur?

Through plasmid-mediated formation of inactivating enzymes called transferases; decreased uptake of the drug or altered target 30S ribosomal subunit.

Are there any toxicities with the aminoglycosides?

Nephrotoxicity—More often seen with **gentamicin** and **tobramycin**. Usually reversible. Severe acute tubular necrosis may occur, especially in the elderly

Ototoxicity—More likely with **amikacin**. **Irreversible** toxicity to vestibular (more common) and auditory nerves. Ototoxicity may be increased by concurrent use of loop diuretics. Ami**NO**glycosides Nephrotoxicity—Ototoxicity

Neuromuscular blockade— Aminoglycosides may cause respiratory paralysis after larger-than-recommended doses due to inhibition of presynaptic release of acetylcholine and postsynaptic sensitization to acetylcholine.

Because of the severe side effects of aminoglycosides, it is absolutely critical to monitor peak and trough plasma levels.

TETRACYCLINES

Give some examples of tetracyclines.

Tetracycline (Sumycin)
Doxycycline (Vibramycin)
Demeclocycline (Declomycin)
Minocycline (Minocin)

Describe the mechanism of action of the tetracyclines.

Tetracyclines bind reversibly to the 30S subunit of bacterial ribosomes, **blocking aminoacyl transfer RNA** from entering the acceptor site on the mRNA-ribosomal complex (see Figure 44–1).

What is the antibiotic spectrum of the tetracyclines?

Tetracyclines are broad-spectrum antibiotics that are bacteriostatic for many Gram-positive and Gram-negative bacteria, including anaerobes, chlamydiae, mycoplasmas, and rickettsiae.

What are the clinical uses of tetracyclines?

They are still considered first-line agents for rickettsial infections, *Mycoplasma pneumoniae, Chlamydia,* and Lyme disease. Demeclocycline has been used in the treatment of the syndrome of inappropriate secretion of antidiuretic hormone (SIADH).

How are the tetracyclines administered and distributed?

They are adequately absorbed after oral administration *except* after the consumption of dairy foods, iron-containing preparations, or antacids that contain Ca^{2+}, Al^{3+}, Mg^{2+}, or Fe^{2+}. Tetracyalines distribute adequately into most tisssues but not the CSF. **Minocycline** is a notable exception which does penetrate the CSF.

Describe the metabolism of the tetracyclines.

Tetracyclines are metabolized in the liver and are ultimately excreted in urine, but **doxycycline** is a notable exception; it is excreted via the GI tract.

How does resistance to tetracyclines develop?

Bacteria can develop resistance through three primary mechanisms:
1. Inability of the drug to accumulate intracellularly, either through an increased efflux by an active transport protein pump or diminished influx. *This mechanism is the most important of the three to remember.*
2. Inability of the drug to bind to the bacterial ribosome
3. Enzymatic destruction of the drug

List the adverse effects of tetracycline administration.

GI effects—Nausea and vomiting are the most common symptoms. However, pseudomembraneous colitis caused by an overgrowth of *C. difficile* is a potentially life-threatening complication. Fortunately, it is rare.

Bony structures and teeth—
Tetracyclines are readily deposited in bone and teeth during calcification, which can lead to discoloration and hypoplasia of teeth in growing children.

Liver toxicity—Patients who are pregnant or who have preexisting liver insufficiency may experience hepatic necrosis when given high doses of tetracyclines.

Photosensitivity—Demeclocycline and **doxycycaline** can induce hypersensitivity to sunlight or ultraviolet light.

Vestibular reactions—Dizziness, nausea, and vomiting can occur with **minocycline** or **doxycycline** administration.

Renal toxicity—Fanconi's syndrome, which is characterized by nausea, vomiting, polyuria, polydipsia, proteinuria, and acidosis has been attributed to the use of outdated and degraded tetracyclines. Pseudotumor cerebri may occur on rare occasions.

Name major contraindications to the use of tetracyclines.	Pregnancy, nursing mothers, young children

SPECTINOMYCIN (TROBICIN)

What is spectinomycin?	An aminocyclitol antibiotic that is structurally related to aminoglycosides
Describe the mechanism of action.	It binds to the 30S ribosomal subunit and inhibits protein synthesis.
What is spectinomycin's route of administration?	IM
State the clinical use of spectinomycin.	This drug is used as an alternative treatment for *Neisseria gonorrhoeae* in patients who are allergic to **ceftriaxone** or who have a resistant strain of gonorrhea.

The **spect**rum of **spect**inomycin is narrow— it covers only *Neisseria.*

What are the adverse effects?	Pain at the injection site Occasional fever with nausea

CHLORAMPHENICOL (CHLOROMYCETIN)

Describe chloramphenicol.

It is a bacterio*static* broad-spectrum antibiotic.

What is its mechanism of action?

It binds reversibly to the 50S ribosomal subunit and inhibits protein synthesis during the peptidyl transferase reaction (see Figure 44–1).

What is chloramphenicol effective against?

It is active against both aerobic and anaerobic Gram-positive and Gram-negative organisms as well as *Rickettsia. Haemophilus influenzae, Neisseria meningitidis,* and *Bacteroides* species are particularly susceptible to **chloramphenicol**. Despite this wide range of coverage, **chloramphenicol** is used very rarely because of its serious side effects.

How does resistance to this drug develop?

Clinically significant resistance is due to bacterial production of chloramphenicol acetyltransferase, an enzyme that inactivates **chloramphenicol** or decreases penetration of the drug.

Describe the absorption and metabolism of this drug.

Chloramphenicol is absorbed orally or through IV and metabolized in the liver. It inhibits the cytochrome P450 system.

Are there adverse reactions?

Yes. The clinical use of **chloramphenicol** has declined because of the serious adverse effects associated with its administration, which include:
"Gray-baby syndrome," which is characterized by cyanosis, vomiting, green stools, and vasomotor collapse

caused by the accumulation of unmetabolized drug. (The neonatal liver has not yet synthesized sufficient glucuronidase to detoxify many drugs.)
Bone marrow suppression
Aplastic anemia (rare but can be fatal)
Hemolytic anemia in G6PD deficiency

MACROLIDES/KETOLIDES

Which drugs are included in this category?

Erythromycin (E-Mycin)—the prototypical macrolide
Clarithromycin (Biaxin)
Azithromycin (Zithromax)
Azithromycin and **clarithromycin** are newer derivatives of **erythromycin**. **Telithromycin** (Protek) belongs to the ketolide class of drugs.

How do macrolides/ketolides work?

By binding to the 50S ribosome and inhibiting the translocation step of protein synthesis (see Figure 44–1). This action is bacteriostatic for some organisms, bactericidal for others. The principle difference of the ketolide is in the structural modification within the ketolide itself that neutralizes the resistance mechanisms that make macrolides ineffective.

Is there a difference between erythromycin's antibacterial activity and that of clarithromycin, azithromycin, and talithromycin?

Yes. **Erythromycin** acts upon many of the same organisms as penicillin and, therefore, can be used as an alternative for penicillin-allergic patients. It is also effective against *Mycoplasma, Legionella, C. trachomatis Corynebacterium diphtheriae,* and *B. pertussis*.
Clarithromycin extends the spectrum by including *H. influenzae* and *N. gonorrhea, Helicobacter pylori* and *Mycobacterium avium intracellulare*.
Azithromycin generally is less effective than erythromycin against Gam positives

but more active against respiratory infections from microbes such as *H. influenzae* and *M. catarrhalis*. It is also first-line for *Mycobacterium avium-intacellulare* complex in AIDS patients.Urethritis as a result from *C. Trachomatis* infection responds very well to azithromycin.

Telithromycin has a spectrum nearly encompassing both clarithromycin and azithromycin. It is primarily used for respiratory tract infections such as bronchitis, acute sinusitis, and drug-resistant *S. pneumonia*.

How does resistance to the macrolides develop?	Through at least two different mechanisms: 1. Defective uptake or efflux of the drug by the microbe 2. Bacterial plasmids coding for enzymes that inactivate these drugs
What is the route of administration?	Oral for all, plus IV for **erythromycin** and **azithromycin**
How are macrolides/ketolides metabolized?	By the cytochrome P-450 system. **Erythromycin** and **telithromycin** in particular inhibit this system.
Are any adverse effects associated with the macrolides?	Yes—epigastric distress (nausea, vomiting, diarrhea), cholestatic hepatitis Cholestatic hepatitis: most commonly seen with the estolate form of erythromycin Allergic reactions have also been noted (skin rashes, eosinophilia).
What are telithromycin's adverse effects?	Nausea and vomiting most common Visual disturbances rarely May worsen myasthenia gravis May cause a significant QTc prolongation and increased risk of arrhythmia
What are the drug-drug interactions?	Avoid using **erythromycin telithromycin** with **theophylline**, oral

anticoagulants, or **cisapride**; it will increase the serum concentrations of these drugs. Many other drugs that are metabolized through the P450 system will interact as well.

LINCOSAMIDES

Name two lincosamides.

Clindamycin—toxic;
Lincomycin—no longer used

What is lincomycin (Lincocin)?

An antibiotic elaborated by *Streptomyces lincolnensis* that resembles **erythromycin**

What is clindamycin (Cleocin)?

A chlorine derivative of **lincomycin**

How does clindamycin work?

This drug is a bacteriostatic agent that binds to the 50S ribosomal subunit and inhibits protein synthesis by interfering with aminoacyl translocation steps (see Figure 44–1).

What is the route of administration for clindamycin?

PO

How is clindamycin metabolized?

Through both renal and hepatic routes

What is clindamycin's clinical use?

It is usually used to treat severe infections by anaerobic bacteria such as *Bacteroides fragilis.* Streptococci, staphylococci, and pneumococci are also inhibited. *Clostridium perfringens* is also affected.

Does this drug readily enter the CNS?

No, but it does penetrate other body fluids well.

What are the side effects?

Pseudomembranous colitis—
Lincosamides destroy the normal intestinal flora, which allows *Clostridium difficile* to grow and secrete its toxin, causing a bloody diarrhea. Treatment of this condition includes **metronidazole** or oral **vancomycin**.

Diarrhea

Granulocytopenia

Skin rashes

45

Quinolones and Drugs Used to Treat Urinary Tract Infections

QUINOLONES

List two members of this drug class.

1. **Nalidixic acid**—1st developed quinolone
2. **Cinoxacin**

Why do the quinolones have limited use?

They are useful only as urinary antiseptics because they do not reach systemic bactericidal levels and rapidly develop resistance. They have largely been replaced by the fluoroquinolones.

FLUOROQUINOLONES

Name several drugs in this class.

1. **Norfloxacin** (Noroxin), the first fluoroquinolone
2. **Levofloxacin** (Levaquin)
3. **Ciprofloxacin** (Cipro)
4. **Ofloxacin** (Floxin)
5. **Sparfloxacin** (Zagam)
6. **Moxifloxacin** (Avelox)
7. **Gatifloxacin** (Tequin)

There are many more; they can be recognized by the "ox" in their names.

What is the advantage of fluoroquinolones over quinolones?

The fluoroquinolones achieve a much higher concentration in the bloodstream and are therefore **bactericidal** against systemic organisms.

What is the pharmacological mechanism of action of fluoroquinolones?

They inhibit DNA gyrase and topoisomerase IV, thus blocking bacterial DNA synthesis.

Describe the distribution of the fluoroquinolones.	These drugs are well absorbed and widely distributed in body fluids, tissue, and bone but not the CNS.
What is the activity of the fluoroquinolones?	They are broad-spectrum agents active against Gram-positive and Gram-negative bacteria, including *Pseudomonas*, *Shigella*, *Campylobacter*, *Neisseria*, *Escherichia coli*, *Chlamydia*, *Mycoplasma*, *Brucella*, and *Legionella*). Methicillin-resistant strains of *Staphylococcus* are not well controlled. Anaerobes are generally resistant except against the newer fluoroquinolones, such as **moxifloxacin** and **gatifloxacin**. These newer agents have excellent activity against Gram-positive organisms while retaining their Gram-negative coverage. They are also effective for *S. pneumoniae* infections
What are the major uses of fluoroquinolones?	Urinary tract infections (UTIs) Respiratory tract infections and ocular infections Gastrointestinal and abdominal infections—diarrhea Skin, bone, and soft tissue infections such as osteomyelitis Prostatitis Sexually transmitted diseases—gonococcal and chlamydial infections Diarrhea due to *Campylobacter*, *Salmonella*, *Shigella* toxin, and *E. coli*. **Trovafloxacin** is reserved for use against life-threatening infection such as pneumonia or intra-abdominal infection.
How are the fluoroquinolones eliminated?	Mainly by tubular secretion through the kidneys, although up to 20% can be metabolized by the liver
What are the adverse effects of fluoroquinolones?	CNS effects—headache, dizziness, insomnia

GI effects—diarrhea, nausea, abnormal liver function tests

Photosensitivity

Tendinitis or tendon rupture in adults. Liver toxicity is associated with **trovafoxacin**.

Can fluoroquinolones be used in children?

No, because they cause cartilage erosion, which also rules out their use during pregnancy and nursing.

What is the route of administration of fluoroquinolones?

IV or PO

Does resistance develop against fluoroquinolones?

Yes, especially by *Staphylococcus, Pseudomonas,* and *Serratia.* Resistance develops through changes to the binding region of the fluoroquinolone target enzyme or because of a change in the penetration of the drug.

Are there any important drug-drug interactions?

Yes. Fluoroquinolones increase plasma theophylline levels. **Cimetidine** interferes with elimination of the fluoroquinolones.

URINARY ANTISEPTICS

NITROFURANTOIN (FURADANTIN)

What is nitrofurantoin?

An agent that is both bacteriostatic and bactericidal (at high doses) against Gram-positive and Gram-negative bacteria except for *Proteus* and *Pseudomonas*

What is its mechanism of action?

Nitrofurantoin alters various bacterial enzymes and bacterial DNA.

What is the clinical indication for nitrofurantoin?

UTI. Especially those caused by *E. coli.* Presently not used very often because of other more effective and less toxic agents.

What is the route of administration?

PO

How is nitrofurantoin metabolized?	It is excreted into the urine through glomerular filtration.

What are the side effects?

Anorexia, nausea, and vomiting—most common effects

Pulmonary infiltrates

Hemolytic anemia in patients with glucose-6-phosphate dehydrogenase deficiency

Neurological disorders such as polyneuropathies

Chronic active hepatitis—rare but serious side effect

Rashes

Brown urine

METHENAMINE

How does methenamine work?

At a pH of 5.5 or less in the urine, it decomposes to formaldehyde, which kills most bacteria.

What is the clinical indication for this drug?

Chronic suppressive treatment of lower urinary tract infections, especially when the organism is *E. coli*

What are the adverse effects?

GI distress

Hematuria and albuminuria at higher dose

46

Folate Antagonists

What is the biological role of folic acid?
It is an essential cofactor in purine, pyrimidine, and amino acid synthesis.

Can human cells absorb preformed folic acid?
Yes.

Can bacteria absorb preformed folic acid?
In general, bacteria must synthesize folic acid from pteridine and para-aminobenzoic acid (PABA). This is the basis for the selective toxicity of sulfonamides and trimethoprim. Some bacteria can use preformed folate and therefore are not affected.

SULFONAMIDES

Describe the structure of a sulfonamide compound.
It resembles PABA (Figure 46–1).

How do sulfonamides work?
Because they resemble PABA, they bind and competitively **inhibit dihydropteroate synthetase**, the enzyme responsible for combining PABA and pteridine. Subsequently, folic acid synthesis is terminated.

Give some examples of sulfonamides.
Sulfamethoxazole
Sulfisoxazole
Sulfamethizole
Sulfasalazine
Sulfacetamide
Silver sulfadiazine
Mafenide
Sulfadiazine

Are sulfonamides bactericidal?
No! They are bacteriostatic and therefore are most effective against rapidly growing organisms.

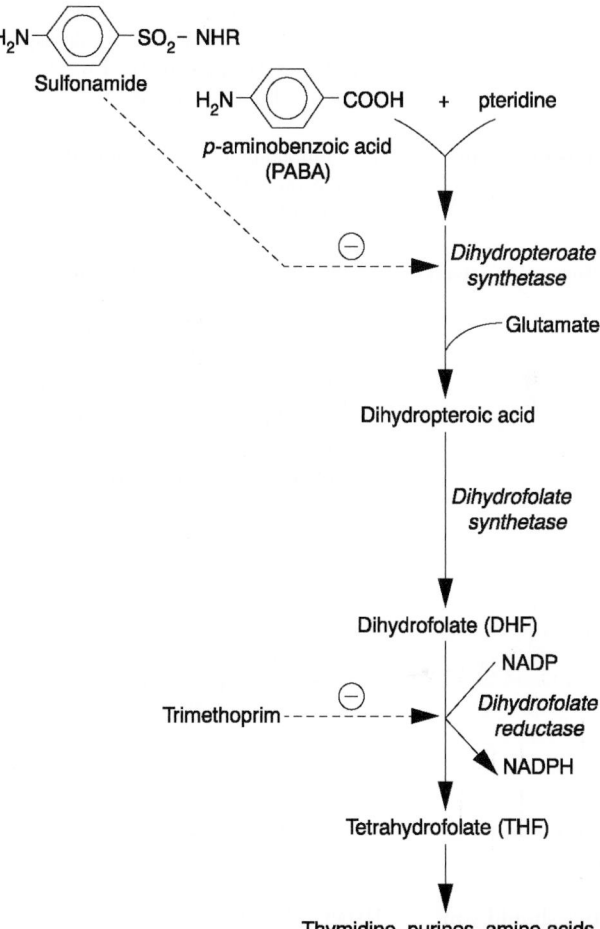

Figure 46–1. Action of folate inhibitors. (Redrawn with permission from Gallia G, Hann CL, Hewson WH: *The Pharmacology Companion.* La Jolla, CA: Alert & Oriented Publishing Company, 1997, p. 176, Fig. 5.3.)

What is the clinical spectrum of sulfonamides?

Gram-positive and Gram-negative organisms, including *Nocardia, Chlamydia, Escherichia coli, Klebsiella, Actinomyces,* and *Enterobacter*

What are the routes of administration and absorption for these drugs?

With few exceptions, all sulfa drugs are well absorbed after oral administration. They also can be given IV. Once absorbed they are largely bound to albumin. Sulfa drugs, in fact, will displace bilirubin and other drugs that were previously bound to albumin.

Do these drugs enter the CNS?

Yes! Sulfonamides easily penetrate the CNS, even in the absence of inflammation.

How are sulfonamides used clinically?

Sulfonamides are used to treat many different diseases, but they are most often used for the following (drugs of choice are indicated):

Simple urinary tract infections due to *E. coli* and *Klebsiella* (they are not effective against *Pseudomonas*)—**sulfisoxazole, sulfamethoxazole**

Ulcerative colitis—**sulfasalazine** (best because it is poorly absorbed)

Burn infections—**silver sulfadiazine**

Ocular infections, especially by *Chlamydia trachomatis*—**sulfacetamide**

Nocardiosis—**sulfisoxazole**

Toxoplasmosis—**sulfadiazine** in combination with **pyrimethamine**, first-line therapy

Where are sulfonamides metabolized?

Sulfonamides are acetylated in the liver.

What toxicities should you watch for in prescribing sulfonamides to your patients?

Hypersensitivity—allergic reactions, rashes, exfoliative dermatitis, photosensitivity

Stevens-Johnson syndrome

Gastrointestinal effects—nausea, vomiting, and diarrhea

Hematotoxicity—Hemolytic anemia may occur in patients with glucose-6-phosphate dehydrogenase deficiency. Agranulocytosis and aplastic anemia have also been reported but are very rare.

Crystalluria/hematuria—Adequate hydration and alkalinization of the urine prevents this problem, which is primarily seen with older sulfonamides such as **sulfadiazine**.

Kernicterus—In newborns, sulfonamides will displace bilirubin from albumin. The excess bilirubin penetrates the CNS and causes this condition.

Remember the mnemonic **CRANK**—**C**rystalluria, **R**ashes, **A**nemia, **N**ausea, **K**ernicterus

Should pregnant women be given sulfonamides?	No! Sulfa drugs will cross into the placenta and breast milk and therefore are contraindicated for pregnant and nursing women.
What drug interactions should you be particularly aware of in prescribing sulfonamides?	Patients who are also taking oral hypoglycemic agents or warfarin may experience a potentiation of effects from these drugs owing to displacement from serum albumin.
How does resistance to sulfonamides occur?	Resistance may occur in one of three ways: 1. Decreased intracellular accumulation of the drug 2. Increased production of PABA 3. A change in the sensitivity of dihydropteroate synthetase to the sulfonamides

TRIMETHOPRIM

How does it work?	**Trimethoprim** stops the conversion of dihydrofolate to tetrahydrofolate by inhibiting the enzyme **dihydrofolate reductase** (see Figure 46–1).
What is the route of administration?	PO
Is this drug commonly used alone?	No. **Trimethoprim** is most often combined with **sulfamethoxazole** or

another **sulfonamide**; together, the two drugs are synergistic.

What can the trimethoprim/sulfamethizole combination drug (Bactrim, Septra) be used for?

The antibacterial spectrum and the clinical indications are greater than when a **sulfonamide** or **trimethoprim** is used alone. The most important uses include:
Complicated or recurrent urinary tract infections (UTIs)
Pneumonia—drug of choice for pneumonia caused by *Pneumocystis carinii;* sometimes given in a nebulized or vaporized form
Bacterial prostatitis
Salmonella infections
Shigella
Gonorrhea
Sinusitis/bronchitis
Acute otitis media
Toxoplasmosis—second-line agent

Can this drug be used for chancroid, shigellosis, typhoid fever (due to *Salmonella typhi*), and nocardiosis?

Yes! **Trimethoprim/sulfamethoxazole** is effective against all these infections.

How do bacteria become resistant to trimethoprim/ sulfamethoxazole?

Several mechanisms could be involved, such as decreased uptake of the drug, increased concentrations of dihydrofolate reductase, or altering the structure of dihydrofolate reductase to reduce its affinity for the drug.

What are the adverse effects of trimethoprim/ sulfamethoxazole?

Dermatologic effects—rash, exfoliative dermatitis, urticaria. AIDS patients are especially susceptible to developing rashes.
Stevens-Johnson syndrome
Gastrointestinal effects—nausea, vomiting, glossitis, stomatitis
Hematological effects—agranulocytosis, megaloblastic anemia (in folate-deficient patients), hemolytic anemia
Headache
Depression

47

Antifungal Drugs

What is the structure of a fungus?	Fungi are eukaryotic organisms with rigid cell walls that contain chitin as well as polysaccharides.
What is a mycosis?	An infectious disease caused by a fungus. The infections can be systemic, subcutaneous, or superficial.

SYSTEMIC AND SUBCUTANEOUS MYCOSES

Name seven drugs used for systemic and subcutaneous mycoses.	1. **Amphotericin** B (Fungizone) 2. **Flucytosine** (Ancobon) 3. **Ketoconazole** (Nizoral) 4. **Fluconazole** (Diflucan) 5. **Itraconazole** (Sporanox) 6. **Voriconazole** (VFEND) 7. **Caspofungin** (Cancidas)

AMPHOTERICIN B

What is the classification of this drug?	**Amphotericin B** is a polyene antibiotic.
What is its importance?	It is the drug of choice for treating many systemic mycotic infections.
How does this drug work?	Fungal cells contain ergosterol, a sterol specific to fungal cell membranes. **Amphotericin B** binds to ergosterol and forms pores or channels within the membrane. This allows electrolytes to leak from the cell, which results in cell death (Figure 47–1).
Does amphotericin B bind to cholesterol?	No. Only ergosterol is affected by this drug.
Does amphotericin B enter the CNS?	No

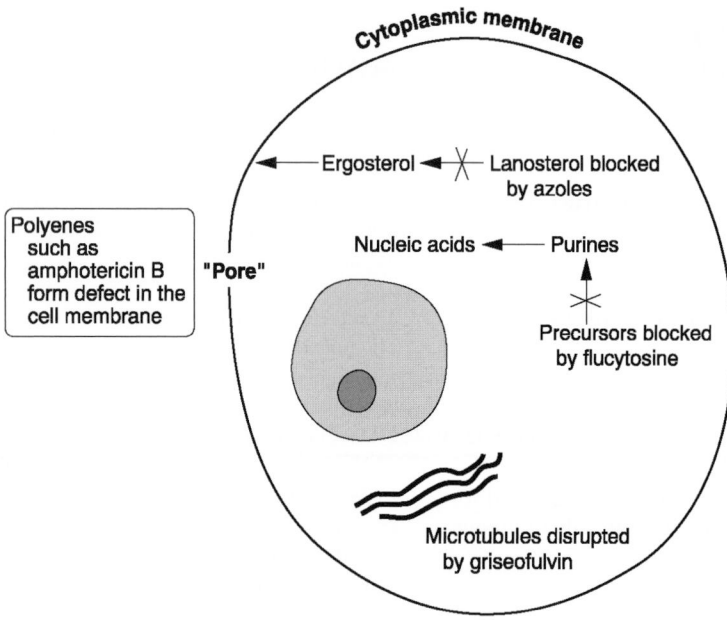

Figure 47–1. Sites of action of antifungal drugs.

What is this drug's antifungal spectrum?	**Amphotericin B** is effective against a broad spectrum of organisms including: *Candida* *Histoplasma capsulatum* *Cryptococcus neoformans* *Blastomyces dermatitidis* *Aspergillus* *Coccidioides immitis* *Mucormycosis*
What is the route of administration?	Usually IV; however, for fungal meningitis, intrathecal administration is required. A topical form of **amphotericin B** also exists.
What are its pharmacokinetics?	Amphotericin B is poorly absorbed from the gastrointestinal tract. Bile is the major route of excretion. A small part of the drug, however, is eliminated in the urine.

How does resistance occur?

Mustants replace ergosterol with other precursor sterols for the cell membrane.

What are adverse signs to watch for during administration?

Renal impairment—80% of patients exhibit a decreased glomerular filtration rate and changes in renal tubular function. This drug can cause a renal tubular acidosis. Newer liposomal formulations of **amphotericin B** can help reduce the renal toxicity.

Hypotension

Fever, chills ("shake and bake" syndrome)

Hypochromic normocytic anemia

Neurological effects

FLUCYTOSINE

What type of drug is flucytosine?

A synthetic pyrimidine antimetabolite. It is related in structure to an anticancer drug called **5-fluorouracil** (5-FU).

When is it used?

Flucytosine is used predominantly in conjunction with **amphotericin B** or **itraconazole**.

How does flucytosine work?

It enters fungal cells through a cytosine-specific permease and is first converted to 5-FU. Subsequently, it is converted to 5-fluorodeoxyuridine monophosphate (5-FdUMP). This acid inhibits thymidylate synthetase, which is an essential enzyme in the production of DNA (Figure 47–2). Mammalian cells do not convert **flucytosine** to 5-FU and therefore are not affected.

Is its antifungal spectrum broad or narrow?

Narrow; it affects only the following:

Candida

Cryptococcus neoformans

Agents causing chromomycosis

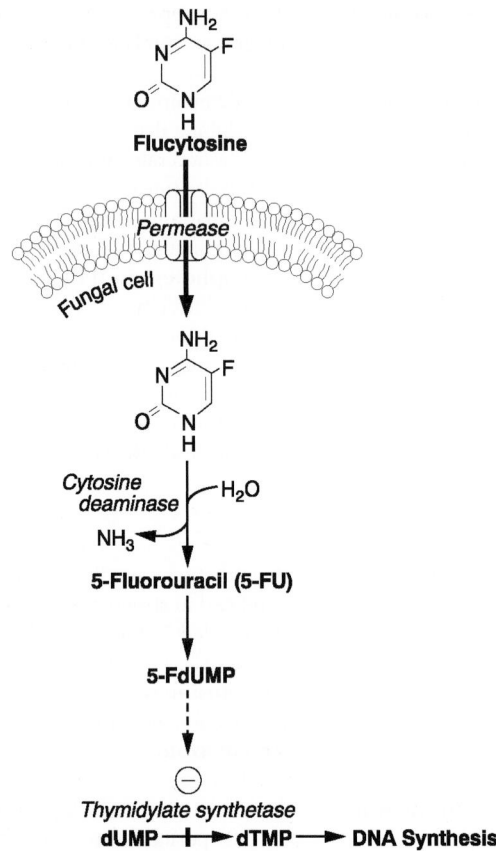

Figure 47–2. Mode of action of flucytosine. 5-FdUMP = 5-fluorodeoxyuridylic acid. dUMP = deoxyuridine monophosphate; dTMP = deoxythymidine monophosphate. (Redrawn with permission from Mycek MJ, Gertner SB, Perper MM [Harvey RA, Champe PC, eds.]. *Lippincott's Illustrated Reviews: Pharmacology,* 2nd ed. Philadelphia: Lippincott-Raven Publishers, 1997, p. 339.)

How is flucytosine usually administered?

PO

What are the pharmacokinetics of flucytosine?

Flucytosine distributes well throughout the tissues, including the cerebrospinal fluid (CSF). It is excreted intact in the urine.

What are the toxicities of this drug?

Hematological—reversible bone marrow depression leading to neutropenia and thrombocytopenia

Elevated hepatic enzymes

Gastrointestinal disturbances—nausea, vomiting, severe enterocolitis

KETOCONAZOLE

Into what category does this drug fit?

Ketoconazole is the prototypical azole used for systemic mycoses. Other drugs in this category include **fluconazole**, **itraconazole**, and **voriconazole**.

They all have the same mechanism of action but different therapeutic indications and pharmacokinetics. Their development provided a way to treat systemic infections orally.

How do the azoles work?

They block cytochrome P-450–mediated lanosterol demethylation to ergosterol. The specific enzyme that is blocked is called C-14-α demethylase.

What is ketoconazole's spectrum?

It is useful and mostly used as a second line agent against *Histoplasma, Candida, Cryptococcus, Blastomyces*, and dermatophytes. It has largely been replaced by **itraconazole** for the treatment of all mycoses because of increased effectiveness and reduced toxicities.

How is this drug administered?

PO only

What are its pharmacokinetics?

Ketoconazole depends on gastric acidity to be dissolved and absorbed; drugs such as **cimetidine** and antacids impair its absorption. **Ketoconazole** is metabolized in the liver and excreted through the bile.

What are ketoconazole's major toxicities?

Gynecomastia and decreased libido due to inhibition of testosterone and cortisol synthesis

GI distress—nausea, vomiting

Hepatic dysfunction—inhibits cytochrome P-450 system

Allergies

State contraindications to the use of this drug.

Never use **ketoconazole** and **amphotericin B** together—they antagonize each other's actions.

FLUCONAZOLE

What are the major advantages of fluconazole over ketoconazole?

Fluconazole can enter the CSF in high concentrations and is not dependent on acidic pH for absorption. It also does not cause the endocrine dysfunction seen with **ketoconazole**.

What are the therapeutic uses of fluconazole?

Disseminated or progressive coccidioidal infections such as meningitis—drug of choice

Disseminated histoplasmosis

Oral, esophageal, and vaginal candidiasis. Also candidemia of the nonimmunosuppressed patient.

Prophylaxis of cryptococcal meningitis in AIDS patients whose infection has been controlled by **amphotericin B**

How is it administered and excreted?

Orally or IV. Eliminated through the kidneys.

What toxicities are associated with fluconazole?

Nausea and vomiting

Headache

Skin rash

Can inhibit the cytochrome P450 system responsible for the metabolism of several other drugs such as cyclosporine, warfarin, and phenytoin.

Similar to most azoles, do not administer to pregnant women.

ITRACONAZOLE

What is itraconazole's therapeutic use?

Itraconazole is the drug of choice for patients with indolent nonmeningeal infections of blastomycosis, histoplasmosis, coccidioidomycosis and cutaneous sporotrichosis.

Is it effective in CNS infections?

No, it does not easily penetrate the blood-brain barrier.

How can this drug be administered?

IV or oral

Where is it metabolized?

In the liver. It is a potent inhibitor of the cytochrome P450 system.

What are the adverse effects of itraconazole?

GI distress, hypertriglyceridemia, rash, hypokalemia, hypertension, and **hepatotoxicity**. It does not have the endocrinological side effects of ketoconazole.

VORICONAZOLE

When is voriconazole used?

This is one of the newer azoles with a broader spectrum than its predecessors. Currently it is reserved for use in invasive Aspergillosis, and life-threatening infections with *Fusarium* or *Scedosporium apiospermum*.

How is it administered?

Oral or IV

How is it metabolized?

Through the cytochrome P450 system. Drugs that induce or inhibit that system can cause dramatic changes in plasma concentrations of voriconazole. Coadministration of **rifampin** or **rifabutin** is contraindicated because of increased **voriconazole** metabolism.

What are its untoward effects?

Transient blurred vision or color perception has been reported shortly after administration. Hepatotoxicity occurs occasionally.
Rash

CASPOFUNGIN

What is it?	This drug is the prototype of a class of antifungals called echinocandins.
How does it work?	It inhibits cell wall synthesis by blocking the formation of $\beta(1,3)$-D-glucan.
How is it administered?	IV only.
What is it used for?	Invasive *Aspergillus* infections for patients who have failed therapy with other agents such as amphotericin B or Voriconazole.
Does it have any adverse effects?	Yes—phlebitis at the injection site and flushing from histamine release

SUPERFICIAL MYCOSES

Identify six major drugs used to treat superficial mycotic infections.	1. **Griseofulvin** (Fulvicin) 2. **Nystatin** (Mycostatin) 3. **Miconazole** (Monistat) 4. **Clotrimazole** (Canesten cream) 5. **Econazole** (Spectazole) 6. **Terbinafine** (Limisil)

GRISEOFULVIN

What is its mode of action?	**Griseofulvin** enters susceptible fungal cells and inhibits microtubule function (see Figure 47–1). With long-term therapy (weeks to months), this drug accumulates in the newly synthesized stratum corneum, making these cells undesirable for fungal growth.
What is the antifungal spectrum of this drug?	It is effective only against dermatophytes, including *Trichophyton, Microsporum,* and *Epidermophyton.* **Griseofulvin** has largely been replaced by **terbinafine** because it requires 6 to 9 months of therapy and is more toxic.

What are the pharmacokinetics of this drug?	**Griseofulvin** is absorbed well orally, especially with a high-fat diet, and distributed to the keratin-containing stratum corneum. It is eliminated through the bile.
State this drug's adverse effects.	Headache Hepatotoxicity GI irritation Rarely teratogenic or carcinogenic

NYSTATIN

What is the structure of drug?	**Nystatin** is a polyene similar in structure to amphotericin B, with the same mechanism of action. It creates pores in the cell membrane of the fungi.
What is the route of administration?	Topical for skin and mucocutaneous infections or oral for thrush
What is nystatin's therapeutic use?	Treatment of superficial *Candida* infections
What are its adverse effects?	Bitter taste, nausea

MICONAZOLE, CLOTRIMAZOLE, AND ECONAZOLE

What is the route of administration for these drugs?	Topical. They are highly toxic if used systemically.
Are other azole drugs used topically?	Yes. New drugs are being developed yearly. **Terconazole** and **butoconazole** are two of the more recently developed drugs, but they are all very similar drugs.
What are the indications for use?	Superficial infections of the skin and mucous membranes (vulvovaginitis). Effective against *Candida* and dermatophytoses
What are the pharmacological properties of these drugs?	They are very similar to **ketoconazole** in mechanism of action and spectrum.

What are the side effects? Since they are only given topically the most common adverse effects include itching, erythema, and burning.

TERBINAFINE

What is it used for? **Terbinafine** is a first-line agent used to treat dermatophyte infections, especially onychomycosis

What is its route of administration? Although it is used to treat superficial infections, it is given orally or topically.

How does it work? Inhibits an enzyme (squalene epoxidase) used to synthesize ergosterol. Accumulation of squalene is toxic to fungi

What are the toxic effects? Rash, headache and GI irritation. Rarely hepatotoxicity and neutropenia may occur. The drug is contraindicated in pregnancy.

48

Antiprotozoal Drugs

What are protozoa?

Unicellular organisms that commonly live as parasites

MALARIA

Which organism causes malaria?

Plasmodium species

Which *Plasmodium* species infect humans?

P. falciparum
P. malariae
P. ovale
P. vivax

What is the vector of transmission?

The female *Anopheles* mosquito

How are antimalarial drugs differentiated?

By the stage in the *Plasmodium* life cycle in which they are effective

What are the five stages in the *Plasmodium* life cycle?

1. A carrier mosquito injects the sporozoite into a human.
2. The sporozoite is transformed into a merozoite in the liver.
3. The merozoite enters into the bloodstream and parasitizes the erythrocytes. (At this stage, the organism is known as a blood schizont.)
4. Erythrocyte lysis occurs with release of gametocytes.
5. A noncarrier mosquito ingests gametocytes by biting an infected human.

Figure 48–1.

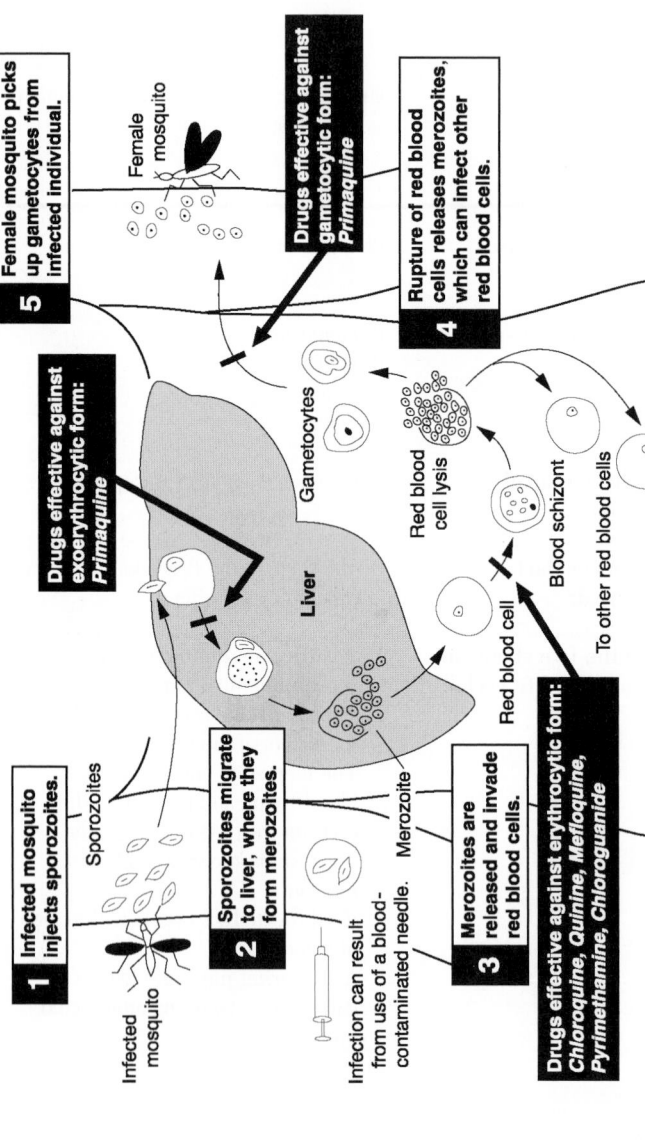

Figure 48–1. Life cycle of the malarial parasite showing the sites of action of antimalarial drugs. (Redrawn with permission from Mycek MJ, Harvey RA, Champe PC [Harvey RA, Champe PC, eds.]. *Lippincott's Illustrated Reviews: Pharmacology,* 2nd ed. Baltimore: Lippincott-Raven Publishers, 1997, p. 350.)

Which *Plasmodium* species have a dormant hepatic (hypnozoite) stage that causes recurrent infections and relapses?

P. ovale and *P. vivax*

What drugs are used to treat malaria?

Chloroquine (Aralen)
Quinine (Quinamm)
Mefloquine (Lariam)
Pyrimethamine (Daraprim)
Pyrimethamine/sulfadoxine (Fansidar)
Atovaquone/proguanil (Malarone)
Primaquine

CHLOROQUINE (Aralen)

How does chloroquine work?

The mechanism of action is not known for certain, but it may include:
—Interfering with DNA and RNA synthesis
—Raising the pH of plasmodial vacuoles, which prevents the parasite from metabolizing red blood cell hemoglobin
—Blockade of plasmodial heme polymerase, which leads to the accumulation of toxic hemoglobin breakdown products

What is the route of administration?

PO

How is chloroquine distributed?

It penetrates the CNS and crosses the placenta. It concentrates in erythrocytes, liver, spleen, kidney, lung, leukocytes, and melanin-containing tissues.

How is chloroquine metabolized?

It is rapidly and completely absorbed and extensively dealkylated by the mixed-function oxidases.

What is its major clinical use?

It is used to treat acute attacks of malaria. Because chloroquine is a blood schizonticide, it will not eradicate hypnozoites and is therefore not useful for the treatment of relapsing malaria caused by *P. ovale* or *P. vivax*.

What other use does this drug have?

Chloroquine has anti-inflammatory effects and is sometimes used in autoimmune disorders.

What are chloroquine's adverse effects?

Low dose—GI upset, headache, rash (should not be used in patients with psoriasis or porphyria)

High dose—peripheral neuropathies, myocardial depression with ECG changes, retinal damage (requires routine ophthalmologic examinations), auditory impairment, and toxic psychosis

Long-term treatment—discoloration of the nail beds and mucous membranes; hemolytic anemia in patients with glucose-6-phosphate dehydrogenase (G-6-PD) deficiency

QUININE (Quinamm)

How does this drug work?

Quinine is a blood schizonticide that forms complexes with double-stranded DNA and prevents strand separation.

What is its route of administration?

Oral

How is quinine metabolized?

It is excreted renally.

What is this drug's clinical use?

It is used to treat malaria due to **chloroquine**-resistant species (usually in combination with **pyrimethamine** and a **sulfonamide**).

What are its adverse effects?

Cinchonism—nausea, vomiting, tinnitus, vertigo, headache, and blurred vision

Hemolytic anemia in G-6-PD–deficient patients

What is a rare complication that can occur in patients who have been sensitized to quinine?	Blackwater fever, in which massive red blood cell lysis leads to hemoglobinuria, which causes dark urine and renal failure. It is potentially fatal.

MEFLOQUINE (Lariam)

How does this drug work?	**Mefloquine** is a blood schizonticide with an unknown mechanism of action.
What is the route of administration?	PO
How is mefloquine distributed?	It concentrates in the liver and the lungs.
How is it metabolized?	It has a long half-life (17 days) owing to extensive enterohepatic recirculation and binding to tissue and plasma proteins. It is excreted in the feces.
What is this drug's clinical use?	It is used in the prophylaxis and treatment of **chloroquine**-resistant *P. falciparum.*
What are its adverse effects?	It is less toxic than **quinine**. However, it may cause nausea, vomiting, and dizziness; at high doses it may cause seizures, hallucinations, and depression.

PYRIMETHAMINE (Daraprim)

How does this drug work?	**Pyrimethamine** is a blood schizonticide that selectively inhibits plasmodial dihydrofolate reductase, thereby depriving the organism of tetrahydrofolate, a cofactor in the biosynthesis of purines and pyrimidines. **Pyrimethamine** can be combined with **sulfadoxine** to produce synergistic effects.
What is its route of administration?	PO

How is this drug metabolized?	It is excreted in the urine after partial metabolism.
What is its clinical use?	When combined with **sulfadiazine**, this drug is the treatment of choice for toxoplasmosis. It is mostly active against *P. falciparum.*
What are the adverse effects?	Folic acid deficiency in high doses Rash GI distress Hemolysis Renal damage

PYRIMETHAMINE/SULFADOXINE (Fansidar)

What is Fansidar's clinical use?	This combination agent is used against chloroquine-resistant species owing to its sequential blockade of two steps in folic acid synthesis.

ATOVAQUONE/PROGUANIL (Malarone)

How does this combination drug work?	The constituents of Malarone, **atovaquone** and **proguanil hydrochloride**, interfere with two different pathways involved in the biosynthesis of pyrimidines required for nucleic acid replication. **Atovaquone** is a selective inhibitor of parasite mitochondrial electron transport. **Proguanil hydrochloride** primarily exerts its effect by means of the metabolite **cycloguanil**, a dihydrofolate reductase inhibitor. Inhibition of dihydrofolate reductase in the malaria parasite disrupts deoxythymidylate synthesis.
What is its route of administration?	PO
How is it metabolized?	**Atovaquone** is excreted largely unchanged in the feces. **Proguanil** is mostly excreted through the urine.

What is chloroguanide's clinical use?	Prophylaxis and treatment of *P. falciparum* malaria.
Are there any adverse effects?	GI distress is the most common (abdominal pain, nausea, diarrhea, vomiting) Headache, dizziness Do not use in patients with severe renal impairment.

PRIMAQUINE

How does this drug work?	**Primaquine** is a tissue schizonticide and gametocide that forms redox compounds that act as cellular oxidants.
What is its route of administration?	It is administered orally.
How is the drug metabolized?	It undergoes rapid oxidative biotransformation. Metabolites exert the schizonticidal effect and are excreted in the urine.
What is its clinical use?	**Primaquine** is used to treat relapsing malaria; it eradicates the liver stages of *P. vivax* and *P. ovale* (primary as well as secondary exoerythrocytic forms). It is also gametocidal for all four *Plasmodium* species and can therefore be used to interrupt transmission of the disease.
Is primaquine effective in treating acute attacks?	No; therefore it must be used in conjunction with a blood schizonticide such as **chloroquine**.
What are its adverse effects?	Methemoglobinemia GI distress Headaches Pruritus Hemolytic anemia in G-6-PD deficiency Granulocytopenia Agranulocytosis (rare)

TOXOPLASMOSIS

What organism causes toxoplasmosis?	*Toxoplasma gondii*
How is it transmitted to humans?	Ingestion of raw or undercooked infected meat Shedding of infectious oocysts by cats Transplacentally
What is the treatment of choice?	**Pyrimethamine** in combination with **sulfadiazine**

LEISHMANIASIS

Which organism causes leishmaniasis?	*Leishmania*
What is the vector of transmission?	Infected sandflies
What is the life cycle of *Leishmania*?	1. A sandfly transfers the flagellated promastigote from an infected animal or human to an uninfected one. 2. The promastigote is phagocytized by macrophages. 3. In the macrophage, the promastigote changes to a nonflagellated amastigote and multiplies, killing the cell. 4. The released amastigotes are phagocytized, and the cycle continues.
What is the drug of choice for the treatment of both mucocutaneous and visceral leishmaniasis?	**Sodium stibogluconate** (Pentostam)
How does this drug work?	Through inhibition of glycolysis at the phosphofructokinase reaction
What is its route of administration?	Parenteral (it is not absorbed orally)
How is this drug metabolized?	There is minimal metabolism, and it is excreted in the urine.

What are its adverse effects?	Pain at the injection site GI distress Cardiac arrhythmias
Which laboratory tests must be ordered during treatment?	Tests to monitor renal and hepatic function
What are alternative agents for the treatment of leishmaniasis?	**Pentamidine**—visceral leishmaniasis **Metronidazole** (Flagyl)—cutaneous lesions **Amphotericin B**—mucocutaneous leishmaniasis

TRYPANOSOMIASIS

Which organisms cause trypanosomiasis?	*Trypanosoma cruzi*—American sleeping sickness (Chagas' disease) *T. brucei* (subspecies *gambiense* and *rhodesiense*)—African sleeping sickness
What drugs are used to treat trypanosomiasis?	**Melarsoprol** (Mel B) **Pentamidine** (Pentam) **Nifurtimox** (Lampit) **Suramin** (Antrypol)

MELARSOPROL (Mel B)

How does this drug work?	**Melarsoprol** inhibits sulfhydryl groups in parasitic enzymes.
What is the route of administration?	IV or PO
How is it distributed?	Into the CNS
What is its metabolism?	It is oxidized by the host to a nontoxic compound. It has a very short half-life and is rapidly excreted in the urine.
What is its clinical use?	It is the drug of choice for the treatment of African sleeping sickness with CNS involvement.

What are the adverse effects?	Encephalopathy GI distress (avoided if patient is fasting during administration) Hypersensitivity reactions Hemolytic anemia in G-6-PD–deficient patients
Are there any contraindications to the use of melarsoprol?	It cannot be used in patients who have influenza.

PENTAMIDINE (Pentam)

How does this drug work?	The mechanism of action is unknown. **Pentamidine** is concentrated in *T. brucei* by a high-affinity uptake system, and the drug is thought to either bind to the organism's DNA or inhibit glycolysis.
What is its route of administration?	IM or aerosol. IV administration may lead to hypotension and tachycardia.
How is pentamidine distributed?	It *does not* enter the CNS but is concentrated in the liver and kidneys.
What is its metabolism?	This drug has a 2- to 4-week half-life and is excreted unchanged in the urine.
What is the major clinical use for pentamidine?	It is the drug of choice for hemolymphatic stages of African sleeping sickness (not effective for the CNS stage).
For what other condition is this drug used?	The aerosol form is used for prophylaxis and treatment of *Pneumocystis carinii* pneumonia that is refractory to trimethoprim/sulfamethoxazole.
List the adverse effects.	Reversible nephrotoxicity Respiratory stimulation followed by depression Pancreatic cell dysfunction

NIFURTIMOX (Lampit)

How does this drug work?

Nifurtimox forms intracellular oxygen radicals which are toxic to the organism.

What is the route of administration?

Oral

How is nifurtimox metabolized?

It is rapidly absorbed and metabolized; by-products are renally excreted.

What is this drug's clinical use?

It is the drug of choice for American sleeping sickness (Chagas' disease); it is also effective for mucocutaneous leishmaniasis.

Does nifurtimox cure Chagas' disease?

No! It is suppressive, not curative.

What are the adverse effects?

Anaphylaxis
Dermatitis and icterus
GI irritation
Peripheral neuropathy
CNS disturbances
Suppression of cell-mediated immunity

SURAMIN (Antrypol)

How does this drug work?

Through inhibition of enzymes involved in energy metabolism

What is the route of administration?

IV

What are suramin's clinical uses?

Prophylaxis and treatment of early stages (without CNS involvement) of African sleeping sickness
In combination with diethylcarbamazine, the drug of choice for treating infection by *Onchocerca volvulus*

What are the adverse effects?

Albuminuria
Rash
GI distress—nausea and vomiting
Urticaria

Neurological complications—
paresthesias, photophobia, palpebral
edema, hyperesthesia
Shock

Are there any indications to discontinue the drug?

Yes—renal casts in the urine

AMEBIASIS

What organism causes amebiasis (amebic dysentery)?

Entamoeba histolytica

Describe the six stages of this organism's life cycle.

1. Ingestion of cysts
2. Formation of trophozoites in the intestinal lumen
3. Trophozoite penetration into the intestinal wall
4. Trophozoite multiplication within the colonic wall
5. Systemic invasion
6. Infective cysts expelled in feces
Figure 48–2

How are amebicides classified?

Mixed—effective against lumenal and systemic disease
Lumenal—effective only in the bowel lumen
Systemic—effective in the intestine and liver

Which amebicides are mixed?

Metronidazole (Flagyl)

Which amebicides are lumenal?

Diloxanide furoate (discontinued in U.S. market)
Paromomycin (Humatin)
Iodoquinol (Diodoquin)
Tetracycline

Which amebicides are systemic?

Emetine
Dehydroemetine
Chloroquine (Aralen)

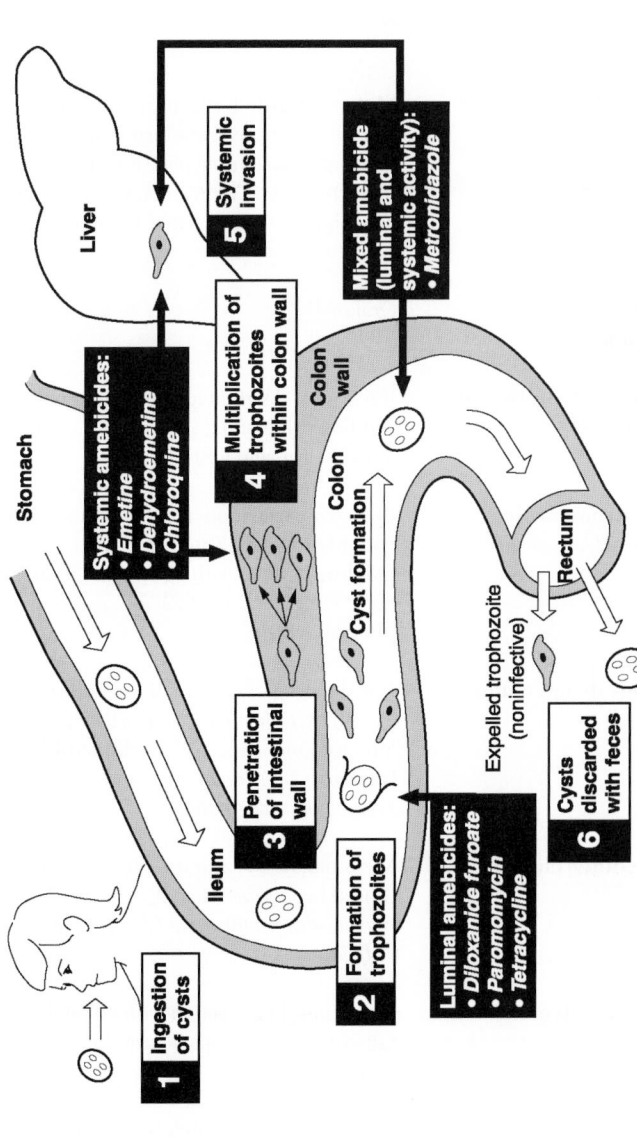

Figure 48–2. Life cycle of *Entamoeba histolytica* showing sites of action of amebicides. (Redrawn from Mycek MJ, Harvey RA, Champe PC [Harvey RA, Champe PC, eds.]. *Lippincott's Illustrated Reviews: Pharmacology*, 2nd ed. Baltimore: Lippincott-Raven Publishers, 1997, p. 346.)

METRONIDAZOLE (FLAGYL)

What action does this drug have?

Metronidazole is selectively toxic to amebae, anaerobes, and anoxic/hypoxic cells.

How does this drug work?

Metronidazole has a nitro group that receives electrons from ferredoxin (present in anaerobic parasites) in a redox reaction. The resultant compound binds both to proteins and DNA and is cytotoxic.

What is the route of administration?

Oral or IV

What is the distribution of metronidazole?

It is widely distributed throughout tissues and fluids, including seminal and vaginal fluids, saliva, and CSF.

How is metronidazole metabolized?

By hepatic oxidation and glucuronidation. Its rate of metabolism is increased when the drug is given with agents that induce hepatic metabolism (such as **phenobarbital**).

What is this drug's major clinical use?

It is the drug of choice for infections caused by *E. histolytica* (usually with a lumenal amebicide such as **diloxanide furoate**), *Giardia lamblia,* and *Trichomonas vaginalis.*

Are there other clinical uses?

Metronidazole is also used for infections caused by *Gardnerella vaginalis, Bacteroides fragilis,* and *Clostridium difficile.*

What are the adverse effects?

Disulfiram-like reaction with ethanol
GI irritation—cramps, nausea, and vomiting
Metallic taste
Potentiation of **warfarin's** (Coumadin's) anticoagulation effects
Discoloration of urine
Oral moniliasis

	CNS disturbances—dizziness, vertigo, numbness, and paresthesias
Is metronidazole safe for pregnant women?	No! **Metronidazole** is teratogenic and should be avoided in pregnant women and nursing mothers.

PAROMOMYCIN (Humatin)

How does this drug work?	**Paromomycin** is an aminoglycoside antibiotic that causes protozoal cell membrane leakage. It also reduces the population of intestinal flora, which is a food source for the amebae.
What is the route of administration?	PO. Because this drug is not significantly absorbed from the GI tract, it only exhibits lumenal effectiveness.
What is this drug's clinical use?	Treatment of lumenal amebiasis
What are the adverse effects?	GI distress and diarrhea. Systemic absorption may result in headaches, dizziness, rash, and arthralgias.

IODOQUINOL (Diodoquin)

What is this drug's mechanism of action?	It is unknown.
What is it used for?	Asymptomatic amebiasis
What are its toxicities?	Headache Fever Diarrhea, nausea, and vomiting

TETRACYCLINE

How does this drug work?	**Tetracycline** is an antibiotic that eliminates the normal intestinal flora and therefore the ameba's main food source; it is not a direct amebicide.

What is the route of administration?	Oral
What substances decrease absorption?	Dairy foods and antacids that contain magnesium and aluminum, because they form nonabsorbable chelates with the drug
Are there any contraindications to the use of tetracycline?	Yes—it is contraindicated in children younger than 8 years of age and in pregnant women.
What is the clinical use for this drug?	**Tetracycline** is not highly effective when used alone; it is used mainly as an adjunct to other amebicides.

EMETINE AND DEHYDROEMETINE

How do these drugs work?	They inhibit protein synthesis by blocking ribosomal movement along mRNA.
Describe their distribution	They are distributed widely to tissues.
How are they metabolized?	By slow renal excretion
What is the clinical use?	Because of their severe toxicity, emetine and dehydroemetine are used only as backup treatment for severe intestinal or hepatic amebiasis in hospitalized patients.
What are the adverse effects?	Cardiotoxicity—arrhythmias, congestive heart failure Neuromuscular weakness Nausea Dizziness Rash Pain at injection site

CHLOROQUINE (Aralen)

What is this antimalarial drug's clinical use as it relates to amebiasis?	Treatment and prevention of amebic liver abscesses in conjunction with **metronidazole** and **diloxanide furoate**

49

Anthelmintic Drugs

What is a helminth?	"Helminth" is a Greek word meaning worm.
What are the classifications of helminths?	There are three classifications: 1. Nematodes (roundworms) 2. Trematodes (flukes) 3. Cestodes (tapeworms) The last two are types of flatworms.
Name six drugs used predominantly in the treatment of nematodes.	1. **Mebendazole** (Vermox) 2. **Thiabendazole** (Mintezol) 3. **Albendazole** (Zentel) 4. **Pyrantel pamoate** (Antiminth) 5. **Diethylcarbamazine** (Hetrazan) 6. **Ivermectin** (Mectizan) Table 49–1
Name a drug used predominantly in the treatment of cestodes and trematodes.	**Praziquantel**

ANTHELMINTICS FOR NEMATODES

MEBENDAZOLE (Vermox)

What infections are treated with mebendazole?	**Mebendazole** is the drug of choice for pinworm (*Enterobius vermicularis*) and whipworm (*Trichuris trichiura*). It is also very effective against *Necator americanus* (hookworm) and *Ascaris lumbricoides* (roundworm).
What is the mechanism of action?	**Mebendazole** interferes with the synthesis of parasite microtubules and decreases glucose uptake.
What is the route of administration?	PO. Very little of the drug is absorbed systemically.

Table 49–1. Drugs for the Treatment of Helminthic Infections

Infecting Organism	Drug of Choice	Alternative Drugs
Roundworms (nematodes)		
Ascaris lumbricoides (roundworm)	Pyrantel pamoate or mebendazole	Albendazole,[2] piperazine, or levamisole[2]
Trichuris trichiura (whipworm)	Mebendazole	Albendazole[2] or oxantel/pyrantel pamoate[1]
Necator americanus (hookworm); *Ancylostoma duodenale* (hookworm)	Pyrantel pamoate[2] or mebendazole	Albendazole[2] or levamisole[2]
Combined infection with *Ascaris*, *Trichuris*, and hookworm	Mebendazole or albendazole[2]	Oxantel/pyrantel pamoate[1]
Combined infection with *Ascaris* and hookworm	Mebendazole or pyrantel pamoate[2]	Albendazole[2]
Strongyloides stercoralis (threadworm)	Ivermectin[3]	Thiabendazole, albendazole[2,4]
Enterobius vermicularis (pinworm)	Mebendazole or pyrantel pamoate	Albendazole[2]
Trichinella spiralis (trichinosis)	Mebendazole[2,4] or thiabendazole[4]; add corticosteroids for severe infection	Albendazole[4,5]; add corticosteroids for severe infection
Cutaneous larva migrans (creeping eruption)	Albendazole[5] or ivermectin[2]	Thiabendazole
Visceral larva migrans	Thiabendazole[8] or albendazole[2]	Mebendazole[2,4] or ivermectin[4]
Angiostrongylus cantonensis	Levamisole[2,4] or thiabendazole[4]	Albendazole[2,4] or mebendazole[2,4]
Wuchereria bancrofti (filariasis); *Brugia malayi* (filariasis); tropical eosinophilia; *Loa loa* (loiasis)	Diethylcarbamazine[6]	Ivermectin[3,7]
Onchocerca volvulus (onchocerciasis)	Ivermectin	Suramin[7]
Dracunculus medinensis (guinea worm)	Metronidazole[2]	Thiabendazole[2] or mebendazole[2]

Flukes (trematodes)

Schistosoma haematobium (bilharziasis)	Praziquantel	Metrifonate[1]
Schistosoma mansoni	Praziquantel	Oxamniquine
Schistosoma japonicum	Praziquantel	
Clonorchis sinensis (liver fluke);	Praziquantel[2]	Albendazole[2,4] or mebendazole[2,4]
Opisthorchis species		
Paragonimus westermani (lung fluke)	Praziquantel[2]	Bithionol[7]
Fasciola hepatica (sheep liver fluke)		Praziquantel[2,8] or emetine or dehydroemetine[7]
Fasciolopsis buski (large intestinal fluke)	Praziquantel[2]	Tetrachloroethylene[1]
Heterophyes heterophyes; Metagoninus	Praziquantel[2]	Tetrachloroethylene[1]
yokogauai (small intestinal flukes)		

Tapeworms (cestodes)

Taenia saginata (beef tapeworm)	Praziquantel[2]	Mebendazole[2,4]
Diphyllobothrium latum (fish tapeworm)	Praziquantel[2]	
Taenia solium (pork tapeworm)	Praziquantel[2]	
Cysticercosis (pork tapeworm larval stage)	Albendazole	Praziquantel[2]
Hymenolepis nana (dwarf tapeworm)	Praziquantel[2]	
Hymenolepis diminuta (rat tapeworm);	Praziquantel[2]	
Dipylidium caninum		
Echinococcus granulosus (hydatid disease);	Albendazole	Mebendazole[2,8,1]
Echinococcus multilocularis		

[1]Not available in the United States but available in some other countries.
[2]Available in the United States but not labeled for this indication.
[3]Available in the United States from Merck Sharpe & Dohme.
[4]Effectiveness not established.
[5]Available in the United States.
[6]Available in the United States from Wyeth-Ayerst Laboratories.
[7]Available in the United States only from the Parasitic Disease Drug Service, Parasitic Diseases Branch, Centers for Disease Control and Prevention, Atlanta.
[8]Effectiveness is low
[9]A veterinary drug, not approved for human use
(Adapted from Katzung BG: *Basic and Clinical Pharmacology,* 7th ed. Stamford, CT, Appleton & Lange, 1998, p 863–864.)

Is mebendazole safe for pregnant women?

No! The drug has proved teratogenic in animal experiments, so it should not be given to pregnant women. In general, most anthelmintic drugs are not considered safe in pregnancy.

What are the adverse effects of mebendazole?

Adverse effects are usually mild. The most frequent complaints are GI disturbances such as nausea and vomiting. Intrahepatic cholestasis has also been reported.

THIABENDAZOLE (Mintezol)

What is this drug's mechanism of action?

Thiabendazole, like **mebendazole**, binds to tubulin and inhibits microtubule polymerization.

What is the route of administration?

PO

What is its therapeutic use?

Thiabendazole can be used for treatment of the following infections:
Strongyloides stercoralis (threadworm)
Cutaneous larva migrans caused by
    Ancylostoma species
Visceral larva migrans caused by *Toxocara*

What are the adverse effects of this drug?

The most important side effects of **thiabendazole** are:
CNS effects—tingling and numbness
GI effects—diarrhea, nausea, vomiting
Reactions caused by dying parasites—
    fever, chills, and lymphadenopathy,
    Stevens-Johnson syndrome (rare)

ALBENDAZOLE (Zentel)

What is this drug?

A relatively new broad-spectrum anthelmintic, which, along with **mebendazole** and **thiabendazole**, belongs to a family of drugs known as benzimidazoles.

What is albendazole's clinical use?	In the United States it is primarily used for cysticercosis and hydatid disease. *Also used to treat infections caused by Toxocara canis.*
How does it work?	**Albendazole** blocks glucose uptake, resulting in eventual depletion of the parasites' energy stores.
What are the adverse effects of albendazole?	The adverse effects are usually mild and include nausea, vomiting, and dizziness. When treating neurocysticercosis, however, mental changes, seizures, and hyperthermia can occur.

PYRANTEL PAMOATE (Antiminth)

What is this drug's therapeutic use?	**Pyrantel pamoate** is used for treating *Ascaris* infections; it can also be used for pinworms and hookworms.
How does it work?	**Pyrantel pamoate** acts as a depolarizing neuromuscular blocking agent that causes persistent activation of nicotinic acetylcholine receptors and thus paralysis of the worm.
What is the toxicity?	Toxic effects are usually transient and may include nausea, vomiting, headache, and rash.

DIETHYLCARBAMAZINE (Hetrazan)

What are the clinical indications for this drug?	**Diethylcarbamazine** is the drug of choice for the treatment of filariasis caused by *Wuchereria bancrofti*. It is also used as an alternative in the treatment of onchocerciasis.
What is its mechanism of action?	The precise mechanism is unknown; **diethylcarbamazine** is thought to decrease the muscular activity of the parasites.

What are the adverse effects?

Toxic effects are usually mild but may include headache, nausea, and vomiting. The Mazzotti reaction may occur in patients receiving treatment for onchocerciasis. This reaction occurs as a result of the effects of dying parasites and is characterized by pruritus, lymphadenopathy, hypotension, and tachycardia.

IVERMECTIN (Mectizan)

What is this drug's therapeutic use?

Ivermectin is the drug of choice for river blindness caused by *Onchocerca volvulus* and for strongyloidiasis caused by *Strongyloides stercoralis* (threadworm).

How does it work?

The drug intensifies GABA-mediated neurotransmission in nematodes and causes immobilization of parasites. **Piperazine** is another antihelmintic that works in a similar fashion to ivermectin. It is used for *Ascaris lumbricoides* infections.

Does ivermectin affect human GABA receptors?

No. In humans GABA receptors are located only in the brain, and ivermectin does not cross the blood-brain barrier.

What toxicities should you watch for?

Fever, headache, dizziness, and pruritus. These symptoms are usually of short duration and can be controlled.

ANTHELMINTICS FOR TREMATODES AND CESTODES

PRAZIQUANTEL (BILTRICIDE)

What is this drug's therapeutic use?

Praziquantel is the drug of choice for treatment of schistosomiasis (all species), certain tapeworm infections such as cysticercosis, and infections by trematodes (flukes).

What is the mechanism of action?

Praziquantel increases permeability of the cell membrane to calcium, which causes tetanic contraction of the trematode muscle and death of the trematode.

What is the route of administration?

PO. **Praziquantel** is rapidly absorbed after administration and distributes readily to the CNS.

How is it metabolized?

Praziquantel is metabolized in the liver and excreted through the urine.

What are the adverse effects?

Drowsiness, dizziness, nausea, headache

NICLOSAMIDE (NICLOCIDE)

What is it?

A drug previously used for cestode infections. Presently it is no longer on the U.S. market because it was found to cause cysticercosis in patients infected with *T. solium*.

50   Antiviral Drugs

Define *virus*.

A virus is an obligate intracellular parasite; its metabolic processes, such as synthesis of proteins and DNA, depend on the host cell.

Can all viruses be pharmacologically treated?

No. Most drugs cannot distinguish between host cell functions and viral functions. Therefore the drugs would cause significant toxicity to both.

List the steps in viral replication.

1. Absorption and penetration of host cells
2. Synthesis of early nonstructural proteins, such as nucleic acid polymerases
3. Synthesis of RNA and DNA
4. Synthesis of late structural proteins
5. Assembly of virus particles

Antiviral drugs usually inhibit one of these steps (Figure 50–1).

What is the easiest way to remember the antiviral drugs?

By classifying them according to which virus they attack

DRUGS USED TO TREAT HERPESVIRUS AND CMV INFECTION

Name five drugs used to treat herpesvirus and CMV infection.

1. Foscarnet
2. Ganciclovir
3. Idoxuridine
4. Vidarabine
5. Acyclovir
6. Cidofovir

"For herpes, **GIV acyclovir.**"

What pathogens are included in the herpesvirus family?

Herpes simplex virus types 1 and 2 (HSV-1 and HSV-2)

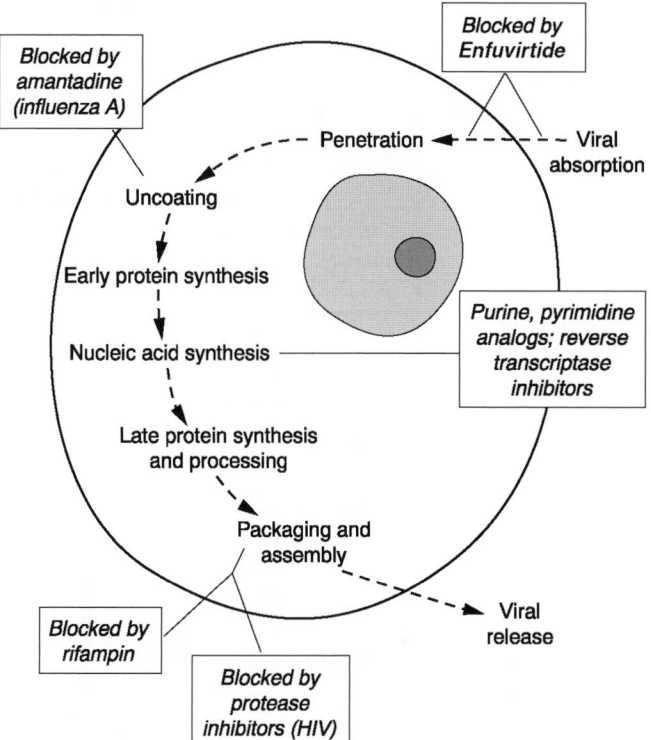

Figure 50–1. Sites of action of some antiviral drugs.

Varicella zoster virus
Cytomegalovirus (CMV)
Epstein-Barr virus

ACYCLOVIR (Zovirax)

What is it?	**Acyclovir** is a guanine analog.
What is its mechanism of action?	Acyclovir is monophosphorylated by a herpes enzyme called thymidine kinase. Later it is di- and triphosphorylated by the host cell. The active triphosphate form of acyclovir is then incorporated into viral DNA, which causes premature DNA-chain termination. (Figure 50–2).

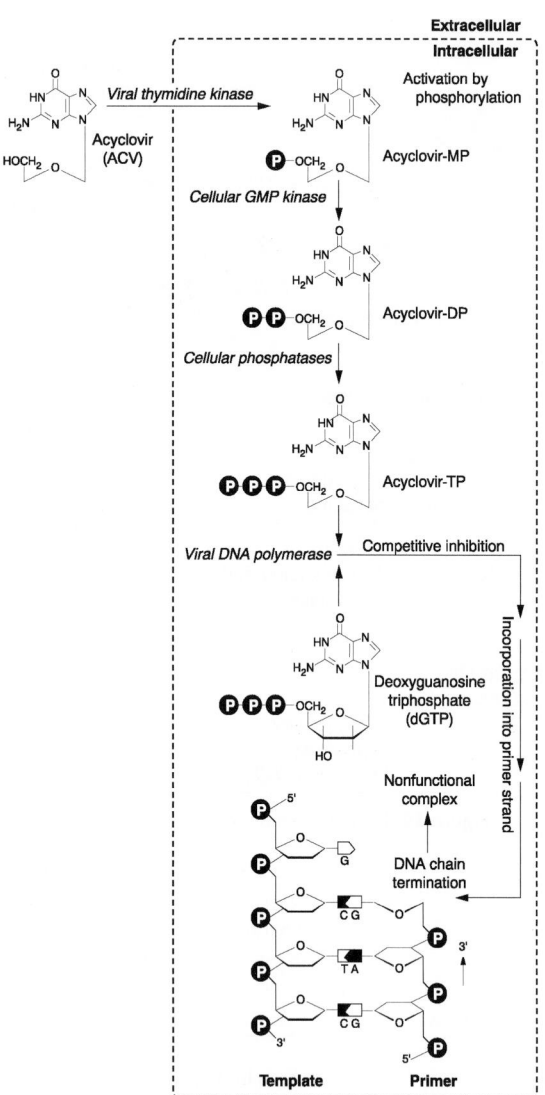

Figure 50–2. Conversion of acyclovir to acyclovir triphosphate, leading to DNA chain termination. Uninfected cells convert very little or no drug to the phosphorylated derivatives. Thus, acyclovir is selectively activated in cells infected with herpesviruses that code for appropriate thymidine kinases. Incorporation of acyclovir-MP from acyclovir-TP into the primer strand during viral DNA replication leads to chain termination and formation of an inactive complex with the viral DNA polymerase. (Redrawn with permission from Hardman JG, Limbird LE [eds.]. *Goodman and Gilman's The Pharmacological Basis of Therapeutics,* 9th ed. New York: McGraw-Hill, 1996, p. 1195.)

Since the initial step occurs through a herpesvirus enzyme, uninfected cells show little activation of the drug. This accounts for **acyclovir's** selective toxicity.

For what would you prescribe acyclovir?	HSV-1, which causes diseases of the mouth, face, eye, skin, esophagus, and brain HSV-2, which causes infections of the genitals, rectum, skin, hands, or meninges Varicella zoster virus

Are there any newer drugs that share similar characteristics to acyclovir?

Yes. They include:
Famciclovir: effective against recurrent genital herpes
Penciclovir: often used topically
Valacyclovir: long duration of action

What is the route of administration?

Intravenous, topical, or oral

What is its metabolism?

Acyclovir is partially metabolized to 9-carboxy methylguanide and excreted by the kidneys.

How does resistance occur?

Through mutations in the viral thymidine kinase.

Is it safe in pregnancy?

No. Acyclovir is secreted in breast milk and is a potential mutagen.

What are acyclovir's adverse effects?

This drug's adverse effects depend on the route of administration:
Intravenous—renal dysfunction and neurotoxicity (delirium, tremor, seizures)
Oral—diarrhea and headache
Topical—local irritation

GANCICLOVIR (Cytovene)

What is it?

Ganciclovir is a guanine analogue similar to acyclovir.
Ganciclovir—**G**uanine analog

How does ganciclovir work?	**Ganciclovir** works very similarly to acyclovir. It is triphosphorylated and then inhibits viral DNA polymerase. It is also incorporated into DNA, terminating chain elongation.
What are ganciclovir's clinical indications?	It is the drug of choice for treating CMV retinitis, pneumonia, and esophagitis. Also used for prophylaxis against CMV in transplant patients.
How is it given to patients?	Orally and IV. It absorbs well into the CNS. **Valganciclovir** is the L-valyl ester prodrug of **ganciclovir** and is preferred when the oral route is chosen.
How is ganciclovir metabolized?	The vast majority of the drug is excreted unchanged in the urine.
What are ganciclovir's adverse effects?	**Bone marrow suppression** CNS toxicity (mild headaches to seizures) Fever Hepatic dysfunction GI disturbances

TRIFLURIDINE (Viroptic)

What is trifluridine?	A thymidine analogue
What is its mechanism of action?	**Trifluridine** is converted into an active triphosphate form by cellular enzymes and is incorporated into DNA, making it more susceptible to breakage.
What are trifluridine's clinical uses?	Treatment of herpes simplex keratitis and vaccinia virus keratitis
What is its route of administration?	**Trifluridine** is administered only by ophthalmic solution or ointment.
What are the adverse effects of trifluridine?	Conjunctival irritation and photophobia

VIDARABINE (Vira-A)

What is it?	**Vidarabine** is an adenosine analog.
What is its mechanism of action?	Like **acyclovir**, **vidarabine** is converted into an active triphosphate form within the host cell and then inhibits viral DNA synthesis.
What is its clinical use?	**Vidarabine** is used to treat HSV-1 keratitis.
What is the route of administration?	**Vidarabine** is only available topically (ophthalmic).
Describe vidarabine's adverse effects.	Ocular irritation

FOSCARNET (Foscavir)

What type of drug is it?	**Foscarnet** is not a nucleoside analogue; it is a pyrophosphonate analogue that does not rely on phosphorylation for activation.
What is foscarnet's mechanism of action?	It inhibits replication by blocking the pyrophosphate binding site of viral DNA polymerase. It also works against HIV reverse transcriptase.
How is foscarnet administered?	Only by the intravenous route. It penetrates into the CNS.
What is its clinical use?	**Foscarnet** is used in the treatment of CMV infections including retinitus when **ganciclovir** fails. It has also been used against acyclovir-resistant HSV and VZV.
How is foscarnet metabolized?	It is excreted largely unchanged through the kidneys.
How does resistance to foscarnet occur?	Through point mutations in viral DNA polymerase.

What are foscarnet's adverse effects?	Nephrotoxicity Electrolyte abnormalities such as hypocalcemia and hypomagnesemia Seizures and other CNS toxicities such as tremor or headache

CIDOFOVIR (Vistide)

State the mechanism of action for cidofovir.	It is a cytosine analogue that is activated by host cell kinases not viral kinases and then incorporates itself into viral DNA. This results in inhibition of chain elongation.
In what clinical situations is cidofovir used?	CMV retinitis in HIV infected patients. It may prove beneficial even when a patient has failed therapy with ganciclovir or foscarnet. Another drug approved for the use CMV retinitis in patients who have failed other therapies is **Fomiversen**. It inhibits viral mRNA. Ocular side effects include vitritis and iritis.
How is it administered?	**Cidofovir's** most common route of administration is IV.
What is cidofovir's toxicity?	Nephrotoxicity and neutropenia. **Probenecid** can be used concomitantly with **cidofovir** to help reduce nephrotoxicity.

DRUGS USED TO TREAT RESPIRATORY VIRUSES

Which drugs are used in the treatment of respiratory viruses?	**Amantadine, rimantadine, ribavirin, oseltamivir, zanamivir**

AMANTADINE AND RIMANTADINE

What are amantadine and rimantadine?	**Amantadine** and its derivative **rimantadine** are uniquely configured tricyclic amines.

What is their mechanism of action?	**Amantadine** and **rimantadine** inhibit viral uncoating.
What is viral uncoating?	Viruses enter cells through endosomes, which are membrane-bound vacuoles that surround the virus particle. Acidification of the endosome is needed for the virus to uncoat and transfer its genetic material to the cytoplasm.
What is the action of these drugs on the viral endosome?	**Amantadine** and **rimantadine** block a viral membrane matrix protein which helps form the endosome. They also act as weak bases to prevent acidification of the endosome.
What is their therapeutic use?	**Amantadine** and **rimantadine** are used mainly for influenza A prophylaxis in elderly and immunosuppressed populations.
What is the route of administration?	**Amantadine** and **rimantadine** are well absorbed orally.
What is their metabolism?	**Amantadine** is not metabolized extensively while **rimantadine** undergoes metabolism in the liver. They are both excreted by the kidneys.
What are their adverse effects?	Insomnia, dizziness, and ataxia. These symptoms are less common with **rimantadine** because it does not cross the blood-brain barrier.

RIBAVIRIN

Describe this drug.	**Ribavirin** is a synthetic guanosine analogue.
What is ribavirin's mechanism of action?	The mechanism of action is not completely clear, but it is thought to decrease synthesis of guanosine triphosphate, inhibit 5′ capping of viral mRNA, and interfere with viral RNA-dependent RNA polymerase of certain viruses.

What is ribavirin's major therapeutic use?

Treatment of infants and young children who are suffering from respiratory syncytial virus bronchiolitis and pneumonia

What other clinical uses does this drug have?

Ribavirin is also a first-line agent used for treating hepatitis C in combination with interferon, severe influenza, and Lassa fever.

How is this drug administered?

Ribavirin is effective when administered orally, intravenously, and by aerosol methods.

What is ribavirin's toxicity?

Dose-dependent transient hemolytic anemia and elevated bilirubin levels

Should this drug be used in pregnant women?

No! It is teratogenic.

OSELTAMIVIR, ZANAMIVIR

When are these drugs used?

These drugs are used to ameliorate the symptoms of both influenza A and B. They are most effective when used within 24 hr of the onset of symptoms.

How do these drugs work?

They inhibit an enzyme called neuraminidase. This ultimately results in decreased viral spread.

What are their toxicities?

oseltamivir: Given orally. GI distress
zanamivir: Inhaled agent therefore may cause bronchospasm.

ANTIHEPATITIS AGENTS

Interferons

What are interferons?

Interferons are a family of naturally existing glycoproteins or cytokines that possess antiviral actions. Their exact mechanism of action is still under investigation.

What are the therapeutic uses for interferons?	Condyloma acuminatum Chronic hepatitis B and C Kaposi's sarcoma Hairy cell leukemia
What are the adverse effects of interferons?	An acute flu-like syndrome including headache, fever, chills, and muscle aches is the most common adverse effect. However, interferons may also cause **neurotoxicity**, cardiotoxicity, thyroid dysfunction, and **bone marrow depression**.
Name three other drugs in addition to interferon used for the treatment of hepatitis.	**Adefovir, lamivudine, ribavarin**
How does adefovir work?	It is triphosphorylated by host cell kinases and then is incorporated into viral DNA, which terminates chain elongation. **Adefovir** has shown success in **lamuvidine**-resistant HBV infections.
What are its adverse effects?	Nephrotoxicity and tubular dysfunction are the most important.

Lamuvidine and ribavarin are discussed elsewhere in this chapter. Interferon is also discussed in Chapter 40.

DRUGS USED TO TREAT HIV INFECTION AND AIDS

Define acquired immunodeficiency syndrome (AIDS).	AIDS, caused by the human immunodeficiency virus (HIV), is characterized by a CD4 count of less than 200 and the presence of opportunistic infections.
How is the CD4 count calculated?	White blood cells (WBCs) × % lymphocytes × % CD4 cells
How does HIV differ from other viruses?	HIV is a retrovirus. After entering the host cell, it undergoes reverse transcription and is then incorporated into the host cell's DNA.

List two *surrogate markers* that help to predict the risk of progression from HIV positive to AIDS.

The CD4 count and HIV RNA PCR (polymerase chain reaction), which is commonly called the *viral load*

What are some uses of the viral load test?

It can predict progression to AIDS, and it is also used for therapeutic monitoring.

What is HAART?

An acronym meaning "highly active antiretroviral therapy." It is a combination of drugs from different classes and is the standard of care today.

Which two viral enzymes do antiretroviral medications inhibit?

1. **Reverse transcriptase**
2. **Protease**

What is the action of reverse transcriptase?

It converts viral RNA into DNA.

What is the action of viral protease?

It cleaves viral protein into infectious virions. Helps with the maturation process.

What are the two types of reverse transcriptase inhibitors (RTIs)?

1. Nucleoside and nucleotide analogues (NRTIs)
2. Nonnucleoside analogues (NNRTIs)

NRTIs

Give examples of nucleoside analog RTIs.

1. **Zidovudine** (AZT)
2. **Didanosine** (ddI)
3. **Zalcitabine** (ddC)
4. **Stavudine** (d4T)
5. **Lamivudine** (3TC)
6. **Abacavir**
7. **Tenofovir**
8. **Emtricitabine**

Describe zidovudine and stavudine.

Structural analogues of **thymidine**.

Describe didanosine.

It is a structural analogue of **adenosine**.

Describe zalcitabine, lamivudine and emtricitabine.

Structural analogues of cytosine. **Emticitabine** is a fluroro-derivative of **lamivudine**.

Describe abacavir.

It is a structural analogue of **guanosine**.

Describe tenofovir.

It is the first approved drug that is a nucleotide analog rather than a nucleoside. In the cell, it is phosphorylated twice rather than three times, since the parent drug already has a phosphate group.

What is the mechanism of action of these drugs?

They are phosphorylated by host cell kinases and subsequently incorporated into viral DNA by reverse transcriptase. They then terminate chain elongation once they are incorporated into the viral DNA. They also have a direct inhibitor effect on HIV reverse transcriptase.

Is hepatoxicity common to all of the NRTIs?

Yes. Except for **lamivudine** and **abacavir**. The toxicity is potentially fatal; therefore monitor LFTs.

How do these drugs differ?

Mainly in their pharmacokinetics. **Emtricitabine** has a long half-life and has once-a-day dosing, which is rather unique among HIV drugs. **Lamivudine** and **emtricitabine** can also be used against hepatitis B virus.

What are the side effects of AZT?

Anemia, neutropenia, headache, myalgia

What are the side effects of didanosine?

Acute pancreatitis, painful peripheral neuropathy, nausea, and vomiting

What are the side effects of zalcitabine and stavudine?

Painful sensory peripheral neuropathy

What are the side effects of lamivudine?

This is one of the least toxic NRTIs. Headaches and neutropenia have been reported.

What are the side effects of abacavir?	Common side effects include GI distress headache and dizziness. Rarely, severe hypersensitivity reactions may occur.
What are the side effects of tenofovir and emtricitabine?	**tenofovir:** GI distress **emcricitabine:** nausea, vomiting and headache most common, but hyperpigmentation of the soles and palms, hepatomegaly, and lactic acidosis can also occur.

NNRTIs

Give some examples of nonnucleoside analogue reverse transcriptase inhibitors (NNRTIs).	**Nevirapine** (Viramune) and **delavirdine** (Rescriptor), **efavirenz** (Sustiva)
State the mechanism of action for the NNRTIs.	These drugs bind to HIV's reverse transcriptase at a different site than NRTI's and block its function. They do not require phosphorylation to be active.
How are NNRTIs administered?	Orally. They are used in combination with other HIV drugs because resistance occurs very rapidly if used as monotherapy.
How are these drugs metabolized?	Cytochrome P450 system. **Nevirapine** induces this system while the others inhibit it. Therefore, all three interact with a wide range of drugs.
Which of these drugs can be used in pregnancy?	**Nevirapine** has been shown to reduce vertical transmission of HIV during pregnancy. The others are contraindicated in pregnancy.
What is the main toxicity associated with all NNRTIs?	Rash.
What other toxicities are associated with NNRTIs?	**Nevirapine:** Severe reactions such as Stevens–Johnson syndrome and toxic epidermal necrosis, hepatotoxicity

Delavirdine: Headache, dizziness, nausea
Efavirenz: CNS effects such as dizziness, headache, nightmares

PROTEASE INHIBITORS

Give some examples of protease inhibitors.

Saquinavir (Invirase)
Ritonavir (Norvir)
Indinavir (Crixivan)
Nelfinavir (Viracept)
Amprenavir (Agenerase)
Fosamprenavir (Lexiva)
Lopinavir/Ritonavir (Kaletra)
Atazanavir (Reytaz)

How do these drugs work?

These agents inhibit HIV protease an enzyme that is needed for cleaving the viral polyprotein into essential structural and enzymatic (reverse transcriptase, protease) components

How are these drugs administered?

Orally. **Lopinavir** is only available as a coformulation with **ritonavir** because of poor bioavailability when given by itself. **Ritonavir** is sometimes given with other protease inhibitors to improve their bioavailability as well. Fatty meals can affect absorption of any of the protease inhibitors.

How are they metabolized?

They are all extensively metabolized by the cytochrome P450 system. They also are potent inhibitors of this system and therefore can cause a great number of drug interactions. **Ritonavir** is the most potent inhibitor.

Name at least four important drugs that should not be given with protease inhibitors.

Warfarin, rifampin, midazolam, phenobarbital

What can be done to limit resistance to these drugs?

Give them in combination. Resistance can occur when a mutation causes a change in the HIV protease enzyme.

Resistance to one protease inhibitor does not mean the patient will be resistant to all of them.

What are the side effects associated with protease inhibitors?

In general, all of them can cause GI distress (nausea, vomiting, diarrhea, abdominal pain), glucose intolerance, hyperlipidemia, paraesthesias and fat redistribution (buffalo hump, truncal obesity) similar to Cushing's disease.

Indinavir can cause an obstructive nephropathy, nephrolithiasis and hyperbilirubinemia. **Amprenavir** is most likely to produce skin eruptions. **Atazanavir** is likely to cause hyperbilirubinemia as well as prolong the PR interval on ECG. However, in contrast to the others, it has a low propensity to raise lipid levels.

ENTRY INHIBITORS

Currently, which drug is the only one capable of preventing HIV from fusing to host cell membranes?

Enfuvirtide (Fuzeon)

How does it work?

For the HIV virus to enter host cells it must go through a conformational change, which is mediated by a gp41 viral trans membrane glycoprotein.

Enfuvirtide blocks this protein so that the virus is no longer able to modify its shape to fuse with and gain entry into the host cell.

Is it a first-line agent?

No. Because of its expense and other factors, this drug is indicated only for patients who have failed all other antiretroviral regimens.

How is it administered?

Must be given subcutaneously twice a day.

What are its untoward effects?	Injection site reactions.

DRUGS USED TO PREVENT INFECTION IN PATIENTS WITH HIV

Which vaccines *should* be given to patients who have HIV?	Pneumococcal, hepatitis, and influenza vaccines
Which vaccines *should not* be given to patients with HIV?	Live vaccines such as the oral polio vaccine and varicella vaccine
Medications are used for primary prophylaxis of which infections?	*Pneumocystis carinii* pneumonia (PCP) *Mycobacterium avium-complex* (MAC) Mycobacterial tuberculosis (TB)
What are the indications for PCP prophylaxis?	Prior PCP infection CD4 count of less than 200 cells per cubic millimeter HIV-associated thrush Unexplained fevers over 100°F for more than 2 weeks
Which medications are used for PCP prophylaxis?	**Trimethoprim/sulfamethoxazole, dapsone,** and aerosolized **pentamidine**
What are the indications for MAC prophylaxis?	A CD4 cell count less than 50 and prior diagnosis of MAC
Which medications are used for MAC prophylaxis?	**Clarithromycin, azithromycin,** and **rifabutin**
What are the indications for TB prophylaxis?	Tuberculin skin test (TST) ≥ 5 mm Prior positive TST results without treatment Contact with active case of TB
Which medications are used for TB prophylaxis?	**Isoniazid** and **rifampin**

DRUG THERAPY FOR OPPORTUNISTIC INFECTIONS IN PATIENTS WITH HIV

What medications are used to treat PCP?	**Trimethoprim/sulfamethoxazole** (drug of choice) **Pentamidine** **Atovaquone**
What medications are used to treat *Toxoplasma* infection?	A combination of **pyrimethamine** and **sulfadiazine** or a combination of **pyrimethamine** and **clindamycin**
What medications are used to treat esophageal *Candida albicans?*	**Fluconazole, ketoconazole,** and **amphotericin B**
What medications are used to treat MAC?	Macrolides (**clarithromycin** or **azithromycin**) plus one of the following: **Ethambutol** **Ciprofloxacin** **Amikacin**
What medications are used to treat *Cryptococcus* infection?	**Amphotericin, fluconazole,** and **itraconazole**
What medications are used to treat *Cytomegalovirus?*	**Ganciclovir** and **foscarnet**

HIV POSTEXPOSURE PROPHYLACTIC MEDICATIONS

Which body fluids have been documented to carry HIV?	Blood, semen, vaginal secretions, cerebrospinal fluid, synovial fluid, pleural fluid, peritoneal fluid, pericardial fluid, and amniotic fluid
Which body fluids have *not* been documented to carry HIV?	Feces, nasal secretions, sputum, saliva, sweat, tears, urine, and vomitus
Which medication has established efficacy when used for postexposure prophylaxis?	**AZT**

Which medications should be prescribed for the recipient of a deeply penetrating hollow-bore needle stick injury from a host who has HIV?

1. **AZT**
2. **Lamivudine**
3. **Indinavir**

How soon after exposure should these medications be started?

As soon as possible; preferably within 1 to 2 hr

51

Drugs Used to Treat Tuberculosis and Leprosy

What is the primary worldwide cause of death from infectious disease?

Tuberculosis (TB)

TUBERCULOSIS

Which organism causes tuberculosis?

Tuberculosis is caused by the bacterium *Mycobacterium tuberculosis.*

What makes tuberculosis difficult to treat?

There are three major complicating factors:
1. *Mycobacterium* tuberculosis is an intracellular organism.
2. The organism grows very slowly. Consequently infections are often chronic, and therapy may be required for as long as 2 years.
3. Resistance to drugs develops rapidly.

Why is tuberculosis treated with multiple drugs?

Multiple drugs are used to delay the emergence of resistant strains of the organism.

What are the five first-line pharmacological treatment options for tuberculosis?

1. **Isoniazid** (INH)
2. **Rifampin**
3. **Pyrazinamide**
4. **Ethambutol**
5. **Streptomycin**

ISONIAZID (Laniazid)

How does this drug work?

Isoniazid is believed to act by inhibiting the enzymes **enoyl acyl carrier protein reductase (InhA)** and a **β-ketoacyl ACP synthase (KasA)**. These enzymes are essential for the synthesis of mycolic acids, which are unique to the mycobacterial cell walls.

What is the route of administration?

The drug is readily absorbed orally and parenterally. Absorption is impaired, however, if **isoniazid** is taken with aluminum-containing antacids.

How does resistance to the drug occur?

A mutation or deletion of the *katG* gene results in underproduction of the mycobacterial enzyme needed for **isoniazid** to become biologically active. A mutation in the InhA enzyme can also cause resistance.

What is this drug's distribution?

Isoniazid penetrates all body fluids, cells, and caseous material. Therefore it is able to act on intracellular mycobacteria.

State the metabolism of the drug.

Isoniazid is metabolized in the liver by *N*-acetylation. The rate of acetylation shows a genetic variance among humans; it can be as fast as 1 hr or as slow as 3 hr.

How does isoniazid affect the cytochrome P-450 system?

Isoniazid inhibits this system; the drug therefore increases plasma levels of drugs such as **phenytoin, benzodiazepines,** and **warfarin**.

State isoniazid's adverse effects.

Peripheral neuritis—Most commonly paraesthesias of the hands and feet. This is thought to be caused by **isoniazid's** action in binding and inactivating pyridoxine (vitamin B_6). Vitamin B_6 supplementation can minimize this problem.

Hepatotoxicity—Jaundice and hepatitis can be severe. LFTs must be monitored.

Rashes and skin eruptions

Neurological problems such as convulsions in patients prone to seizures

When is isoniazid given alone?

In most cases **isoniazid** is given along with other drugs. However, for prophylactic treatment of skin test converters and for close contacts of patients who have active disease, **isoniazid** is given alone.

Can you use isoniazid in pregnant patients?

No! This drug crosses the placenta and may cause peripheral neuritis in newborns.

RIFAMPIN (Rifadin)

What is its mechanism of action?

Rifampin inhibits the β-subunit of DNA-dependent RNA polymerase. It suppresses RNA synthesis by blocking chain initiation. **Rifabutin** and **rifapentine** are in the same family of drugs as **rifampin** and work similarly to **rifampin**.

What is the metabolism of this drug?

Rifampin is metabolized by and **induces** the cytochrome P-450 system. Therefore other drugs such as **ketoconazole** and **warfarin** may require higher dosages to maintain therapeutic concentrations. **Rifabutin** does not induce the cytochrome P-450 system as much as **rifampin** and therefore is used in tuberculosis-infected HIV patients who are taking protease inhibitors.

In what other setting is rifabutin used?

It is used as prophylaxis against Mycobacterium Avium Complex (MAC). MAC also can be treated with a combination of **ethambutol, rifabutin** and **clarithromycin** or **azithromycin**.

State the clinical indications for rifampin in addition to the treatment of tuberculosis.

Prophylaxis of meningitis caused by *Haemophilus influenzae* and *Neisseria meningitidis*
Leprosy—used in combination with dapsone
Legionnaires' disease—used in combination with **erythromycin**

What is the absorption and distribution of the drug?

Rifampin is orally absorbed. It easily penetrates into all tissue cells and fluids, including the CNS.

How does resistance to rifampin occur?

Through decreased permeability or a mutation in the mycobacterial DNA-dependent RNA polymerase.

State the adverse effects.

Urine, sweat, tears, and other secretions may become red-orange in color. (**R**ifampin—**R**ed-orange)

Rash, fever, nausea, and vomiting are common.

A flu-like syndrome with chills, fever, and myalgias may develop in patients who use **rifampin** once or twice weekly.

PYRAZINAMIDE

When is this drug used?

For short-course ($\leq$ 6 months) treatment of tuberculosis in combination with **isoniazid** and **rifampin**

What is the absorption and distribution of this drug?

Pyrazinamide is orally absorbed and distributed to most body tissues, including the CNS.

State the mechanism of action.

The target of pyrazinamide appears to be the mycobacterial fatty acid synthase I gene involved mycolic acid synthesis.

What are pyrazinamide's adverse effects?

Hepatotoxicity

Gout due to the inhibition of uric acid secretion

Arthralgia and myalgia (most common)

ETHAMBUTOL (Myambutol)

What is the clinical use of this drug?

Ethambutol is almost always used against *M. tuberculosis*, but it can be used against *M. avium* and *M. kansasii* as well.

How does it work?

Ethambutol inhibits the enzyme **arabinosyl transferase**, which is involved in the synthesis of arabinogalactan, an essential component of the mycobacterial cell wall.

State the absorption and distribution of the drug.

It is well absorbed orally and distributes into all cells, including the CNS.

Is this drug bacteriostatic or bacteriocidal?

Ethambutol is the only first-line drug that is bacteriostatic.

What are the adverse effects?

Optic neuritis or other visual disturbances (decreased visual acuity, red-green color blindness)
Gout due to a decrease in uric acid secretion
Rash, fever

STREPTOMYCIN

See *Chapter 44—Protein Synthesis Inhibitors,* for more detailed information on **streptomycin**.

What is the classification of this drug?

Streptomycin is an aminoglycoside.

What is its mechanism of action?

Streptomycin binds to the 30S ribosomal subunit, causing a misinterpretation of the genetic code.

State the clinical indication for streptomycin.

Treatment of life-threatening tuberculosis in combination with other first-line drugs

What are streptomycin's adverse effects?

Ototoxicity
Nephrotoxicity—usually reversible

TREATMENT GUIDELINES

What is the preferred recommendation for the initial treatment of active TB?

A 2-month regimen of **pyrazinamide, INH, ethambutol** and **rifampin** and a 4-month regimen of **INH** and **rifampin** for a total of 6 months

Name the second-line agents used in the treatment of tuberculosis.	1. **Ethionamide**
	2. **Aminosalicylic acid** (PAS)
	3. **Cycloserine**
	4. **Fluoroquinolones (moxi or gatifloxacin)**
	5. **Macrolides (Azithromycin)**
Why are these drugs second-line agents?	They are lower in efficacy and higher in toxicity or they are active against atypical strains of mycobacterium. They are used only if the patient cannot tolerate the first-line drugs or if the strain is resistant to them.

DRUGS USED TO TREAT LEPROSY

What organism causes leprosy?	*Mycobacterium leprae*
What are the pharmacological treatment options for leprosy?	**Dapsone, clofazimine**, and **rifampin**. Usually all three of them are used concomitantly.

DAPSONE

How does dapsone work?	It is related to the sulfonamides and inhibits folate biosynthesis by acting as a competitive antagonist of PABA.
What is this drug's route of administration?	PO
What is the metabolism of this drug?	It undergoes acetylation in the liver.
How is it used?	**Dapsone** is used in combination with **rifampin** and **clofazimine** to treat leprosy. It is also used in the treatment and prophylaxis of *Pneumocystis carinii* pneumonia.
What are the adverse reactions?	GI irritation Methemoglobinemia Hemolysis (*dose-related*) especially in patients with GGPD deficiency Drug-induced lupus erythematosus

CLOFAZIMINE (Lamprene)

How does this drug work?	**Clofazimine** binds to DNA and inhibits its replication.
How is this drug given?	Orally
What are the adverse effects?	A distinctive reddish-brown discoloration of the skin GI irritation (nausea, vomiting, diarrhea)

Section XI   Toxicology

52

Toxicology

What is toxicology?	The study of the adverse effects of chemicals and physical agents on biological systems
Name the six steps in managing a poisoned patient.	1. Stabilize the patient (use the ABCs of first aid). 2. Identify the toxin (by toxicology screen). 3. Prevent toxin absorption (by gastric lavage, activated charcoal, and other such techniques). 4. Institute specific antidotal therapy. 5. Enhance toxin elimination (by changing urine pH, hemodialysis). 6. Monitor the patient.

TOXICITIES AND TREATMENTS OF COMMONLY USED DRUGS AND CHEMICALS

ACETAMINOPHEN

What are the signs and symptoms of acetaminophen toxicity?	Nausea, vomiting, anorexia, and diaphoresis. **Acetaminophen** toxicity is often asymptomatic until 24 to 48 hr after ingestion, when hepatotoxicity becomes evident.
What is the Rumack-Matthew nomogram?	A graph used to indicate possible hepatotoxicity and the need for antidotal therapy based on a patient's serum **acetaminophen** level
How long after ingestion should a serum acetaminophen level be drawn for correlation on the nomogram?	Between 4 to 24 hr after ingestion

How is acetaminophen toxicity treated?	Supportive care with cardiac monitoring Activated charcoal administration if patient presents within 1 to 2 hr of ingestion. Administration of *N*-acetylcysteine if indicated by the Rumack-Matthew nomogram
How is *N*-acetylcysteine administered?	Loading dose of 140 mg/kg orally Maintenance dose of 70 mg/kg orally every 4 hr for 17 doses

β-ADRENERGIC BLOCKERS

Name the signs and symptoms of β-adrenergic blocker toxicity.	Nausea Vomiting Hypotension Bradycardia CNS depression
How do you treat β-adrenergic blocker toxicity?	1. Perform gastric lavage. *whole intest lavage (c Golitely)* 2. Administer **glucagon** 5 to 10 mg IV, then 1 to 5 mg /hr IV. 3. Administer **atropine** or cardiac pacing if hemodynamically significant bradycardia exists. 4. Give IV fluids and vasopressors for treatment of hypotension.

BENZODIAZEPINES

glucagon → CaCl → Insulin / N. epi +/- pacing

What are the signs and symptoms of benzodiazepine toxicity?	Weakness, ataxia, and (in severe cases) coma and respiratory depression. **Benzodiazepine** overdose rarely causes death.
How do you treat benzodiazepine toxicity?	1. Supportive therapy (oxygen, IV fluids) 2. Activated charcoal if patient presents within 4 hr of ingestion. 3. Administer **flumazenil**, a competitive **benzodiazepine** receptor antagonist.
How is flumazenil administered?	In incremental doses of 0.2, 0.3, and 0.5 mg IV at 1-min intervals until the desired

effect is achieved or a maximum dose of
3 to 5 mg has been given

Why shouldn't flumazenil be administered in cases of benzodiazepine overdose associated with polypharmacy overdose?	Because it may cause seizures in patients who have coingested stimulants. **Flumazenil** may also cause seizures in patients who have a history of chronic **benzodiazepine** use.

CALCIUM CHANNEL BLOCKERS

What are the signs and symptoms of calcium channel blocker toxicity?	Bradycardia Hypotension CNS depression Constipation
How do you treat calcium channel blocker toxicity?	1. Supportive therapy. 2. Gastric lavage followed by activated charcoal. Avoid ~~ipecac syrup~~ (induces emesis). *∅ ipecac !* 3. Administer calcium chloride 10% IV at 0.2 mL/kg over 5 min. 4. Administer **atropine, glucagon**, or cardiac pacing for hemodynamically significant bradycardia. 5. Use vasopressors, or an intra-aortic balloon pump in refractory cases of hypotension.

CYANIDE

How does cyanide affect human cells?	It inhibits cytochrome oxidase and therefore blocks electron transport, which results in decreased aerobic energy production.
What are the signs and symptoms of cyanide toxicity?	Nausea Vomiting Tachycardia Hypertension Arrhythmias Apnea Acute respiratory distress syndrome Coma

What odor can sometimes be detected on the breath of a person who has cyanide poisoning?

A bitter almond odor

How is cyanide toxicity treated?

1. Gastric lavage
2. Lilly cyanide antidote kit—amyl nitrite pearls for inhalation, 3% sodium nitrite IV, and 25% sodium thiosulfate IV
3. High-dose oxygen therapy

How does the nitrite therapy work?

Nitrites induce methemoglobinemia. **Cyanide** has a higher affinity for methemoglobin than cytochrome oxidase; therefore, the **cyanide** dissociates from the cytochrome oxidase, which allows aerobic energy production to continue.

ETHYLENE GLYCOL

Where is ethylene glycol commonly found?

In antifreeze and windshield de-icers.

What are the signs and symptoms of ethylene glycol toxicity?

Nausea
Vomiting
Abdominal pain
Ataxia
Seizures
Coma

How do you treat ethylene glycol toxicity?

1. Give ethanol 5% to 10% in 5% dextrose in water (D5W) IV, or 20% to 30% solution orally. Maintain blood alcohol level > 100 mg/dL.
2. Use hemodialysis in severe cases of renal failure.
3. Give **pyridoxine** (vitamin B_6), 50 mg IV every 6 hr.
4. Give **thiamine** 100 mg IM every 6 hr.
5. Give **folic acid** 1 mg orally every day.

Activated charcoal is *not* effective in adsorbing ethylene glycol.

ISONIAZID

What are the signs and symptoms of isoniazid toxicity?	Nausea Vomiting Dizziness Slurred speech Lethargy Hepatic injury Seizures Coma
How is isoniazid toxicity treated?	1. Gastric lavage 2. Activated charcoal administration 3. **Pyridoxine** (5 g IV) and **diazepam** to control seizures 4. Hemodialysis in severe cases

ISOPROPYL ALCOHOL

Where is isopropyl alcohol commonly found?	In antifreeze and rubbing alcohol
What are the signs and symptoms of isopropyl alcohol toxicity?	Nausea Vomiting Abdominal pain Ataxia Respiratory depression
How is isopropyl alcohol toxicity treated?	1. Gastric lavage 2. Supportive therapy—IV fluids and bicarbonate administration to correct acidosis 3. Hemodialysis in severe cases with renal failure Activated charcoal is *not* effective in adsorbing isopropyl alcohol.

LITHIUM

What are the signs and symptoms of lithium toxicity?	Lethargy Dysarthria Delirium Seizures Coma

How is lithium toxicity treated?	1. Gastric lavage and irrigation of the entire bowel 2. Administration of IV fluids 3. Administration of **sodium polystyrene sulfonate** 4. Hemodialysis in severe cases Activated charcoal is *not* effective in adsorbing **lithium**.

METHANOL

Where is methanol commonly found?	In antifreeze, solvents, and bootleg (homemade) alcohol ("moonshine")
What are the signs and symptoms of methanol toxicity?	Nausea Vomiting Abdominal pain Blurred vision Blindness Seizures Coma
How is methanol toxicity treated?	1. Use ethanol 5% to 10% in D5W IV or 20% to 30% solution orally. Maintain blood alcohol level > 100 mg/dL. 2. Use hemodialysis in severe cases of renal failure. 3. Administer thiamine and **folate**. Activated charcoal is *not* effective in adsorbing methanol.

OPIOIDS

What are the signs and symptoms of opioid toxicity?	Miosis *"to close the eyes"—constrict.* Altered mental status Bradycardia Respiratory depression Hypothermia
How is opioid toxicity treated?	With **naloxone** 2 mg IV, which is short-acting and therefore may require a continuous infusion

SALICYLATES

What are the early- and late-stage acid-base disorders associated with salicylate toxicity?	Early stage—respiratory alkalosis secondary to tachypnea Late stage—metabolic acidosis
What are the signs and symptoms of salicylate toxicity?	Nausea Vomiting ⭐Tinnitus Hyperthermia Coagulopathy Hypoglycemia Acute renal failure Coma
How can the severity of a patient's toxicity be determined?	A serum level can be collected. A peak level < 3 mmol/L is associated with no symptoms; a level of 3 to 7 mmol/L is associated with mild-to-moderate symptoms; and a level > 7 mmol/L is associated with severe toxicity.
What is the treatment for salicylate toxicity?	1. Gastric lavage 2. Activated charcoal 3. Saline diuresis and alkalinization of the urine to a pH of 8 to increase HCO₃ urinary excretion of salicylates 4. Hemodialysis in severe cases

THEOPHYLLINE

What are the signs and symptoms of theophylline toxicity?	Nausea Vomiting Irritability Tachypnea Tachycardia Hypotension Arrhythmias ≥ seizures
At what serum level do seizures and cardiac arrhythmias typically occur?	At 40 to 60 mg/L (normal = 10 to 20 mg/L)

How is theophylline toxicity treated?

1. Gastric lavage
2. Activated charcoal
3. Hemodialysis in severe cases—acute ingestion with serum level > 80 mg/L or chronic ingestion with serum level > 60 mg/L
4. β-adrenergic blockers to reverse tachycardia and hypotension

TRICYCLIC ANTIDEPRESSANTS

Name the signs and symptoms of tricyclic antidepressant toxicity.

Mild overdose—predominance of anticholinergic side effects, such as mydriasis, hallucinations, urinary retention, hypertension, and tachycardia (wronppose symp.)

Severe overdose—CNS depression along with seizures, hypotension, and cardiotoxicity

wide **QRS complex > 0.10 s** on the ECG correlates with an increased risk of seizures and cardiac arrhythmias.

How can one determine the severity of a patient's overdose?

Serum levels can be used for diagnosis as well as determining severity:
—Serum level < 1000 nmol/L = therapeutic
—Serum level > 3300 nmol/L = severe overdose

Name the steps for treating tricyclic antidepressant toxicity.

1. Gastric lavage
2. Activated charcoal
3. Supportive therapy—airway protection (intubation), ECG monitoring, and IV fluids
4. **Norepinephrine, phenylephrine,** or **dopamine** for hypotension
5. **Phenytoin** or **diazepam** for seizures

The use of ipecac syrup to induce emesis is contraindicated in treating tricyclic antidepressant toxicity.

CHELATORS AND HEAVY METALS

What is a chelator (chelating agent)?	A chelator is a molecule with two or more electronegative groups that is used to bind toxic metals in stable complexes. These complexes have relatively low toxicity and enhanced fecal and renal excretion. Chelators are used in the treatment of heavy metal toxicities.
Name the five most commonly used chelators.	1. **Ethylenediamine tetra-acetic acid** (EDTA) *Pb* 2. **Dimercaprol** (also known as BAL) *Hg Arsenic* 3. **Penicillamine** *Copper Au As Pb* *Pb Cd* 4. **Deferoxamine** *Fe* 5. **Succimer** *Pb*

EDTA

What is the primary use of EDTA?	Treating lead poisoning
How is it administered?	Parenterally (IV or IM)
What is the most important adverse effect of EDTA?	Nephrotoxicity (reversible)
Why must the calcium disodium salt of EDTA be used?	Because the sodium salt of EDTA can cause severe hypocalcemia

DIMERCAPROL

For what reason was dimercaprol first developed?	As an antidote for lewisite, an arsenical war gas. It was first named BAL (British antilewisite).
What is dimercaprol used to treat?	Mercury, arsenic, lead, and cadmium toxicities
How must it be administered?	Parenterally (IM)

What are the contraindications to dimercaprol administration?	Concurrent use of iron therapy (iron forms a toxic complex with **dimercaprol**) Glucose-6-phosphate dehydrogenase (G-6-PD) deficiency Allergy to peanut oil (**dimercaprol** is administered intramuscularly in a solution of peanut oil)

PENICILLAMINE

What is it used to treat?	Poisoning by copper (Wilson's disease), lead, arsenic, mercury, and gold as well as rheumatoid arthritis and cystinuria
How is penicillamine administered?	Enterally. (**Penicillamine** is the only commercially available oral chelating agent for adults.)
What adverse effects can result from administration of this chelating agent?	Rash Fever Leukopenia Thrombocytopenia resembling a penicillin hypersensitivity reaction *Rare side effects include the following:* Aplastic anemia Stevens-Johnson syndrome Lupus erythematosus

DEFEROXAMINE

What is this chelator used to treat?	Acute iron (ferrous salts) intoxication
How is deferoxamine administered?	Parenterally
Does it compete for heme iron in hemoglobin and cytochromes?	Yes, but very poorly
What adverse effects are associated with deferoxamine administration?	Neurotoxicity Hepatic and renal dysfunction Severe coagulopathies Histamine release and hypotensive shock when given by rapid IV infusion

SUCCIMER

Succimer is an oral congener of which of the other chelating agents?	**Dimercaprol**
What is the only FDA-approved use of this chelating agent?	Treatment of childhood lead intoxication with serum levels > 45 µg/dL
Name the adverse effects associated with succimer administration.	Transient increase in hepatic transaminase levels Skin rash GI distress

HEAVY METALS

ARSENIC

Where is arsenic commonly found?	**Organic arsenic**—ubiquitous in the environment **Inorganic arsenic**—insecticides, *pesticides* fungicides, rodenticides, and compounds used in glass manufacturing **Arsine gas**—produced in smelting of metals and making of silicon microchips and lead plating
How does arsenic cause toxicity?	It interferes with oxidative phosphorylation.
What are the signs and symptoms of acute arsenic toxicity?	**GI distress**—nausea, vomiting, rice-water stools **Cardiovascular effects**—hypotension and arrhythmias **CNS effects**—seizure and coma **Hematological effects**—hemolysis and bone marrow depression **Renal effects**—acute tubular necrosis and oliguria
List the signs and symptoms of chronic arsenic toxicity.	Polyneuritis Skin changes—erythroderma, hyperkeratosis, Aldrich-Mees lines

(transverse white striae of the fingernails)

What is the characteristic smell of the breath of a patient who is experiencing acute arsenic toxicity?

A sweet, garlicky odor

How can arsenic intoxication be detected?

Through serum arsenic levels

What is the treatment for acute arsenic toxicity?

1. Gastric lavage
2. **Dimercaprol** or **penicillamine**
3. Hemodialysis if the patient has renal failure

LEAD

Where is lead commonly found?

It is ubiquitous in nature. Lead salts may be found in paints made before 1978.

How is lead absorbed?

Through ingestion or inhalation

Are the toxic effects of chronic lead exposure different between children and adults?

In some respects, yes:
Childhood form—abdominal pain, anemia, and subclinical CNS effects, such as mental retardation and learning disabilities
Adult form—abdominal pain, anemia, peripheral neuropathy, ataxia, memory loss, and renal disease

Which is more common, acute or chronic lead toxicity?

Chronic lead toxicity

How can lead intoxication be detected?

Through serum lead levels

What is the treatment for lead toxicity?

1. Remove the source of lead exposure.
2. Perform gastric lavage if the lead was ingested.
3. Administer **EDTA, dimercaprol, penicillamine,** or **succimer**. (**Deferoxamine** is the *only* chelator

that *cannot* be used to treat lead toxicity.)

MERCURY

Where is mercury commonly found?	In batteries, thermometers, and dental fillings
Has a correlation between dental fillings and mercury intoxication been scientifically proved?	No
Through what route does mercury intoxication commonly occur?	Through inhalation. However, this metal may be ingested or absorbed through the skin.
What are the signs and symptoms of acute mercury intoxication?	GI distress—nausea and vomiting Chest pain and shortness of breath secondary to inflammation of airways and interstitial pneumonitis CNS effects—intention tremor, increased excitability, and delirium
List the signs and symptoms of chronic mercury intoxication.	CNS effects as with acute toxicity Loosening of the teeth, gingivitis, and stomatitis Excessive salivation
How is mercury toxicity detected?	Through serum mercury levels
What is the treatment for mercury toxicity?	1. Removal of the source of mercury exposure 2. Gastric lavage if the mercury was ingested 3. **Dimercaprol, penicillamine,** or **succimer**

AIR POLLUTANTS

List the major air pollutants in industrialized countries and briefly describe them.	Carbon monoxide (50%)—colorless, odorless Sulfur oxides—colorless Nitrogen oxides—brownish gas

Ozone

Hydrocarbons—colorless

CARBON MONOXIDE (CO)

What commonly produces CO?

Combustion of fossil fuels and cigarette smoking

How does carbon monoxide adversely affect the human body?

CO causes tissue hypoxia because the affinity of CO for hemoglobin is more than *200-fold greater* than that of oxygen.

What are some symptoms of CO toxicity?

Headache
Confusion
Loss of visual acuity
Syncope (occurs when approximately 40% of hemoglobin has been converted to carboxyhemoglobin)
Coma

How do you treat carbon monoxide exposure?

1. Remove the patient from the CO source.
2. Have the patient breathe 100% oxygen. *Hyperbaric oxygen* accelerates the clearance of CO.

SULFUR DIOXIDE (SO$_2$)

What commonly produces sulfur dioxide?

Combustion of fossil fuels
Manufacturing of sulfuric acid
Refrigerants

How does SO$_2$ adversely affect the human body?

It forms sulfurous acid on contact with moist mucous membranes.

What signs and symptoms result from SO$_2$ exposure?

Conjunctival and bronchial irritation
Epistaxis
Delayed pulmonary edema (severe exposure)

How do you treat sulfur dioxide exposure?

1. Remove the patient from the source of exposure.
2. Relieve irritation and inflammation with supportive therapies.

NITROGEN DIOXIDE (NO₂)

What occupations involve increased risk of NO₂ exposure?	Farming and firefighting would both increase the risk of exposure. NO₂ is formed in silage on farms and is also a by-product of fires.
How does nitrogen dioxide adversely affect the human body?	It causes deep lung irritation and pulmonary edema and may also cause irritation of the eyes, nose, and throat.
How do you treat NO₂ exposure?	There is no specific treatment, but measures should be taken to reduce the risk of exposure.

OZONE (O₃)

What commonly produces O₃?	Ozone is produced in water and air purification devices as well as arc welding.
How does O₃ adversely affect the human body?	**Acute exposure**—irritation and dryness of mucous membranes **Chronic exposure**—can lead to emphysema, bronchitis, bronchiolitis, and pulmonary fibrosis
How do you treat O₃ exposure?	There is no specific treatment, but symptomatic therapies to decrease inflammation and pulmonary edema should be attempted. Also, the patient should be removed from the source of exposure.

HYDROCARBONS

What commonly produces hydrocarbons?	Industrial and cleaning solvents
Name some common examples of everyday hydrocarbons.	Benzene Toluene Carbon tetrachloride
How do hydrocarbons adversely affect the human body?	They are potent CNS depressants and thus can cause nausea, vertigo, headache, and coma.

What ill effects can benzene cause?	Bone marrow suppression with pancytopenia
How do you treat hydrocarbon exposure?	Remove the patient from the source of exposure and provide supportive therapies.

INSECTICIDES

What are the three major classes of insecticides?	1. Chlorinated hydrocarbons—DDT 2. Organophosphorus insecticides 3. Botanical agents—nicotine, rotenone, pyrethrum

CHLORINATED HYDROCARBONS

How do chlorinated hydrocarbons adversely affect the human body?	They block physiologic inactivation of nerve membranes in the sodium channels, thus causing uncontrollable firing of action potentials.
How do you treat chlorinated hydrocarbon exposure?	There is no specific treatment, but measures should be taken to remove the person from the exposure.
Are the chlorinated hydrocarbons still available as insecticides?	No. They were removed from the market because of their long half-lives (years) and their severe environmental toxicity.

ORGANOPHOSPHATES

How do organophosphates function?	They irreversibly inhibit acetylcholinesterase and increase the levels of acetylcholine at the muscarinic and nicotinic synapses.
What are the signs and symptoms of organophosphate toxicity?	**Nicotinic effects**—fasciculations, weakness, hypertension, and tachycardia **Muscarinic effects**—nausea, vomiting, abdominal cramps, urinary and fecal incontinence, sweating, salivation, and miosis. If the toxicity is severe,

bradycardia, respiratory failure, and hypotension may also occur.

How is organophosphate toxicity treated?

Initial treatment depends on the mode of exposure:

If absorbed through the skin—All contaminated clothes should be removed and the skin should be washed thoroughly.

If inhaled—The patient should be removed from the site of exposure.

If ingested—Gastric lavage should be initiated, followed by activated charcoal treatment.

After initial treatment:

Atropine (0.5 to 2 mg IV every 15 to 20 min until desired effect) can be used for treating muscarinic side effects.

Pralidoxime (1 to 2 g IV over 5 to 20 min every 4 to 6 hr until desired effect) can be used for treating nicotinic side effects.

Airway management and **supportive therapy** are initiated.

BOTANICAL INSECTICIDES

Name three botanical insecticides.

1. Nicotine
2. Rotenone
3. Pyrethrum

How does nicotine function as an insecticide?

Nicotine causes excitation of nicotinic receptors, followed by paralysis of ganglionic, CNS, and neuromuscular transmission.

How is nicotine toxicity treated?

Treatment is supportive with special attention paid to avoiding convulsions.

What adverse effects are caused by rotenone?

GI irritation, conjunctivitis, and dermatitis

How is rotenone toxicity treated?

Treatment is symptomatic.

What symptoms occur if high doses of pyrethrum are inhaled or absorbed?

Contact dermatitis, excitation, and convulsions

How is pyrethrum toxicity treated?

Treatment is symptomatic.

HERBICIDES

What are the two major agents used as herbicides?

1. Paraquat
2. Chlorophenoxyacetic acid

By what route of exposure does paraquat cause toxicity to the human body?

Ingestion

What are the manifestations of paraquat toxicity?

GI irritation with bloody stools and vomiting

Pulmonary impairment that usually leads to pulmonary fibrosis and death, which typically occurs within 1 to 2 days of exposure

Is there an antidote for paraquat exposure?

No

What is the mortality rate after ingestion of 5 mL or more of paraquat?

Greater than 50%

How do you treat paraquat exposure?

With supportive therapies, gastric lavage, and activated charcoal

What are the major signs of chlorophenoxyacetic acid toxicity?

Coma, muscle hypotonia, and dermatitis

How is the toxicity treated?

Treatment consists of gastric lavage and supportive therapy.

SPECIFIC ANTIDOTES

What are the specific antidotes for the following drugs?

Opioids	**Naloxone**
Carbon monoxide	100% oxygen
β-adrenergic blockers	**Glucagon**
Benzodiazepines	**Flumazenil**
Theophylline	**Esmolol**
Isoniazid	**Pyridoxine**
Ethylene glycol and methanol	**Ethanol**
Digoxin	Digoxin-specific antibodies
Acetylcholinesterase inhibitors (organophosphates)	**Atropine** and **pralidoxime** Sx reactivator.
Acetaminophen	N-acetylcysteine
Calcium channel blockers	**Calcium chloride** and **glucagon**
Cyanide	**Nitrites** and **thiosulfate**
Iron	**Deferoxamine**
Mercury, arsenic, and gold	**Dimercaprol**
Warfarin (Coumadin)	Vitamin K and fresh frozen plasma
Heparin	**Protamine sulfate**
Nitrites	**Methylene blue**
Copper	**Penicillamine**

Lead	**EDTA, succimer**
Salicylates	Alkalinize urine

IMPORTANT DRUG TOXICITIES

What are the causal agents for the following drug toxicities?

Pulmonary fibrosis	**Bleomycin, amiodarone, busulfan**
Hepatitis	**Isoniazid** (INH), **halothane**
Focal to massive hepatic necrosis	**Halothane, valproic acid, acetaminophen,** *Amanita phalloides*
Anaphylaxis	**Penicillin**
SLE-like syndrome	**H**ydralazine, **I**NG, **P**rocainamide, **P**henytoin (it's not **HIPP** to have lupus)
Hemolysis in G6PD-deficient patients	Sulfonamides, **INH, aspirin, ibuprofen, primaquine, nitrofurantoin, pyrimethamine, chloramphenicol**
Thrombotic complications	OCPs (e.g., estrogens and progestins)
Adrenocortical insufficiency	Withdrawal of glucocorticoids (HPA suppression)
Photosensitivity reactions	**S**ulfonamides, **A**miodarone, **T**etracycline (**SAT** for a photo!)
Tubulointerstitial nephritis	Sulfonamides, **furosemide, methicillin, rifampin**, NSAIDs (except **aspirin**)
Hot flashes	**Tamoxifen**
Cutaneous flushing	**Niacin**, Ca^{2+} channel blockers, **adenosine, vancomycin**

Cardiac toxicity	**Doxorubicin** (Adriamycin), **daunorubicin**
Agranulocytosis	**Clozapine, carbamazepine, colchicine**
Stevens-Johnson syndrome	**Ethosuximide**, sulfonamides, **lamotrigine**
Cinchonism	**Quinidine, quinine**
Tendonitis, tendon ruptures, and cartilage damage (kids)	Fluoroquinolones
Disulfiram-like reaction	**Metronidazole**, certain cephalosporins, **procarbazine**, sulfonylureas
Ototoxicity and nephro-toxicity	Aminoglycosides, loop diuretics, **cisplatin**
Drug-induced Parkinson's	**Haloperidol, chlorpromazine, reserpine, MPTP**
Torsades de pointes	Class III (**sotalol**), class IA (**quinidine**) antiarrhythmics
Aplastic anemia	**Chloramphenicol, benzene**, NSAIDs
Neuro- and nephro-toxicity	Polymyxins
Pseudomembranous colitis	**Clindamycin, ampicillin**
Gynecomastia	**S**pironolactone, **D**igitalis, **C**imetidine, chronic **A**lcohol use, estrogens, **K**etoconazole (**S**ome **D**rugs **C**reate **A**wesome **K**nockers)
Atropine-like side effects	Tricyclics
Cough	ACE inhibitors (**losartan** → no cough)

Gingival hyperplasia	**Phenytoin**
Diabetes insipidus	**Lithium**
Tardive dyskinesia	Antipsychotics
Fanconi's syndrome	Expired tetracyclines
Gray-baby syndrome	**Chloramphenicol**
Extrapyramidal side effects	**Chlorpromazine, thioridazine, haloperidol**
Osteoporosis	**Corticosteroids, heparin**
Coronary vasospasm	**Cocaine**

(With permission from Bhushan V, Le T. *First Aid for the USMLE Step 1.* New York: McGraw-Hill, 2005, pp. 334–335.)

53

Pharmacology Power Review

The Pharmacology Power Review follows this general format:

drug name	Mechanism of action. ***Rx:*** Therapeutic uses. ***Tox:*** Side effects. ***Other:*** Additional important or unique properties of a drug such as contraindications, metabolism, or drug interactions (included only for some drugs).

Only high-yield drugs and facts are discussed in the Pharmacology Power Review. For further details, refer to the chapters in parentheses.

CHOLINERGIC AGONISTS (CHAPTER 6)

DIRECT-ACTING AGONISTS

acetylcholine	An endogenous cholinomimetic that acts on both muscarinic and nicotinic receptors. ***Rx:*** Occasionally used intraocularly for miosis in cataract surgery. In general it is used infrequently because it is rapidly hydrolyzed, but synthetic derivatives of acetylcholine such as **bethanechol** are used. ***Tox:*** Excessive cholinergic stimulation—remember *dumbels* <u>d</u>iarrhea, <u>u</u>rination, <u>m</u>iosis, <u>b</u>ronchoconstriction, <u>Bradycardia</u> <u>e</u>xcitation (of CNS and skeletal muscle), <u>l</u>acrimation, and <u>s</u>alivation.
bethanechol	A carbamic acid ester with little nicotinic activity but strong muscarinic activity that increases smooth muscle contractions of bowel and bladder. ***Rx:*** Bowel or bladder atony. ***Tox:*** dumbels.

carbachol

A carbamic acid ester that stimulates both muscarinic and nicotinic receptors. ***Rx:*** Open-angle glaucoma. ***Tox:*** dumbels.

pilocarpine

Primarily a muscarinic agonist. ***Rx:*** Glaucoma. ***Tox:*** CNS disturbances (headache, visual difficulties) along with excessive cholinergic stimulation (dumbels).

methacholine

A choline ester that stimulates primarily muscarinic receptors. ***Rx:*** Used to test for asthma and bronchial hyperreactivity. ***Tox:*** Generalized cholinergic stimulation.

INDIRECT-ACTING AGONISTS

isoflurophate, echothiophate, parathion

Organophosphates *irreversibly* bind to and inhibit acetylcholinesterase, the enzyme responsible for metabolizing acetylcholine. ***Rx:*** Parathion is used as an insecticide. **Isoflurophate** and **echothiophate** are used occasionally for glaucoma and accommodative esotropia. ***Tox:*** Excessive cholinergic stimulation (dumbels).

physostigmine

A reversible cholinesterase inhibitor that **can enter the CNS.** ***Rx:*** Glaucoma, accommodative esotropia, bowel and bladder atony; overdoses of **atropine**, phenothiazines, and tricyclic antidepressants. ***Tox:*** Convulsions, muscle paralysis, excessive cholinergic stimulation.

neostigmine

A reversible cholinesterase inhibitor that does not enter the CNS. ***Rx:*** Treatment of myasthenia gravis, paralytic ileus, urinary retention; antidote for nondepolarizing neuromuscular blockade as with **tubocurarine**. ***Tox:*** Excessive cholinergic stimulation (dumbels).

edrophonium

A reversible cholinesterase inhibitor. **Rx:** Diagnosis of myasthenia. **Tox:** Excessive cholinergic stimulation.

pyridostigmine

A reversible cholinesterase inhibitor similar to **edrophonium** but with a longer half-life. **Rx:** Therapy of myasthenia gravis. **Tox:** Excessive cholinergic stimulation (dumbels).

CHOLINERGIC ANTAGONISTS (CHAPTER 7)

atropine, homatropine

These drugs are primarily muscarinic blockers. **Rx: Atropine** is used to treat bradycardia and serves as an antidote for organophosphate poisoning. Both agents are used in ophthalmology as cycloplegics and mydriatics. **Tox:** Decreased secretion, decreased vision, delusions, hyperthermia, dilation of cutaneous vessels. "Dry as a bone, blind as a bat, mad as a hatter, hot as a hare, and red as a beet."

scopolamine

Nonselective cholinergic blocker. **Rx:** Similar to **atropine** but particularly beneficial in the treatment of motion sickness. **Tox:** Similar to **atropine**.

NEUROMUSCULAR BLOCKERS

tubocurarine, pancuronium

Nondepolarizing neuromuscular agents that competitively inhibit acetylcholine at nicotinic receptors. **Rx:** Used as adjuvant drugs in anesthesia; with these agents, less anesthetic is required to produce muscle relaxation. **Tubocurarine** is used by hunters to cause muscle paralysis in prey. **Tox:** Ganglionic blockade, histamine release; may result in hypotension and bronchospasm.

succinylcholine

A **depolarizing** neuromuscular blocking agent that reversibly binds acetylcholine receptors. *Rx:* Skeletal muscle relaxation for surgical procedures. *Tox:* Hypotension, arrhythmias; can cause respiratory collapse, malignant hyperthermia.

GANGLIONIC BLOCKERS

hexamethonium, trimethaphan, nicotine

Ganglionic inhibitors block the nicotinic receptors of both the parasympathetic and sympathetic ganglia. *Rx:* Used in the past for hypertensive emergencies. *Tox:* Nonselective parasympathetic and sympathetic blockade.

ADRENERGIC AGONISTS (CHAPTER 8)

α AGONISTS

phenylephrine

An α_1 agonist that activates the PIP_2 cascade. *Rx:* Nasal decongestant, mydriatic (no cycloplegia), and hypotension. *Tox:* Rebound mucosal swelling, hypertensive headache.

methoxamine

Similar to **phenylephrine**; binds α_1 receptors and activates the PIP_2 cascade. *Rx:* Hypotension, paroxysmal atrial tachycardia; also used as a mydriatic. *Tox:* Elevated blood pressure may lead to pulmonary edema, cerebral hemorrhage, or cardiac necrosis.

clonidine

Stimulates presynaptic α_2 receptors on sympathetic neurons. *Rx:* Hypertension, withdrawal from benzodiazepines and opiates. *Tox:* Orthostatic hypotension, dry mouth, sexual dysfunction.

β AGONISTS

Dobutamine

A synthetic analog of **dopamine** that stimulates primarily β_1 receptors but has some activity at β_2 receptors. *Rx:* Short-term management of acute CHF. *Tox:*

cardio shock

Arrhythmias, headache, hypertension, palpitations.

isoproterenol

Stimulates β_1 and β_2 receptors. **Rx:** Treatment of bradycardia or heart block. **Tox:** Tachycardia, headache, flushing of skin, anginal pain.

albuterol, metaproterenol, terbutaline

Stimulate both types of β receptors but preferentially β_2 over β_1. **Rx:** Treatment of asthma and COPD, suppression of premature labor (**terbutaline**). **Tox:** Tremor, restlessness, tachycardia. **Other:** Systemic side effects are minimal since these drugs are usually inhaled.

α AND β AGONISTS

norepinephrine

Acts on α_1, α_2, and β_1 receptors; vasoconstricts, increases blood pressure and cardiac output, and causes reflex bradycardia due to vagal responses. **Rx:** Severe hypotension, as in shock. **Tox:** Arrhythmias, respiratory distress, *septic* . headache.

epinephrine

Acts on all α and β receptors. **Rx:** Anaphylaxis, bronchospasm; used as a nasal decongestant and ophthalmic vasoconstrictor, and as an adjuvant with local anesthetics. **Tox:** Hypertension, cardiac arrhythmias, headache. **Other:** Contraindicated in patients who are on nonselective β blockers because the unopposed α response may lead to severe hypertension.

dopamine

A neurotransmitter and agonist at dopamine, α_1, β_1, and β_2 receptors. **Rx:** Used to increase renal blood flow and to increase blood pressure in cases of shock. **Tox:** Arrhythmias, respiratory distress.

adjuvant "last ditch"

INDIRECT AGONISTS

amphetamine
Releases stored norepinephrine and dopamine from the presynaptic nerve terminal. **Rx:** Used to treat ADHD and narcolepsy and as an appetite suppressant. **Tox:** Confusion, insomnia, headache, restlessness, palpitation.

ephedrine
Stimulates release of norepinephrine from nerve terminals but can directly stimulate adrenergic receptors as well. **Rx:** Treatment of enuresis, hypotension. **Tox:** Arrhythmias, insomnia.

ADRENERGIC ANTAGONISTS (CHAPTER 9)

α BLOCKERS

prazosin, terazosin, doxazosin
α_1-selective blockers decrease peripheral vascular resistance and relax smooth muscle in the prostate. **Rx:** Treatment of hypertension, benign prostatic hypertrophy. **Tox:** First-dose hypotension, syncope, sexual dysfunction, lethargy, dry mouth.

phentolamine
A reversible nonselective α blocker. **Rx:** Short-term management of pheochromocytoma-induced hypertension. **Tox:** Orthostatic hypotension, reflex tachycardia, impotence.

1st before β Blocker

phenoxybenzamine
An **irreversible** α_1 and α_2 blocker. **Rx:** Treatment of pheochromocytoma-induced hypertension, carcinoid syndrome, Raynaud's phenomenon. **Tox:** Orthostatic hypotension.

β BLOCKERS

propranolol
Nonselective β-blocker prototype. **Rx:** Myocardial infarction, migraine, hypertension, and tachycardia; also used

as an antianginal and antiarrhythmic, and to treat thyrotoxicosis. ***Tox:*** Bradycardia, heart block, fatigue, impotence; may mask signs of hypoglycemia in diabetics. ***Other:*** Contraindicated in asthmatics because it induces bronchoconstriction.

timolol

A nonselective competitive β antagonist given only as an ophthalmic solution. ***Rx:*** Glaucoma. ***Tox:*** Similar to **propranolol** but milder because there is less systemic absorption.

pindolol

A nonselective β antagonist with intrinsic sympathomimetic activity, which means that it acts as a partial agonist at β receptors. ***Rx:*** Hypertension in patients with a propensity for bradycardia. ***Tox:*** Similar to **propranolol**.

metoprolol, atenolol, esmolol, acebutolol

β_1 selective blockers. ***Rx:*** Treatment of hypertension, angina, and arrhythmias. **Atenolol** is similar to **metoprolol** but longer-acting. **Esmolol** is similar to **metoprolol** but very short-acting; it is often given IV in surgical situations. ***Tox:*** Similar to **propranolol** but less bronchoconstriction.

labetalol

β blocker that also has β_1 selective blockade. ***Rx:*** Hypertension, atrial fibrillation. ***Tox:*** Hypotension, fatigue.

POSTGANGLIONIC ADRENERGIC NEURONAL BLOCKERS

guanethidine

Enters peripheral nerves via the reuptake mechanism for norepinephrine and blocks the release of norepinephrine from storage vesicles. ***Rx:*** Treatment of hypertension in the past. ***Tox:*** Orthostatic hypotension, sexual dysfunction.

reserpine

A *Rauwolfia* alkaloid that blocks a nerve terminal's ability to store norepinephrine by blocking its transport from cytoplasm into intracellular storage vesicles. ***Rx:*** Hypertension (very rarely used). ***Tox:*** Sedation mental depression, bradycardia.

ANXIOLYTICS, HYPNOTICS, AND SEDATIVES (CHAPTER 11)

BENZODIAZEPINES

diazepam, triazolam, temazepam, alprazolam, flurazepam

Benzodiazepines stimulate the binding of GABA to the $GABA_A$ receptor, which results in hyperpolarization of the cell membrane and decreased neuronal excitability. ***Rx:*** Anxiety, seizures, insomnia, alcohol withdrawal. ***Tox:*** Drowsiness, ataxia, dizziness. ***Other:*** Individual benzodiazepines differ mainly in half-life.

BENZODIAZEPINE ANTAGONISTS

flumazenil

Competitive antagonist of benzodiazepines at the $GABA_A$ receptor. ***Rx:*** Reversal of **benzodiazepine** sedation or overdose. ***Tox:*** Well tolerated.

AZAPIRONES

buspirone

A partial agonist at serotonin ($5HT_{1A}$) receptors. ***Rx:*** Relieves anxiety with minimal sedation. ***Tox:*** Headache, nausea, dizziness.

CARBAMATES

meprobamate

Mechanism of action is unknown but does act as a CNS depressant. ***Rx:*** Anxiolytic. ***Tox:*** Respiratory depression, ataxia.

BARBITURATES

phenobarbital,
pentobarbital, thiopental

Barbiturates increase GABA neuronal transmission, which subsequently increases Cl⁻ channel activity and decreases neuronal excitability. ***Rx:*** Treatment of seizures and agitation and as an adjuvant in anesthesia. ***Tox:*** Psychological and physical dependence, CNS depression, cough, and bronchospasm.

ANTIPSYCHOTICS (CHAPTER 12)

PHENOTHIAZINES   *low potency...*

chlorpromazine,
promethazine, thioridazine,
fluphenazine, trifluoperazine

These agents block dopamine D_2 receptors in the mesolimbic and mesocortical paths. ***Rx:*** Used to treat schizophrenia, intractable hiccups (**chlorpromazine**), and as antiemetic and antipruritic agents. ***Tox:*** Sedation, hypotension, anticholinergic effects.

THIOXANTHENES

thiothixene

Blocks dopamine D_2 receptors. ***Rx:*** Treatment of schizophrenia. ***Tox:*** Extrapyramidal effects, tardive dyskinesia, hypotension, anticholinergic effects.

BUTYROPHENONES

haloperidol, droperidol

These agents are high-potency dopamine D_2 receptor blockers in the CNS. ***Rx:*** Schizophrenia and other psychotic disorders, agitation; used as antipruritics. ***Tox:*** Extrapyramidal effects (parkinsonism, dystonia, akathisia), tardive dyskinesia, weight gain, infertility, anticholinergic effects.

ATYPICAL AGENTS

clozapine

Blocks dopamine D_1 and D_2 receptors. **Rx:** Schizophrenia. **Tox:** Agranulocytosis, convulsions, hypotension, sedation. **Other:** Atypical agents have a lower likelihood of causing extrapyramidal symptoms.

risperidone

Antagonist at serotonin 5-HT_2 receptors. **Rx:** Schizophrenia. **Tox:** Hypotension.

DRUGS USED TO TREAT DEPRESSION AND MANIA (CHAPTER 13)

TRICYCLICS

imipramine, amitriptyline, amoxapine, desipramine, doxepin, trimipramine, nortriptyline, clomipramine

These agents inhibit the reuptake of norepinephrine and serotonin. **Imipramine** and **amitriptyline** are prototypes. **Rx:** Clinically significant depression, phobias, and obsessive-compulsive disorder. **Tox:** Postural hypotension, sedation, anticholinergic effects (dry mouth, urinary retention, tachycardia), arrhythmias. **Other: Imipramine** is used to treat enuresis in children.

SSRI INHIBITORS

fluoxetine, sertraline, paroxetine, fluvoxamine, trazodone, citalopram, escitalopram

These agents preferentially inhibit reuptake of serotonin over norepinephrine and dopamine. **Rx:** Often first-line agents for clinical depression. **Fluoxetine** is also used for obsessive-compulsive disorder. **Tox:** Usually well tolerated. May cause sedation, postural hypotension, tachycardia.

MAO INHIBITORS

isocarboxazid, tranylcypromine, phenelzine

These drugs block MAO-A, which is responsible for the metabolism of serotonin, norepinephrine, and tyrosine.

Rx: Second-line agents for depression.
Tox: Overdose can lead to hyperthermia, hepatotoxicity, impotence, and hypertensive crisis if consumed with large amounts of tyrosine.

ATYPICAL ANTIDEPRESSANTS

bupropion

Mechanism of action not well understood. *Rx:* Treatment of depression. *Tox:* Headache, nausea, tachycardia, restlessness.

DRUGS USED TO TREAT MANIA

lithium

Unclear mechanism of action; believed to block the enzyme inositol-1-phosphatase. *Rx:* Treatment of bipolar disease, SIADH. *Tox:* Tremor, vomiting, abdominal cramps, nephrogenic diabetes insipidus, ataxia, seizures, thyroid enlargement. *Other:* Contraindicated in pregnancy. Thiazides increase **lithium** concentration.

ANTICONVULSANTS (CHAPTER 14)

phenytoin

Binds to and prolongs the inactivated states of Na$^+$ channels; increases GABA-mediated inhibitory postsynaptic potentials. *Rx:* Treatment of tonic-clonic and partial seizures, status epilepticus after administration of **diazepam, digitalis**-induced arrhythmias. *Tox:* Gingival hyperplasia, nystagmus, diplopia, ataxia, fetal hydantoin syndrome (characterized by abnormal growth and development). *Other:* Contraindicated in sinus bradycardia or AV block. Significantly increases the cytochrome P-450 system.

valproic acid

Like **phenytoin**, it appears to prolong the inactivated states of Na$^+$ channels; it also may increase GABA concentrations. **Rx:** Treatment of absence, myoclonic, and partial seizures. **Tox:** Nausea, vomiting, sedation, hepatotoxicity, neural tube defects. **Other:** Contraindicated in pregnancy.

phenobarbital

Long-acting barbiturate that potentiates synaptic inhibition through an action on the GABA receptor. **Rx:** Treatment of febrile seizures in children and partial and tonic-clonic seizures. **Tox:** Respiratory, cardiac, and mental sedation; nystagmus; psychotic reactions; hypersensitivity reactions.

primidone

Works similarly to **phenytoin** by blocking Na^+ channels from repolarizing. **Rx:** An alternative choice for adults with partial seizures (both simple and complex) and generalized tonic-clonic seizures. **Tox:** Sedation, ataxia, nausea, vomiting, drowsiness. Rarely, Stevens-Johnson syndrome.

carbamazepine

Potentiates synaptic inhibition by blocking Na^+ channels. **Rx:** Drug of choice for partial and tonic-clonic seizures and for trigeminal neuralgia. **Tox:** Severe liver toxicity—patients need frequent liver function tests while on the drug; aplastic anemia; agranulocytosis.

ethosuximide

Inhibits Ca^{2+} influx through low-threshold T-type channels in thalamic neurons. **Rx:** Drug of choice for absence seizures. **Tox:** GI disturbances.

diazepam, clonazepam

Benzodiazepines potentiate GABA transmission. **Rx: Diazepam**—status epilepticus. **Clonazepam**—absence and myoclonic seizures. **Tox:** Drowsiness, sedation.

DRUGS USED TO TREAT CNS DEGENERATIVE DISORDERS (CHAPTER 15)

levodopa/carbidopa

Levodopa crosses the blood-brain barrier and is converted to dopamine. **Carbidopa** increases CNS concentration of **levodopa**: it inhibits conversion of **levodopa** to **dopamine** in the periphery by blocking dopa decarboxylase. ***Rx:*** Parkinson's disease. ***Tox:*** Confusion, delusion, hallucination, dyskinesias, anorexia, nausea, tachycardia, postural hypotension.

selegiline

Selectively inhibits MAO-B and therefore increases dopamine concentration. ***Rx:*** Parkinson's disease. ***Tox:*** Dyskinesia, mood alterations.

amantadine

This antiviral agent works by both increasing release and delaying reuptake of dopamine in the substantia nigra. ***Rx:*** Parkinson's disease. ***Tox:*** Restlessness; a bluish discoloration of the legs known as livedo reticularis.

bromocriptine

An ergot alkaloid that acts as a strong **agonist** at presynaptic D_2 receptors. ***Rx:*** Treatment of Parkinson's disease, acromegaly, and conditions involving hyperprolactinemia such as amenorrhea, galactorrhea, and infertility. ***Tox:*** Hypotension, GI distress, and mental confusion and delusions.

benztropine

A tertiary amine alkaloid that blocks cholinergic output of neurons in the corpus striatum. ***Rx:*** Parkinson's disease. ***Tox:*** Anticholinergic effects.

NONERGOT DOPAMINE AGONISTS

pramipexole, ropinirole

Rx: First line or adjuncts for Parkinson's disease. **Tox:** Somnolence dyskinesia, postural hypotension, hallucination.

CATECHOL-O-METHYLTRANSFERASE INHIBITORS

entacapone, tolcapone

Rx: Adjunctive use in Parkinson's disease. **Tox:** Dyskinesia, hallucination, sleep disorders. **Tolcapone** can cause acute liver necrosis.

ANESTHETICS (CHAPTER 16)

INHALED AGENTS

halothane, isoflurane, enflurane

The mechanism of action of these agents is unclear, but they are thought to increase the threshold for activating CNS neurons. **Rx:** Anesthesia. **Tox:** Malignant hyperthermia, hepatotoxicity.

INTRAVENOUS AGENTS

thiopental, thiamylal

Ultra–short-acting barbiturates that, like other barbiturates, enhance GABA transmission. **Rx:** Induction of anesthesia. **Tox:** Bronchospasm, cough. **Other:** Contraindicated in acute intermittent porphyria because this condition predisposes to widespread demyelination of the CNS and PNS.

diazepam, midazolam, lorazepam

These benzodiazepines potentiate GABA transmission. **Rx:** Can be used as the sole anesthetic agents for procedures that do not require analgesia (e.g., cardiac catheterization, endoscopy, cardioversion), or in combination with other agents to induce anesthesia. **Tox:** Severe drowsiness.

propofol

Unclear mechanism of action. **Rx:** Induction and maintenance of anesthesia, and sedation during intensive care. ***Tox:*** Apnea, severe hypotension.

morphine, fentanyl	Opioid analgesics. See *Chapter 18—Opioid Analgesics and Antagonists,* for discussion of mechanisms of action. ***Rx:*** Used in combination with inhaled agents to produce general anesthesia. ***Tox:*** Severe respiratory and cardiac depression.
ketamine	Structurally similar to **phencyclidine** (PCP); known as a dissociative anesthetic that blocks *N*-methyl-D-aspartate (NMDA) receptors. ***Rx:*** Emergency surgical procedures, trauma. ***Tox:*** Hallucinations.

LOCAL AGENTS

lidocaine, tetracaine, procaine, bupivacaine, benzocaine	These compounds are weak bases that block nerve transmission by inhibiting Na^+ channels. ***Rx:*** Surface anesthesia, nerve block, epidural anesthesia. ***Tox:*** Paraesthesias, allergic reactions, bradycardia.

CNS STIMULANTS (CHAPTER 17)

METHYLXANTHINES

caffeine, theophylline, theobromine	These agents increase cGMP and cAMP by inhibiting phosphodiesterase and blocking adenosine receptors. ***Rx:*** Theophylline is used in asthma treatment. ***Tox:*** Insomnia, agitation, tremor, convulsions, arrhythmias.

AMPHETAMINES

methylphenidate, methamphetamine, dextroamphetamine	Amphetamines release neuronal stores of catecholamines, especially norepinephrine and dopamine. ***Rx:*** Used to decrease fatigue and insomnia; also used for appetite control and in ADHD.

Tox: Irritability, anorexia, nausea, palpitations, angina.

ALCOHOL AND OTHER DRUGS OF ABUSE (CHAPTER 18)

ethanol

Ethanol is a CNS depressant that works through GABA receptors to enhance GABA-mediated synaptic transmission. *Rx:* Treatment of **methanol** overdose, **ethylene glycol** overdose. *Tox:* Euphoria, disinhibition, slurred speech, decreased liver function (hepatitis and cirrhosis may develop), GI irritation, inflammation, gynecomastia, testicular atrophy.

PCP

Phencyclidine, also known as "angel dust," is a dissociative anesthetic (loss of pain without loss of consciousness) that blocks NMDA (N-methyl-D-aspartate) receptors. *Rx:* None. *Tox:* Schizophrenia-like psychosis, increased blood pressure and heart rate, limb numbness, ataxia, hypersalivation, and seizures that may be fatal.

marijuana

Also known as "weed" or "hash"; the active component is α-9THC (tetrahydrocannabinol), which acts upon its own specific receptors. *Rx:* Treatment of nausea in patients undergoing chemotherapy. *Tox:* Increased heart rate and blood pressure, injected conjunctiva, dry mouth, bronchodilation, and hunger.
ch = Apathy.

LSD

Lysergic acid diethylamide interacts with serotonin 5-HT receptors in the midbrain. *Rx:* None. *Tox:* Mydriasis, tachycardia, flushing, increased blood pressure.

cocaine

Blocks reuptake of norepinephrine by inhibiting presynaptic α_2 receptors. *Rx:*

Can be used for surface anesthesia. ***Tox:*** Fatal coronary vasospasm or arrhythmias; seizures.

OPIOID ANALGESICS AND ANTAGONISTS (CHAPTER 19)

FULL AGONISTS

morphine, hydromorphone	Binds primarily to μ receptors. ***Rx:*** Used for severe, constant pain; sometimes used in acute pulmonary edema. ***Tox:*** Respiratory depression, constipation, histamine release, psychological and physiological dependence.
meperidine	Binds to μ receptors. ***Rx:*** Treatment of acute pancreatitis, because it does not induce GI spasms. ***Tox:*** Similar to **morphine**.
fentanyl	Similar to morphine (binds to μ receptors) but 80 × more potent. ***Rx:*** Used as an anesthetic. ***Tox:*** Same as **morphine**.
heroin	An illicit narcotic. ***Rx:*** None. ***Tox:*** Coma, respiratory depression, pinpoint pupils.
codeine	Binds to μ and δ receptors; approximately 10 × less potent than **morphine**. ***Rx:*** Antitussive, mild analgesia. ***Tox:*** Similar to **morphine**.
methadone	Works similarly to **morphine** (binds to μ receptors) but has a longer duration of action. ***Rx:*** Treatment of opioid withdrawal syndromes. ***Tox:*** Similar to **morphine**.

MIXED AGONIST/ANTAGONIST AND PARTIAL AGONISTS

buprenorphine, pentazocine	Agonist at κ and δ receptors, and antagonist at μ receptors. ***Rx:*** Analgesia—relief of moderate to severe pain. ***Tox:*** Psychotomimetic effects, respiratory depression.
nalbuphine	Agonist at κ receptors, antagonist at μ receptors. ***Rx:*** Relief of moderate to severe pain. ***Tox:*** Similar to morphine.

OPIOID ANTAGONISTS

naloxone	Competitive antagonist at μ receptors. ***Rx:*** Reverses the effects of acute opiate overdose (pupil constriction, respiratory depression, constipation). ***Tox:*** Transient tachypnea.
naltrexone	Competitive antagonist at μ receptors. ***Rx:*** For opiate overdose. ***Tox:*** Same as **naloxone**. ***Other:*** Unlike **naloxone**, **naltrexone** can be given orally and is longer acting; therefore, it is better for outpatient management of opiate abuse.

ANTIHYPERTENSIVE DRUGS (CHAPTER 20)

CENTRALLY ACTING DRUGS

methyldopa, clonidine	Cause peripheral vasodilation and reduction in cardiac output through stimulation of central α_2 receptors. ***Rx:*** Treatment of moderate to severe hypertension. ***Tox:*** Drowsiness, headache, decreased libido, hepatotoxicity. **Clonidine** is associated with rebound hypertension after sudden withdrawal.

α BLOCKERS

prazosin, terazosin, doxazosin	α_1-selective blockers that decrease peripheral vascular resistance and relax

smooth muscle in the prostate. *Rx:*
Treatment of hypertension. *Tox:* First-
dose hypotension, syncope, sexual
dysfunction, lethargy, benign prostatic
hypertrophy, dry mouth.

β BLOCKERS

propranolol

Nonselective β blocker prototype. *Rx:*
Used to treat hypertension and
tachycardia; as an antianginal and
antiarrhythmic; for MI prophylaxis; and
to treat thyrotoxicosis. *Tox:* Bradycardia,
heart block, fatigue, impotence; may
mask signs of hypoglycemia in patients
with diabetes. *Other:* Contraindicated in
asthmatics because it induces
bronchoconstriction.

metoprolol, atenolol,
esmolol, acebutolol

β_1-selective blockers. *Rx:* Treatment of
hypertension, angina, and arrhythmias.
Atenolol is similar to **metoprolol** but
longer-acting. **Esmolol** is similar to
metoprolol but very short-acting; it is
often given IV in surgical situations. *Tox:*
Similar to **propranolol** but less
bronchoconstriction.

labetalol

β blocker that also has α_1 selective
blockade. *Rx:* Hypertension, atrial
fibrillation. *Tox:* Hypotension, fatigue.

GANGLIONIC BLOCKERS

trimethaphan,
hexamethonium

Ganglionic inhibitors block the nicotinic
receptors of both the parasympathetic
and sympathetic ganglia. *Rx:* Used in the
past for hypertensive emergencies. *Tox:*
Nonselective parasympathetic and
sympathetic blockade.

POSTGANGLIONIC ADRENERGIC NEURONAL BLOCKERS

guanethidine   Enters peripheral nerves via the reuptake mechanism for norepinephrine and blocks the release of norepinephrine from storage vesicles. ***Rx:*** Used in the past for treatment of hypertension. ***Tox:*** Orthostatic hypotension, sexual dysfunction.

reserpine   A *Rauwolfia* alkaloid that blocks a nerve terminal's ability to store norepinephrine by blocking its transport from cytoplasm into intracellular storage vesicles. ***Rx:*** Hypertension (very rarely used). ***Tox:*** mental depression, bradycardia.

DIRECT VASODILATORS

hydralazine   Increases cGMP, which leads to dephosphorylation of myosin and relaxation of arteriolar smooth muscle. ***Rx:*** Treatment of moderate hypertension, CHF. ***Tox:*** Lupus-like syndrome (✎ board question), hypotension, reflex tachycardia, palpitations, angina, nausea, diarrhea.

minoxidil   A potent arterial vasodilator that works by opening K^+ channels, which results in hyperpolarization and relaxation of smooth muscle cells. ***Rx:*** Treatment of severe hypertension. ***Tox:*** Edema due to sodium and water retention, reflex tachycardia, flushing, pericardial lesions.

sodium nitroprusside   Increases intracellular cGMP, which subsequently leads to diminished intracellular Ca^{2+} ions, causing vasodilation of both arteries and veins. ***Rx:*** Used in hypertensive emergencies. ***Tox:*** Hypotension, arrhythmias, cyanide toxicity.

diazoxide

Opens K^+ channels, causing hyperpolarization and relaxation of arterial smooth muscle cells. ***Rx:*** Used in hypertensive emergencies. ***Tox:*** Hypotension, edema, hyperglycemia secondary to inhibition of insulin release, tachycardia.

CALCIUM CHANNEL BLOCKERS

verapamil, diltiazem, nifedipine

These agents bind to and inhibit L-type Ca^{2+} channels. ***Rx:*** Treatment of hypertension, angina, arrhythmias. ***Tox:*** Headache, heart block, dizziness, CHF, peripheral edema, flushing. ***Other:*** **Verapamil** has the greatest negative inotropic effect; **nifedipine** has the least.

DIURETICS

hydrochlorothiazide, furosemide, ethacrynic acid, bumetanide

See listing in this Power Review under **Diuretics (Chapter 23).**

ACE INHIBITORS

captopril, lisinopril, enalapril, benazepril

These agents block the conversion of angiotensin I to angiotensin II. ***Rx:*** Treatment of mild to moderate hypertension, CHF. ***Tox:*** Cough, hyperkalemia, and dizziness; proteinuria and renal failure in patients with bilateral renal artery stenosis.

ANGIOTENSIN RECEPTOR BLOCKERS

losartan, valsartan, candesartan, irbesartan

Angiotensin II receptor antagonists. ***Rx:*** Hypertension. ***Tox:*** Hypotension, hyperkalemia, headache.

NB

ANTIARRHYTHMIC DRUGS (CHAPTER 21)

CLASS IA

quinidine

Binds to open Na^+ channels, preventing Na^+ influx and thus decreasing the slopes of phase 0 and phase 4. ***Rx:*** Treatment of ventricular and supraventricular arrhythmias. ***Tox:*** Diarrhea, nausea, vomiting, cinchonism (fever, vertigo, tinnitus), increased QT interval, increased digoxin levels, widening of the QRS duration.

disopyramide

Mechanism of action similar to that of **quinidine**. ***Rx:*** Ventricular arrhythmias. ***Tox:*** Significant negative inotrope properties and antimuscarinic properties (dry mouth, blurred vision, constipation)

procainamide

Mechanism of action similar to that of **quinidine**. ***Rx:*** Second-line agent for treatment of ventricular arrhythmias. ***Tox:*** Lupus-like effect (✎ board question), increased QT interval.

CLASS IB

lidocaine

Blocks Na^+ channels and shortens phase 0 of the action potential. ***Rx:*** Treatment of ventricular arrhythmias, especially post-MI. ***Tox:*** Drowsiness, slurred speech, paraesthesias, agitation.

phenytoin

Works similarly to **lidocaine**. ***Rx:*** Treatment of **digitalis**-induced arrhythmias. ***Tox:*** Gingival hyperplasia, nystagmus, diplopia, ataxia, fetal hydantoin syndrome (characterized by abnormal growth and development).

tocainide

Works similarly to **lidocaine**. ***Rx:*** Treatment of ventricular arrhythmias. ***Tox:*** Pulmonary fibrosis.

mexiletine	Works similarly to **lidocaine**. **Rx:** Treatment of ventricular arrhythmias. **Tox:** Tremor, blurred vision, lethargy.

CLASS IC

flecainide, propafenone, moricizine	Class 1C drugs block Na^+ channels and suppress phase 0 upstroke. **Rx:** Treatment of refractory ventricular arrhythmias. **Tox:** Proarrhythmogenic dizziness, nausea. **Other:** **Propafenone** displays some β-blockade activity.

CLASS II (β BLOCKERS)

propranolol, metoprolol, atenolol, esmolol	These agents diminish phase 4 depolarization and thus decrease automaticity, prolong AV conduction, and decrease heart rate. **Rx:** Treatment of tachyarrhythmias. **Tox:** Bradycardia, heart block, fatigue, impotence; may mask signs of hypoglycemia in diabetics. **Other:** **Propranolol** is contraindicated in asthmatics because it induces bronchoconstriction.

CLASS III (K-CHANNEL BLOCKERS)

amiodarone	Has properties of more than one antiarrhythmic class but is usually categorized as a class III agent. In addition to prolonging repolarization, **amiodarone** acts as a vasodilator and negative inotrope. **Rx:** Treatment of atrial fibrillation, atrial flutter, ventricular tachycardia. **Tox:** Pulmonary fibrosis, hepatotoxicity, microcystic deposits on the cornea, thyroid dysfunction (hypo- or hyperthyroidism).
ibutilide/dofetilide	Class III blocks K^+ channels. **Rx:** conversion of atrial flutter/fibrillation. **Tox:** Torsades de pointes.

CLASS IV (CA^{2+} CHANNEL BLOCKERS)

verapamil, diltiazem

These agents bind to L-type Ca^{2+} channels and result in decreased Ca^{2+} influx; this slows the response of the SA and AV nodes. *Rx:* These drugs control ventricular rate in atrial flutter or fibrillation. *Tox:* CHF, peripheral edema, hypotension. *Other:* **Nifedipine** is not used as an antiarrhythmic.

DRUGS USED TO TREAT CONGESTIVE HEART FAILURE (CHAPTER 22)

CARDIAC GLYCOSIDES

digitalis, digitoxin

These agents inhibit the Na$^+$/K$^+$-ATPase pump, which ultimately results in more intracellular Ca^{2+} and a positive inotropic effect. They also slow conduction through the AV node. *Rx:* CHF, atrial fibrillation, or atrial flutter. *Tox:* Nausea, vomiting, blurred vision, headache.

BIPYRIDINE DERIVATIVES

amrinone, milrinone

These agents inhibit phosphodiesterase, which subsequently results in increased cardiac contractility. *Rx:* Treatment of acute CHF. *Tox:* Nausea, vomiting, thrombocytopenia, arrhythmias.

VASODILATORS

isosorbide dinitrate

Nitrates cause the release of nitric oxide, which relaxes veins and arteries; veins are dilated predominantly. *Rx:* Treatment of hypertension, CHF, and angina. *Tox:* Tachycardia, orthostatic hypotension.

hydralazine	Increases cGMP, which leads to dephosphorylation of myosin and relaxation of arteriolar smooth muscle. ***Rx:*** Treatment of moderate hypertension, CHF. ***Tox:*** Lupus-like syndrome (✎ board question), hypotension, reflex tachycardia, palpitations, angina, nausea, diarrhea.

β AGONISTS

dobutamine	Increases cardiac contractility by stimulating β receptors. ***Rx:*** Treatment of acute CHF. ***Tox:*** Arrhythmias.
dopamine	Stimulates β and dopamine receptors. ***Rx:*** CHF, shock, and hypotension. ***Tox:*** Arrhythmias.

β BLOCKERS

Carvedilol, metaprolol	***Rx:*** Improves mortality in patients with chronic heart failure not used in acute setting. ***Tox:*** similar to other beta blockers.

ACE INHIBITORS

captopril, enalapril	These agents block the conversion of angiotensin I to angiotensin II. ***Rx:*** Treatment of mild to moderate hypertension, CHF. ***Tox:*** Cough, hyperkalemia, dizziness; proteinuria and renal failure in patients with bilateral renal artery stenosis.

DIURETICS

furosemide, ethacrynic acid, hydrochlorothiazide	See listing below under **Diuretics (Chapter 23)**.

DIURETICS (CHAPTER 23)

CARBONIC ANHYDRASE INHIBITORS

acetazolamide	Inhibits carbonic anhydrase in the proximal convoluted tubule. ***Rx:***

Treatment of glaucoma, mountain sickness, metabolic alkalosis. ***Tox:*** Paraesthesias, metabolic acidosis, interstitial nephritis. ***Other:*** Contraindicated in patients with hepatic or renal disease.

LOOP DIURETICS

furosemide, ethacrynic acid, bumetanide

These agents inhibit the Na^+,K^+-2Cl^- cotransporter in the thick ascending limb of the loop of Henle. ***Rx:*** Treatment of edematous states such as congestive heart failure. ***Tox:*** Hypokalemia, hypocalcemia, hyperuricemia.

THIAZIDES

hydrochlorothiazide

Inhibits the Na^+,Cl^- transporter in the early segment of the distal convoluted tubule. ***Rx:*** Treatment of hypertension, edema, CHF, nephrogenic diabetes insipidus. ***Tox:*** Hypokalemia, hyperglycemia, hyponatremia, hyperlipidemia, hyperuricemia.

K^+-SPARING DIURETICS

amiloride, triamterene

These K^+-sparing diuretics work by inhibiting luminal Na^+ from entering the principal cells of the late distal convoluted tubule and collecting tubule. ***Rx:*** Hypertension, CHF. ***Tox:*** Hyperkalemia, hyponatremia, gynecomastia. ***Other:*** Very weak efficacy; usually used in conjunction with another diuretic.

spironolactone

Competitive antagonist of aldosterone at the aldosterone receptor in the distal convoluted tubule and collecting tubule. ***Rx:*** Treatment of edema due to CHF, cirrhosis, primary aldosteronism. ***Tox:*** Hyperkalemia, gynecomastia, hyponatremia.

OSMOTIC DIURETICS

mannitol	Increases oncotic pressure intravascularly and therefore pulls fluid away from tissues. ***Rx:*** Rapid decrease of intracranial or intraocular pressure; maintenance of urine output. ***Tox:*** Pulmonary edema, dehydration, hypernatremia. ***Other:*** Given IV only because of poor absorption.

ANTIANGINAL DRUGS (CHAPTER 24)

NITRATES

nitroglycerin, isosorbide nitrate, amyl nitrate	Nitrates cause the release of nitric oxide, which relaxes veins and arteries (veins are dilated predominantly). ***Rx:*** Treatment of hypertension, CHF, angina, and cyanide poisoning. ***Tox:*** Tachycardia, orthostatic hypotension.

CALCIUM CHANNEL BLOCKERS

diltiazem, verapamil, nifedipine	These agents bind to L-type Ca^{2+} channels and result in decreased Ca^{2+} influx, which slows the response of the SA and AV nodes. ***Rx:*** Beneficial in angina because they reduce afterload and decrease heart rate; also used to treat hypertension, arrhythmias. ***Tox:*** Heart block, CHF, peripheral edema, hypotension.

β BLOCKERS

propranolol, timolol, metoprolol, atenolol	See previous listing in this Power Review under **Adrenergic Antagonists (Chapter 9).**

ANTICOAGULANT, FIBRINOLYTIC, AND ANTIPLATELET DRUGS (CHAPTER 25)

heparin	Enhances the activity of antithrombin III more than 1000-fold by binding to antithrombin III and inducing a structural change that exposes the active site of antithrombin III. ***Rx:*** Used in pulmonary embolism, stroke, MI, unstable angina, DVT. ***Tox:*** Bleeding, thrombocytopenia. ***Other:*** Effects of heparin are reversed with protamine sulfate.
warfarin	An oral anticoagulant that interferes with vitamin K–dependent clotting factors (II, VII, IX, X). ***Rx:*** Treatment of venous thrombosis, pulmonary emboli, atrial fibrillation, and other conditions requiring long-term anticoagulation. ***Tox:*** Hemorrhage. ***Other:*** Contraindicated in pregnancy. Effects of **warfarin** are reversed with vitamin K or fresh frozen plasma.
tissue plasminogen activator (TPA, alteplase)	A "second-generation" recombinant human thrombolytic enzyme that activates plasminogen bound to fibrin; this, in theory, limits systemic bleeding. ***Rx:*** Acute MI resulting from coronary thrombosis, DVT, pulmonary emboli. ***Tox:*** Hemorrhage.
urokinase	An enzyme generated by the human kidney that directly converts plasminogen to plasmin. ***Rx:*** Treatment of acute pulmonary embolism. ***Tox:*** Systemic bleeding.
streptokinase	Binds with plasminogen, causing a conformational change that then catalyzes the conversion of other plasminogen molecules into plasmin. ***Rx:*** Coronary thrombolysis, acute MI, severe pulmonary emboli. ***Tox:*** Bleeding, fever, hypersensitivity with continued use.

aminocaproic acid	Binds to plasmin and plasminogen; this prevents plasmin from binding to fibrin and therefore inhibits clot lysis. *Rx:* Used for control of hemorrhage due to hypofibrinogenemia; counteracts the effects of **urokinase, TPA,** and **streptokinase**. *Tox:* Myopathy, hypotension, intravascular thrombosis.

ANTIHYPERLIPIDEMIC DRUGS (CHAPTER 26)

BILE ACID RESINS

cholestyramine, colestipol	These bile acid resins prevent absorption of dietary cholesterol and bile acids; they also increase hepatic LDL receptors. *Rx:* Used to lower LDL plasma levels. *Tox:* Indigestion, nausea, lipid-soluble vitamin deficiency.

HMG-COA INHIBITORS

lovastatin, simvastatin, pravastatin	These HMG-CoA reductase inhibitors block endogenous cholesterol synthesis, forcing hepatocytes to increase LDL receptors. *Rx:* Hypercholesterolemia. *Tox:* GI distress. *Other:* Rhabdomyolysis may occur when these agents are used with **niacin** or **gemfibrozil**.

NIACIN

niacin	Mechanism of action not well understood; appears to decrease adipose tissue lipolysis, which in turn reduces circulating free fatty acids. *Rx:* Hypertriglyceridemia. *Tox:* A cutaneous flush and pruritus are the most common problems. Liver toxicity—must monitor LFTs at least every 6 months. Hyperglycemia, hyperuricemia, nausea, constipation.

fibric acid derivatives

clofibrate, gemfibrozil

Mechanism of action not well understood. These drugs increase activity of lipoprotein lipase, a plasma enzyme that degrades chylomicrons and VLDL. ***Rx:*** Very effective for hypertriglyceridemia. ***Tox:*** Skin rash is common with gemfibrozil. Clofibrate has been associated with an increase in hepatobiliary and GI neoplasms. ***Other:*** These drugs also potentiate the effects of anticoagulant drugs.

AGENTS USED TO TREAT ANEMIA (CHAPTER 27)

iron

Most commonly given through oral ferrous iron supplementation. ***Rx:*** Treatment of iron-deficient microcytic anemia. ***Tox:*** GI disturbances are the most common side effects. If the dose is sufficiently high, shock, metabolic acidosis, and even death can occur.

Cyanocobalamin (vitamin B_{12})

A cofactor in the transfer of one-carbon units, which is a step necessary in the synthesis of DNA. ***Rx:*** Treatment of megaloblastic anemia, pernicious anemia, tabes dorsalis. ***Tox:*** None.

folic acid

Necessary for the transfer of one-carbon fragments in the synthesis of purine and pyrimidine bases. ***Rx:*** Treatment of megaloblastic anemia; critical in pregnancy to reduce risk of neural tube defects. ***Tox:*** No known adverse effects.

erythropoietin

A glycoprotein produced by the kidney. ***Rx:*** Treatment of anemias associated with end-stage renal failure and bone marrow failure. ***Tox:*** The only toxicity is associated with an excessive increase in red blood cell count.

DRUGS USED TO TREAT ASTHMA, COUGHS, AND COLDS (CHAPTER 28)

SYMPATHOMIMETICS

metaproterenol, terbutaline, albuterol, salmeterol

These β_2 agonists work by increasing cyclic AMP, which results in bronchodilation. ***Rx:*** Drugs of choice for acute relief of bronchospasm. ***Tox:*** Tremor, tachycardia.

CORTICOSTEROIDS

beclomethasone, flunisolide, triamcinolone, fluticasone

These glucocorticoids reduce inflammation by reversing mucosal edema, decreasing the permeability of capillaries, and inhibiting the release of leukotrienes. ***Rx:*** Treatment of asthma and other reactive airway diseases. ***Tox:*** Minimal toxicities if given through aerosol; rarely, adrenal suppression.

ANTICHOLINERGICS

ipratropium

Inhibits acetylcholine receptors found in smooth muscle; minimizes bronchial secretion and bronchoconstriction. ***Rx:*** Treatment of asthma, COPD. ***Tox:*** Dry mouth, sedation.

METHYLXANTHINES

theophylline

Phosphodiesterase inhibitor that increases cAMP and results in bronchodilation; also has some anti-inflammatory effects. ***Rx:*** Treatment of asthma, COPD. ***Tox:*** Palpitations, tachycardias, arrhythmias, headaches.

LEUKOTRIENE INHIBITORS

zileuton, zafirlukast

Zileuton is a 5-lipoxygenase inhibitor; **zafirlukast** is an LTD4 receptor antagonist. *Rx:* Treatment of asthma. *Tox:* With **zileuton**, some cases of hepatitis have been reported; with **zafirlukast**, drug allergy has been reported.

cromolyn sodium

An effective drug that stabilizes the membrane of mast cells and prevents histamine and leukotriene release, probably by blocking calcium gates. *Rx:* Prophylaxis against asthmatic attacks. *Tox:* Well tolerated but can cause cough or wheezing.

HYPOTHALAMIC AND PITUITARY HORMONES (CHAPTER 29)

oxytocin

Stimulates the force and frequency of uterine contractions; causes milk ejection by contracting myoepithelial cells surrounding mammary alveoli. *Rx:* Induction of labor in patients with delivery complications; control of postpartum and postabortal uterine hemorrhage. *Tox:* Hypertensive episodes, uterine rupture.

vasopressin

Activates receptors on the renal tubular cells to increase the number and insertion of water channels in the kidney collecting tubule; also vasoconstricts vessels. *Rx:* Used in the treatment of central diabetes insipidus; infused to stop variceal bleeding. *Tox:* Headache, nausea, abdominal cramps, hypertension, bradycardia.

THYROID AND ANTITHYROID DRUGS (CHAPTER 30)

DRUGS USED TO TREAT HYPOTHYROIDISM

levothyroxine sodium

A synthetic analogue of thyroxine (T_4). *Rx:* Treatment of hypothyroidism. *Tox:* Cardiac effects (palpitations, hypertension, arrhythmias), thyrotoxicosis heat intolerance.

liothyronine sodium

A synthetic analogue of triiodothyronine (T_3). *Rx:* Treatment of hypothyroidism; adjuvant in the treatment of myxedema coma because of its rapid onset of action. *Tox:* Palpitations, hypertension, arrhythmias, thyrotoxicosis.

DRUGS USED TO TREAT HYPERTHYROIDISM

propylthiouracil, methimazole

These thioamides stop the iodination and coupling of the thyroglobulin molecule; therefore, monoiodotyrosine (MIT) and diiodotyrosine (DIT) cannot be produced. Without MIT and DIT, it is impossible to produce T_3 and T_4. *Rx:* Treatment of hyperthyroidism. *Tox:* Agranulocytosis—rare but most important side effect to watch for; also rash, edema, joint pain.

perchlorate, thiocyanate

These ionic inhibitors competitively inhibit the concentration of iodide in the thyroid gland by blocking the iodide transport mechanism. *Rx:* Previously used to treat Graves' disease, their use today has diminished. *Tox:* **Perchlorate** has caused fatal aplastic anemia.

potassium iodide

Inhibits release of T_3 and T_4. *Iodide* also decreases the vascularity and size of the thyroid gland. *Rx:* Rarely used today as sole therapy; most often used prior to surgery or in conjunction with a thioamide and **propranolol** in thyrotoxic crisis. *Tox:* Anaphylactoid reaction— angioedema and swelling of the larynx. Chronic **iodide** intoxication (iodism)— brassy taste and burning in the mouth, soreness of the teeth and gum, swelling of the eyelids, coryza and sneezing that simulates a cold, respiratory problems, enlarged parotid and submaxillary glands.

SEX STEROIDS AND REPRODUCTIVE DRUGS (CHAPTER 31)

ESTROGENS

estradiol, ethinyl estradiol, estrone, mestranol	These agents bind to cytosolic receptors and travel to the nucleus where they regulate estrogen-sensitive gene transcription. *Rx:* Used in the treatment of dysmenorrhea, in oral contraceptives, and in hormone replacement therapy. *Tox:* Hypertension, thrombophlebitis, thromboembolism, endometrial hyperplasia.

ESTROGEN ANTAGONISTS

tamoxifen, raloxifene	Blocks estrogen receptors. *Rx:* Treatment of breast cancer. *Tox:* Hot flashes.
clomiphene	Blocks estrogen receptors. *Rx:* Treatment of female infertility. *Tox:* Multiple births, excessive enlargement of ovaries.

PROGESTINS

medroxyprogesterone, norethindrone	These agents bind to cytosolic receptors and travel to the nucleus, where they stimulate transcription of progestin-responsive genes. *Rx:* Used in the treatment of dysfunctional uterine bleeding and endometriosis, and in contraception. *Tox:* Decreased HDL, increased blood pressure, thrombophlebitis and weight gain.

PROGESTIN ANTAGONISTS

danazol	An agonist at progestin, glucocorticoid, and androgen receptors. *Rx:* Treatment of endometriosis. *Tox:* Edema, acne, weight gain.
mifepristone	Inhibits progestin by blocking receptors. *Rx:* Abortifacient. *Tox:* Heavy bleeding.

ANDROGENS

methyltestosterone, fluoxymesterone, oxymetholone	These agents bind to cytosolic receptors and then migrate to the nucleus, where they stimulate transcription of testosterone-responsive genes. ***Rx:*** Treatment of hypogonadism and anemia; chemotherapy for estrogen-sensitive breast cancers. ***Tox:*** Prostatic hypertrophy, priapism, cholestatic jaundice, hepatocellular carcinoma.

CORTICOSTEROIDS AND INHIBITORS (CHAPTER 32)

GLUCOCORTICOIDS

cortisol, prednisone, triamcinolone, dexamethasone, betamethasone	These agents bind to cytosolic receptors and then are taken to the nucleus, where they simulate transcription of glucocorticoid-responsive genes. ***Rx:*** Anti-inflammatory agents; used in the treatment of autoimmune disease and adrenocortical insufficiency. ***Tox:*** Adrenal suppression, immunosuppression, osteoporosis, salt retention, hyperglycemia, steroid psychosis. ***Other:*** **Dexamethasone** is used for treatment of cerebral edema and diagnosis of Cushing's disease. **Betamethasone** is used for induction of surfactant synthesis in premature newborns.

MINERALOCORTICOIDS

fludrocortisone, deoxycorticosterone	Synthetic analogues of aldosterone. ***Rx:*** Treatment of Addison's disease; replacement therapy after adrenalectomy. ***Tox:*** CHF, hypokalemia, anaphylaxis.

INSULINS AND ORAL HYPOGLYCEMIC DRUGS (CHAPTER 33)

INSULINS

regular insulin, NPH, ultralente	**Insulin** binds to tyrosine kinase receptors on cell membranes; it does not enter the nucleus. ***Rx:*** Insulin-dependent diabetes. ***Tox:*** Hypoglycemia, insulin allergy,

insulin antibody, lipodystrophy. ***Other:*** The three forms of **insulin** differ in their onset of action and duration of action.

SULFONYLUREAS

tolbutamide, glyburide, glipizide, glimepiride

These agents stimulate the release of endogenous insulin from β cells of the pancreas, and increase binding of insulin to target tissues and receptors. The initial step in the facilitation of endogenous insulin release is binding and blocking ATP-sensitive K^+ channels. ***Rx:*** Type II diabetes. ***Tox:*** Hypoglycemia, GI distress, pruritus, agranulocytosis (rare).

MEGLITINIDES

repaglinide

Stimulates the release of insulin from pancreatic β cells. ***Rx:*** Type II diabetes. ***Tox:*** hypoglycemia.

BIGUANIDES

metformin

Decreases hepatic glucose production and intestinal glucose absorption, and increases peripheral glucose uptake; also, improves insulin sensitivity. ***Rx:*** Treatment of type II diabetes. ***Tox:*** Lactic acidosis, diarrhea, nausea, upset stomach.

α-GLUCOSIDASE INHIBITORS

acarbose, miglitol

Delays the absorption of glucose from the GI tract. The advantage of this drug is that it does not cause a reactive hypoglycemia. ***Rx:*** Type II diabetes. ***Tox:*** GI distress (abdominal pain, diarrhea).

THIAZOLIDINEDIONES

rosiglitazone, pioglitazone

These drugs improve target cell response to insulin by binding to nuclear receptors that regulate the transcription of a number of insulin-responsive genes. They

are dependent upon insulin for activity.
Rx: Type II diabetes. *Tox:* Hepatotoxicity,
hypoglycemia.

DRUGS AFFECTING CALCIUM HOMEOSTASIS AND BONE METABOLISM (CHAPTER 34)

DRUGS USED TO TREAT HYPOCALCEMIA

calcium gluconate, calcium chloride
Calcium supplements. *Rx:* Treatment of hypocalcemia. *Tox:* Hypercalcemia.

ergocalciferol
Vitamin D agent that increases calcium absorption from the intestine. *Rx:* Treatment of hypocalcemia. *Tox:* Hypercalcemia.

DRUGS USED TO TREAT HYPERCALCEMIA

calcitonin
Decreases osteoclastic bone resorption and calcium reabsorption from the kidney; does not usually affect bone formation. *Rx:* Paget's disease of the bone, hypercalcemia. *Tox:* GI effects, flushing, redness or tingling of the face.

BISPHOSPHATES

etidronate, pamidronate, alendronate
Short-chain compounds that act on osteoclasts to reduce both the formation and dissolution of hydroxyapatite crystals. *Rx:* Postmenopausal osteoporosis, treatment of Paget's disease of the bone, malignancy-induced hypercalcemia. *Tox:* Esophageal erosion, osteomalacia, nausea, diarrhea.

MISCELLANEOUS AGENTS

plicamycin
Inhibits the effect of parathyroid hormone (PTH) on osteoclasts or blocks the effects of vitamin D. *Rx:* Paget's disease of the bone, hypercalcemia. *Tox:* Nausea, vomiting, loss of appetite, hypocalcemia.

ANTI-INFLAMMATORY DRUGS AND ACETAMINOPHEN (CHAPTER 35)

NONSTEROIDAL ANTI-INFLAMMATORY DRUGS (NSAIDS)

acetylsalicylic acid (aspirin)

Irreversibly inhibits cyclooxygenase, blocking production of prostaglandin and thromboxane. ***Rx:*** Used in the treatment of a wide variety of diseases involving inflammation, fever, or pain (arthritis, headache, dysmenorrhea); MI prophylaxis (antiplatelet effects). ***Tox:*** Renal failure, salicylism (tinnitus, decreased hearing, vertigo), GI bleeding, respiratory alkalosis, and metabolic acidosis.

ibuprofen, indomethacin, naproxen (many more examples)

These agents *reversibly* inhibit cyclooxygenase. ***Rx:*** Used to reduce fever and inflammation; as analgesics for arthritis, gout, and muscle aches and pains; and as anticoagulants secondary to antiplatelet activity. ***Tox:*** GI bleeding, interstitial nephritis, papillary necrosis.

PARA-AMINOPHENOL DERIVATIVES

acetaminophen

Acts by inhibiting prostaglandin synthesis in the CNS. It has little effect on cyclooxygenase in peripheral tissues, which accounts for its weak anti-inflammatory effects. ***Rx:*** Used for fever, mild to moderate pain. Patients with peptic ulcer disease or hemophilia tolerate acetaminophen better then aspirin. ***Tox:*** Hepatotoxicity. ***Other:*** Treat overdoses with *N*-acetylcysteine.

DRUGS USED TO TREAT GOUT (CHAPTER 36)

colchicine

Inhibits microtubulin function; this, in turn, prevents migration of neutrophils to areas of inflammation. ***Rx:*** Both for treatment of acute attacks and for prophylaxis. **Tox:** GI distress (vomiting diarrhea, abdominal pain), alopecia. With chronic use: leukopenia, agranulocytosis aplastic anemia are possible.

indomethacin

Reversibly inhibits cyclooxygenase; consequently, the production of prostaglandins and thromboxane, which are responsible for inflammation, are reduced. **Rx:** Drug of choice for acute gout. **Tox:** Headache, vertigo, abdominal distress, renal toxicity, rash.

probenecid, sulfinpyrazone

At therapeutic concentrations, these uricosuric agents increase uric acid excretion by inhibiting uric acid reabsorption in the proximal tubule. **Rx:** Treatment of chronic gout and asymptomatic hyperuricemia. These drugs are not indicated in acute attacks of gout. **Tox:** These agents can precipitate an acute attack of gouty arthritis in the early stages of treatment. Other side effects are GI distress and occasional hypersensitivity reactions.

allopurinol

Inhibits the enzyme xanthine oxidase. **Rx:** Gout, recurrent renal stones, tumor lysis syndrome. **Tox:** Usually well tolerated but can cause hypersensitivity reactions (allergic dermatitis, fever), GI distress (diarrhea, abdominal pain). Peripheral vasculitis and neuritis are rare complications.

AUTACOIDS AND AUTACOID ANTAGONISTS (CHAPTER 37)

SEROTONIN AGONISTS

buspirone, sumatriptan

These agents stimulate serotonin (5-HT) receptors. **Rx: Buspirone**—anxiolytic; **sumatriptan**—treatment of migraine headaches. **Tox: Buspirone**—drowsiness; **sumatriptan**—dizziness and tingling.

SEROTONIN ANTAGONISTS

ondansetron, cyproheptadine

These agents competitively bind and inhibit serotonin (5-HT) receptors. ***Rx:*** **Ondansetron** is used in the treatment of nausea and vomiting associated with surgery. **Cyproheptadine** is used in the treatment of carcinoid tumor and postgastrectomy dumping syndrome as well as allergic conditions. ***Tox:*** **Ondansetron**—hepatotoxicity, constipation. **Cyproheptadine**—anticholinergic effects.

ERGOT ALKALOIDS

bromocriptine, ergonovine, ergotamine

These agents act on 5-HT, dopamine, and α-adrenoreceptors; they diminish cerebral vascular pulsations. ***Rx:*** Treatment of hyperprolactinemia (**bromocriptine**), migraine (**ergotamine**), postpartum hemorrhage (**ergonovine** and **ergotamine**), motion sickness, nausea and vomiting, insomnia. ***Tox:*** GI disturbances; ergotism (St. Anthony's fire), which consists of vasospasm possibly resulting in gangrene; CNS psychosis; abortion if patient is pregnant.

DRUGS USED TO TREAT GI DISORDERS (CHAPTER 38)

ANTACIDS

calcium carbonate

Neutralizes gastric acid. ***Rx:*** Treatment of peptic ulcer and reflux disease. ***Tox:*** Constipation, diarrhea.

PROTON PUMP INHIBITORS

omeprazole, lansoprazole, rabeprazole, pantoprazole, esomeprazole

Parietal cell proton pump inhibitors. ***Rx:*** Treatment of Zollinger-Ellison syndrome, peptic ulcer disease. ***Tox:*** Diarrhea, abdominal pain, headache.

MUCOSAL PROTECTORS

sucralfate

Binds to necrotic peptic ulcer tissue and acts as a barrier to acid and other destructive substances. **Rx:** Peptic ulcer disease. **Tox:** GI discomfort, constipation.

misoprostol

A prostaglandin E_1 analogue thought to stimulate gastric secretion of mucus. **Rx:** Peptic ulcer disease. **Tox:** Diarrhea; can cause unwanted uterine contractions leading to abortion.

HISTAMINE BLOCKERS

cimetidine, ranitidine, famotidine, nizatidine

These agents competitively block histamine at H_2 receptors. **Rx:** Treatment of peptic ulcer disease, Zollinger-Ellison syndrome. **Tox:** Mental status changes, antiandrogen effects; inhibits P_{450} system. **Other: Famotidine** and **nizatidine** have similar effects but do not cause mental status changes in the elderly.

PROKINETIC AGENTS

metoclopramide

Antagonist at D_2 receptors in gastric smooth muscle. **Rx:** Treatment of gastropareses, gastroesophageal reflux. **Tox:** Extrapyramidal side effects, diarrhea, agranulocytosis.

ANTINEOPLASTIC DRUGS (CHAPTER 39)

ANTIBIOTICS

dactinomycin

Binds to the double helix of DNA and forms a **dactinomycin**-DNA complex that inhibits DNA-dependent RNA polymerase. **Rx:** Treatment of Wilms' tumor, rhabdomyosarcoma. **Tox:** Bone marrow depression, nausea, vomiting, dermatological effects, sensitization to radiation.

doxorubicin, daunorubicin

These agents intercalate with the sugar-phosphate backbone of DNA, causing DNA breaks. This results in inhibition of DNA and RNA synthesis. **Rx: Doxorubicin**—ALL and AML, breast and lung cancer. **Daunorubicin**—AML and ALL. **Tox:** Irreversible cardiotoxicity (✎ board question), myelosuppression, nausea, vomiting, alopecia.

bleomycin

Combines with iron and forms a complex that reacts with oxygen to produce free radicals. This causes strand scission and DNA fragmentation. **Rx:** Testicular carcinoma, squamous carcinomas, Hodgkin's disease. **Tox:** Pulmonary fibrosis (✎ board question), fever and chills, mucocutaneous toxicity, hypersensitivity.

mitomycin

Reduces to a bi- or trifunctional alkylating agent that inhibits DNA synthesis. **Rx:** Cervical carcinoma, bladder carcinoma. **Tox:** Nausea, vomiting, loss of appetite, bone marrow suppression, hemolytic-uremic syndrome (rare).

ANTIMETABOLITES

6-mercaptopurine

A purine antimetabolite that inhibits DNA and RNA synthesis. **Rx:** ALL, AML. **Tox:** Bone marrow suppression, hepatotoxicity, GI mucositis.

methotrexate

Folic acid analogue that inhibits dihydrofolate reductase. **Rx:** Treatment of ALL; carcinomas of the breast, lung, ovary, bladder, and neck; choriocarcinoma; psoriasis; and rheumatoid arthritis. **Tox:** Myelosuppression, GI hemorrhagic enteritis, neurotoxicity.

5-fluorouracil	Converted to 5F-dUMP, which inhibits RNA synthesis. ***Rx:*** Breast carcinoma, colon carcinoma. ***Tox:*** Leukopenia, diarrhea, infection, esophagitis, stomatitis.

ALKYLATING AGENTS

mechlorethamine	Forms an ethylene ammonium that cross-links strands of RNA and DNA. ***Rx:*** Used for Hodgkin's disease. ***Tox:*** Myelosuppression, nausea, vomiting, amenorrhea, phlebitis at site of injection.
cyclophosphamide	The metabolite of this drug, called phosphoramide mustard, cross-links DNA and RNA strands. ***Rx:*** Ovarian and breast carcinoma, Hodgkin's and non-Hodgkin's lymphoma, all of the leukemias. ***Tox:*** Nausea, hemorrhagic cystitis, skin pigmentation, hair loss, gonadal and bone marrow suppression.
lomustine	Inhibits DNA, RNA, and protein synthesis by causing DNA strand disruption. ***Rx:*** Melanoma, GI cancers, brain tumors. ***Tox:*** Nausea, vomiting, bone marrow suppression.
streptozocin	Alkylating agent that inhibits DNA synthesis by cross-linking strands of DNA. ***Rx:*** Pancreatic carcinomas. ***Tox:*** Renal failure, nausea, vomiting.
cisplatin	Cross-links DNA and causes strand disruption. ***Rx:*** Testicular and bladder carcinomas. ***Tox:*** Nephrotoxicity, ototoxicity, bone marrow suppression.
carboplatin	Same mechanism of action as cisplatin. ***Rx:*** Ovarian carcinomas. ***Tox:*** Bone marrow suppression, anemia.
busulfan	Cross-links strands of DNA. ***Rx:*** Drug of choice for chronic myelocytic leukemia (CML). ***Tox:*** Bone marrow suppression.

carmustine

Inhibits DNA, RNA, and protein synthesis. ***Rx:*** Brain tumors, Hodgkin's and non-Hodgkin's lymphomas, GI cancers, multiple myeloma. ***Tox:*** Bone marrow suppression, pulmonary fibrosis.

dacarbazine

Inhibits DNA and RNA synthesis via formation of carbonium ions. ***Rx:*** Hodgkin's lymphoma. ***Tox:*** Nausea, vomiting, bone marrow suppression, hepatotoxicity.

MITOTIC INHIBITORS

vinblastine

Binds to tubulin and inhibits the polymerization of microtubules. ***Rx:*** Testicular tumors, lymphomas. ***Tox:*** Myelosuppression.

vincristine

Binds to tubulin and inhibits the polymerization of microtubules. ***Rx:*** Lymphomas, Wilms' tumor, leukemias. ***Tox:*** Peripheral neuropathy, alopecia.

HORMONES

glucocorticoids

These agents bind to nuclear receptors that code for glucocorticoid-responsive genes. ***Rx:*** Hodgkin's lymphoma, acute leukemia. ***Tox:*** Hyperglycemia, increased number of infections, osteoporosis, cataracts, hypertension.

tamoxifen

A competitive antagonist at estrogen receptors. ***Rx:*** Estrogen receptor–positive breast cancer. ***Tox:*** Hot flashes, nausea, vomiting.

leuprolide

Gonadotropin-releasing hormone (GnRH) analogue that inhibits the release of follicle-stimulating hormone (FSH) and luteinizing hormone (LH). ***Rx:*** Endometriosis, prostatic carcinoma. ***Tox:*** Hot flashes, impotence.

PENICILLINS (CHAPTER 42)

NATURAL PENICILLINS

penicillin G, penicillin V	These agents inhibit cell wall synthesis by blocking peptidoglycan translocation. **Rx:** Treatment of Gram-positive cocci, Gram-positive bacilli, spirochetes, *Neisseria*, and most anaerobic infections (except *Bacteroides fragilis*). **Tox:** Hypersensitivity reactions (anaphylaxis, urticaria, nephritis), Coombs'-positive hemolytic anemia. GI distress, cation toxicity

AMINOPENICILLINS

ampicillin	Like natural penicillins, it inhibits cell wall synthesis by interfering with the cross-linking of peptidoglycans. **Rx:** Drug of choice for enterococcus and *Listeria;* also used to treat infections by Gram-positive and some Gram-negative organisms such as *E. coli, Salmonella, Shigella.* **Tox:** Drug-induced hemolytic anemia, allergic reactions (rashes, anaphylaxis, fever, urticaria, joint swelling).
amoxicillin	An oral equivalent of ampicillin.

ANTIPSEUDOMONAL PENICILLINS

ticarcillin, piperacillin	Mechanism of action similar to natural penicillin. **Rx:** Treatment of Gram-negative bacilli infections, especially *Pseudomonas, Proteus*, and *Serratia.* **Tox:** Same as for natural penicillins.

ANTISTAPHYLOCOCCAL PENICILLINS

nafcillin, oxacillin, dicloxacillin, cloxacillin	Mechanism of action similar to that of natural penicillins; however, these drugs are resistant to penicillinase. **Rx:** Treatment of methicillin-sensitive

staphylococci. **_Tox:_** Methicillin in particular induces interstitial nephritis. Most of these drugs can induce a granulocytopenia and Coombs'-positive hemolytic anemia.

CEPHALOSPORINS AND OTHER CELL WALL SYNTHESIS INHIBITORS (CHAPTER 43)

FIRST-GENERATION CEPHALOSPORINS

cefadroxil, cephradine, cephalexin, cefazolin

These agents inhibit cell wall synthesis by blocking cross-linking of peptidoglycans. **_Rx:_** Excellent Gram-positive coverage. **_Tox:_** Hypersensitivity reactions, potential nephrotoxicity.

SECOND-GENERATION CEPHALOSPORINS

cefotetan, cefprozil, cefaclor, cefuroxime, loracarbef, cefoxitin

Mechanism of action similar to that of first-generation cephalosporins. **_Rx:_** Increased Gram-negative coverage and decreased Gram-positive coverage as compared with first-generation cephalosporins; also some anaerobic coverage. **_Tox:_** Hypersensitivity reactions, alcohol intolerance; bleeding with cefamandole and cefotetan.

THIRD-GENERATION CEPHALOSPORINS

cefoperazone, ceftazidime, ceftriaxone, ceftizoxime cefotaxime

Mechanism of action similar to that of first-generation cephalosporins. **_Rx:_** Greatest Gram-negative coverage of the cephalosporin group; least Gram-positive coverage. **_Tox:_** Ceftriaxone causes biliary stasis, Coombs'-positive hemolytic anemia, hypersensitivity reactions.

OTHER CELL WALL INHIBITORS

vancomycin

Binds to cell wall precursors and prevents polymerization of peptidoglycans. **_Rx:_**

Used against methicillin-resistant *Staphylococcus aureus* (MRSA), for serious Gram-positive infections, in penicillin-allergic patients, and for pseudomembranous colitis caused by *Clostridium difficile*. **Tox:** Ototoxicity, nephrotoxicity; flushing of face when infused rapidly (known as "red man syndrome").

imipenem/cilastatin

Imipenem inhibits cell wall synthesis, while **cilastatin** inhibits metabolism of the drug in the proximal convoluted tubule by renal dehydropeptidase. **Rx:** Effective against aerobic and anaerobic Gram-positive and Gram-negative organisms. **Tox:** Seizures in patients with renal dysfunction; cross-allergy with penicillin. **Other: Imipenem** is an extremely broad-spectrum antibiotic but does *not* cover MRSA.

aztreonam

Inhibits peptidoglycan synthesis. **Rx:** Used against Gram-negative aerobic rods; *not* effective against Gram-positive or anaerobic bacteria. **Tox:** GI distress. elevated liver enzymes. skin rashes. **Other:** Minimal cross-reactivity with penicillins.

PROTEIN SYNTHESIS INHIBITORS (CHAPTER 44)

chloramphenicol

Binds reversibly to the 50S ribosomal subunit and inhibits protein synthesis at the peptidyl transferase step. **Rx:** Treatment of typhoid fever caused by *Salmonella;* topical treatment of eye infections; effective against both Gram-positive and Gram-negative organisms. **Tox:** Aplastic anemia. Bone marrow depression causes dose-related nausea and vomiting. The drug is toxic for newborn infants; ingestion by the mother during late pregnancy may result in gray-baby syndrome with vomiting, flaccidity, hypothermia, and possibly death.

MACROLIDES

erythromycin, clarithromycin, azithromycin

These agents bind to the 50S ribosome and prevent the translocation step of protein synthesis. *Rx:* Chlamydial infections and diphtheria due to *Corynebacterium diphtheriae.* Drugs of choice for community-acquired *Mycoplasma* and *Legionella* pneumonias. Also used against streptococcal and pneumococcal infection in penicillin-allergic patients. *Tox:* Epigastric distress, cholestatic jaundice, hypersensitivity reactions (fever, rashes, eosinophilia). *Other:* **Azithromycin** and **clarithromycin** are second-generation macrolides with increased activity against *Haemophilus influenzae* and *Mycobacterium avium* complex.

LINCOSAMIDES

clindamycin

A bacteriostatic agent that binds to the 50S ribosomal subunit and inhibits protein synthesis by interfering with translocation (similar to **erythromycin**). *Rx:* Anaerobic infections that cause diseases such as empyema, lung abscess, and aspiration pneumonia; Gram-positive cocci. *Tox:* **Pseudomembranous colitis,** granulocytopenia, erythema multiforme, skin rashes, inhibition of neuromuscular transmission.

AMINOGLYCOSIDES

gentamicin, streptomycin, tobramycin, amikacin, netilmicin, spectinomycin

Bind to the 30S ribosome and inhibit protein synthesis by blocking the formation of an initiation complex or causing the misreading mRNA. **Rx:** Life-threatening Gram-negative microbial infections; especially effective against *Pseudomonas aeruginosa, Enterobacter* species, *Klebsiella* species. **Tox:** Ototoxicity, nephrotoxicity. **Other:** Spectinomycin is effective only for gonorrhea. Amikacin is uniquely resistant to inactivating enzymes.

neomycin, kanamycin

These agents work the same way as the other aminoglycosides. **Rx:** Given orally for treatment of bacteria in the intestinal lumen. Treatment of hepatic encephalopathy. **Tox:** Ototoxicity, nephrotoxicity; intestinal malabsorption, neuromuscular blockade, respiratory paralysis.

TETRACYCLINES

doxycycline, minocycline, demeclocycline

These agents bind reversibly to the 30S subunit of the bacterial ribosome, blocking the binding site of amino acyl tRNA to its acceptor site on the mRNA. **Rx:** Tetracyclines are broad-spectrum antibiotics. They are bacteriostatic for Gram-positive and Gram-negative organisms, including *Borrelia* (cause of Lyme disease), chlamydiae, mycoplasmas, *Treponema* species, *Vibrio cholera, Francisella tularensis* (cause of tularemia), and *Rickettsia* species. Also used for acne. **Tox:** GI distress; tooth discoloration in children younger than 7 years; liver toxicity; photosensitivity; vestibular reactions (dizziness, nausea, and vomiting can occur with **minocycline**). **Other:** Contraindicated in pregnant women and nursing mothers. Ca^{2+}-containing substances impair absorption.

QUINOLONES AND DRUGS USED TO TREAT URINARY TRACT INFECTIONS (CHAPTER 45)

ofloxacin, ciprofloxacin, norfloxacin, moxifloxacin, gatifloxacin

Bactericidal agents that inhibit bacterial DNA topoisomerase II (DNA gyrase). **Rx:** Active against many Gram-negative organisms but not anaerobes; used to treat UTIs, respiratory infections caused by *Haemophilus influenzae*, *Legionella*, and *Pseudomonas*, GI infections, prostatitis, and gonorrhea. **Tox:** May cause cartilage damage in children; can cause nausea, headache, dizziness, crystalluria, and photosensitivity. **Other:** Can increase levels of theophylline.

nitrofurantoin

Nitrofurantoin alters various bacterial enzymes and DNA **Rx:** Treatment of UTIs, especially those caused by *E. coli* and enterococci. **Tox:** Nausea, vomiting, acute pneumonitis, neuropathies, hemolytic anemia in patients with glucose-6-phosphate dehydrogenase (G6PD) deficiency.

FOLATE ANTAGONISTS (CHAPTER 46)

sulfamethoxazole, sulfisoxazole, silver sulfadiazine, sulfasalazine, sulfacetamide

The sulfonamides, because they resemble PABA, bind and competitively inhibit dihydropteroate synthetase, the enzyme responsible for combining PABA and pteridine. **Rx:** Simple UTIs due to *E. coli* and *Klebsiella* species; ulcerative colitis (**sulfasalazine** is best because it is poorly absorbed); burn infections (**mafenide, silver sulfadiazine**); ocular infections, especially *Chlamydia trachomatis* (sulfacetamide); nocardiosis; *Pneumocystis carinii* pneumonia. **Tox:** Rashes, angioedema, Stevens-Johnson syndrome, GI distress (nausea and vomiting), hemolytic anemia in patient with G6PD deficiency, crystalluria/hematuria, kernicterus in infants, phototoxicity. ***Other:*** Contraindicated in pregnant women and newborns because of the risk of kernicterus.

trimethoprim Stops the conversion of dihydrofolate to tetrahydrofolate by inhibiting the enzyme dihydrofolate reductase. **Trimethoprim** is very often combined with **sulfamethoxazole**; this compound is know as cotrimoxazole. ***Rx:*** Effective in treating complicated or recurrent UTIs. Treatment of bacterial prostatitis, gonorrhea, acute chronic bronchitis, acute otitis media, toxoplasmosis. Drug of choice for *Pneumocystis carinii* pneumonia. Sometimes given in a nebulized or vaporized form. ***Tox:*** Dermatological effects, GI effects (nausea, vomiting), hematological effects (leukopenia, megaloblastic anemia), renal impairment in patients with renal disease, headache, depression. AIDS patients are especially likely to develop rashes.

ANTIFUNGAL DRUGS (CHAPTER 47)

amphotericin B Amphotericin B binds to ergosterol and forms pores or channels within the cell membrane. This allows electrolytes to leak from the cell, resulting in cell death. ***Rx:*** Treatment of aspergillosis and infection by *Candida, Blastomyces dermatitidis, Histoplasma, Cryptococcus,* and *Coccidioides.* ***Tox:*** Renal impairment (80% of patients exhibit decreased GFR and changes in renal tubular function), hypotension, fever, chills, anemia. Because of its high toxicity, **amphotericin** is nicknamed "amphoterrible."

ketoconazole, fluconazole, miconazole, itraconazole

These agents block conversion of lanosterol into ergosterol by blocking a P_{450} enzyme. ***Rx: Ketoconazole***—Most commonly used to treat histoplasmosis; effective against most of the same fungi as **amphotericin B**; can also be used against **griseofulvin**-resistant dermatophytes. ***Fluconazole***—Very effective for oral candidiasis, cryptococcosis, and coccidioidomycosis. ***Itraconazole***—Drug of choice for blastomycosis; has similar spectrum of action as **ketoconazole**. ***Tox: Ketoconazole***—GI irritation, endocrine abnormalities due to inhibition of steroid synthesis (gynecomastia, impotence, decreased libido, menstrual irregularities), hepatic dysfunction. ***Fluconazole***—Has no endocrinological effects but can cause GI irritation and rashes. ***Itraconazole***—Can cause GI irritation, hypokalemia, headache. ***Other:*** **Miconazole** and **clotrimazole** are very similar to **ketoconazole** in their mechanism of action and clinical uses. However, these agents are usually given only topically and therefore do not have systemic side effects. **Fluconazole** penetrates the CNS; the others do not.

flucytosine

Enters fungal cells through a cytosine-specific permease and is first converted to 5-fluorouracil (5-FU). Subsequently it is converted to 5-fluorodeoxyuridylic acid (5F-dUMP). This acid inhibits thymidylate synthetase, an essential enzyme in the production of DNA. ***Rx:*** Given in combination with **amphotericin B** for treatment of systemic *Candida* and *Cryptococcus* infections. ***Tox:*** Hematological effects (reversible neutropenia, thrombocytopenia, bone marrow depression), hepatic dysfunction, GI disturbances (nausea, vomiting).

griseofulvin

Enters susceptible fungal cells and inhibits microtubule function; may also inhibit synthesis and polymerization of nucleic acids. Accumulates in the newly synthesized keratin-containing tissues and is fungistatic. ***Rx:*** Effective only against dermatophytes, including *Trichophyton, Microsporum,* and *Epidermophyton.* ***Tox:*** GI irritation, headache, hepatotoxicity. ***Other:*** Contraindicated in acute intermittent porphyria; induces P-450 system activity; may be teratogenic.

nystatin

Binds to ergosterol in fungal cell membranes and creates pores. ***Rx:*** Used topically for local *Candida* infections. ***Tox:*** Very mild side effects (local irritation).

ANTIPROTOZOAL DRUGS (CHAPTER 48)

primaquine

A tissue schizonticide and gametocide that forms cellular oxidants that are toxic to the protozoa. ***Rx:*** Eradicates the liver stages of *P. vivax* and *P. ovale* (primary as well as secondary exoerythrocytic forms); *not* effective against the erythrocytic stage of malaria. Gametocidal for all four *Plasmodium* species and can therefore be used to interrupt transmission of the disease. ***Tox:*** Methemoglobinemia, GI distress, headaches, pruritus, hemolytic anemia in G6PD-deficient patients. Granulocytopenia and agranulocytosis can occur in patients who have lupus or arthritis.

chloroquine

Multiple mechanisms of action: (1) increases the pH of plasmodial food vacuoles, which results in an inability of the parasite to digest hemoglobin; (2) inhibits the plasmodial enzyme heme polymerase, which is responsible for eliminating toxic hemoglobin breakdown by-products; (3) disrupts plasmodial

DNA. **Rx:** Acts against erythrocyte forms of *Plasmodium falciparum, P. vivax,* and *P. ovale.* Since it is a blood schizonticide, it will not eradicate hypnozoites and is therefore not useful for the treatment of relapsing malaria caused by *P. ovale* or *P. vivax.* Also has anti-inflammatory effects and is sometimes used in autoimmune disorders. **Tox:** Peripheral neuropathies, myocardial depression with ECG changes, retinal damage (requires routine ophthalmological exams), auditory impairment, toxic psychosis.

quinine

A blood schizonticide that complexes with dsDNA and prevents strand separation. **Rx:** Useful against malarial strains resistant to other agents such as **chloroquine**. **Tox:** GI distress. Cinchonism (tinnitus, headache, dizziness). Hemolytic anemia. **Other:** Elevates digoxin levels.

mefloquine

Structural analogue of quinine. **Rx:** Treatment of malaria secondary to *Plasmodium*. **Tox:** GI distress, headache, dizziness, hallucinations.

pyrimethamine

Selectively inhibits plasmodial dihydrofolate reductase, thereby depriving the organism of tetrahydrofolate, a cofactor in the biosynthesis of purines and pyrimidines. **Rx:** Effective alone against *P. falciparum;* used in the treatment of toxoplasmosis when combined with **sulfadiazine**. **Tox:** Folic acid deficiency in high doses, rash, GI distress, hemolysis, renal damage.

sodium stibogluconate

Unclear mechanism of action. **Rx:** Treatment of leishmaniasis. **Tox:** GI distress, cardiac arrhythmias.

suramin

Inhibits enzymes involved in energy metabolixm. **Rx:** Treatment of African sleeping sickness before CNS involvement (use melarsoprol if CNS is involved). *Tox:* GI effects (nausea, vomiting).

metronidazole

Forms a cytotoxic metabolite that interacts with protozoal DNA and RNA. *Rx:* Treatment of pseudomembranous colitis, *Giardia* and *Trichomonas vaginalis* infection, and amebiasis. Also used in triple therapy with bismuth and **amoxicillin** against *H. pylori*. *Tox:* GI distress, CNS effects, paraesthesias, discoloration of urine. *Other:* Will cause a **disulfiram**-like reaction when used with **ethanol**.

pentamidine

Binds DNA and may inhibit replication, but exact mechanism is unknown. *Rx:* Treatment of *Pneumocystis carinii* pneumonia. *Tox:* Nephrotoxicity, pancreatitis, hypotension.

ANTIHELMINTIC DRUGS (CHAPTER 49)

mebendazole, thiabendazole

These agents interfere with the synthesis of microtubules and decreases glucose uptake. *Rx:* Drugs of choice for pinworm (*Enterobius vermicularis*), whipworm (*Trichuris trichiura*). Also used against *Necator americanus* and *Ascaris lumbricoides. Tox:* Nausea and vomiting.

pyrantel pamoate

Acts as a depolarizing neuromuscular blocking agent, causing persistent activation of nicotinic acetylcholine receptors and thus paralysis of the worm. *Rx:* Drug of choice in *Ascaris* infections; can also be used for pinworm and hookworm. *Tox:* Nausea, vomiting, headaches, rash.

diethylcarbamazine

Precise mechanism of action is unknown. *Rx:* Treatment of filariasis. *Tox:* Usually mild but may include headache, nausea and vomiting, lymphadenopathy, hypotension, and tachycardia.

ivermectin

Increases GABA transmission, which results in paralysis of parasites. **Rx:** Treatment of river blindness caused by *Onchocerca volvulus.* **Tox:** Intense itching, skin rashes.

praziquantel

Causes tetanic muscle contraction by increasing the permeability of cell membranes to Ca^{2+}. **Rx:** Schistosomiasis, trematode infections and cysticercosis. **Tox:** GI distress, dizziness, drowsiness. **Other:** Contraindicated in pregnant women and nursing mothers.

ANTIVIRAL DRUGS (CHAPTER 50)

acyclovir

Monophosphorylated by a herpes enzyme called thymidine kinase. Later it is di- and triphosphorylated by the host cell. The active triphosphate form is then incorporated into viral DNA, causing premature DNA-chain termination. **Rx:** Treatment of herpes simplex, varicella zoster virus, and Epstein-Barr virus. **Tox:** Renal dysfunction, neurotoxicity (delirium, tremor, seizures), diarrhea, headache, local irritation.

trifluridine

A thymidine analog. **Rx:** Used topically for eye infections, HSV types 1 and 2. **Tox:** Minimal due to topical application.

amantadine, rimantadine

These agents inhibit viral uncoating. **Rx:** Prophylaxis of influenza A in elderly and immunosuppressed. **Tox:** Insomnia, dizziness, ataxia; these symptoms are less common with **rimantadine** because it does not cross the blood-brain barrier.

foscarnet

Inhibits viral replication by blocking viral DNA polymerase, which prevents chain elongation. **Rx:** Treatment of CMV retinitis in immunocompromised patients. **Tox:** Nephrotoxicity; electrolyte abnormalities such as hypocalcemia and hypomagnesemia; seizures; and fever.

ganciclovir

This drug is triphosphorylated into its active form and then inhibits viral DNA polymerase. Incorporation into DNA also terminates chain elongation. **Rx:** Drug of choice for cytomegalovirus. **Tox:** Bone marrow suppression, seizures, renal dysfunction.

zidovudine (AZT)

After being triphosphorylated into its active form, this drug inhibits viral reverse transcriptase and causes chain termination. **Rx:** HIV. **Tox:** Bone marrow suppression, (thrombocytopenia, granulocytopenia), headaches, occasionally seizures. **Other:** Side effects are potentiated if **zidovudine** is given with drugs, such as **acetaminophen, probenecid,** or **indomethacin,** that decrease glucuronidation.

didanosine (ddI), zalacitabine (ddC)

Inhibits viral reverse transcriptase and, after incorporation into DNA, acts as a chain terminator. **Rx:** Treatment of HIV. **Tox:** Peripheral neuropathy, pancreatitis.

ribavirin

Mechanism of action not fully elucidated, but is thought to be related to decreasing the intracellular stores of guanosine triphosphate and inhibiting 5-cap formation of viral mRNA. **Rx:** Treatment of infants and young children who are suffering from bronchiolitis and pneumonia due to respiratory syncytial virus (RSV). Also used occasionally for treating influenza A and Lassa fever B. **Tox:** Dose-dependent hemolytic anemia, elevated bilirubin.

DRUGS USED TO TREAT TUBERCULOSIS AND LEPROSY (CHAPTER 51)

isoniazid

Inhibits the synthesis of mycolic acids, which are unique to the mycobacterial cell walls. **Rx:** Treatment of active tuberculosis; tuberculosis prophylaxis in those who are close contacts of TB patients or who have a positive PPD. **Tox:** Potentially fatal hepatitis, peripheral neuropathy, rashes, skin eruptions. **Other:** Half-life depends on whether patient is a slow or fast acetylator.

rifampin

Inhibits the β-subunit of DNA-dependent RNA polymerase; suppresses RNA synthesis by blocking chain initiation. **Rx:** Treatment of tuberculosis; used in combination with **dapsone** to treat leprosy; used in combination with **erythromycin** to treat Legionnaire's disease. Also used prophylactically for close contacts of patients diagnosed with *Haemophilus influenzae* meningitis. **Tox:** Causes urine, sweat, tears, and other secretions to become red-orange in color; rash, fever, nausea and vomiting, hepatic dysfunction. **Other: Rifampin** significantly induces the P-450 system.

ethambutol

Mechanism of action not known for certain, but it is thought to inhibit incorporation of mycolic acid into the mycobacterial cell wall. **Rx:** Treatment of tuberculosis in combination with **isoniazid** (INH), **pyrazinamide**, and **rifampin**. **Tox:** Optic neuritis, decreased visual acuity, and loss of red-green discrimination; may precipitate a gout attack.

pyrazinamide

Not known. **Rx:** Treatment of tuberculosis in combination with **isonicotinic acid hydrazide (INH), pyrazinamide,** and **rifampin**. **Tox:** Hepatotoxicity; gout due to the inhibition of uric acid secretion arthralgia, and myalgia.

streptomycin

See aminoglycosides in this power review.

dapsone   Inhibits folate synthesis by acting as a competitive antagonist of paraaminobenzoic acid. ***Rx:*** Leprosy; *Pneumocystis carinii* pneumonia in HIV patients. ***Tox:*** Hemolysis in patients with G6PD deficiency, lupus erythematosus, methemoglobinemia.

Appendices

Appendices

Appendix A   Sample Problems

PROBLEM #1

The graph in **Figure A** plots the results of an experiment in which a 30-mg
IV bolus of drug Y was given at time 0 and measurements of plasma
concentration of the drug were taken over the next 5 days. The labeled data
points indicate the actual **plasma concentration in micrograms per
milliliter** for each of the 5 days.

Using the information contained in the graph, answer the questions below
concerning the pharmacokinetic parameters of drug Y. Assume that drug Y is
distributed instantly throughout its volume of distribution. *Remember:* 1
$\mu g/mL$ = 1 mg/L; 1 day = 1440 min.

1. Determine the half-life ($t_{1/2}$).
2. Determine the volume of distribution (V_D)
3. Determine the clearance (Cl).
4. An infusion pump is set to deliver a constant 2.88 mg/min of drug Y into
   an identical experimental subject. Assuming that no initial bolus was
   given, predict the average plasma concentration (C_{av}) at steady state for
   drug Y. How long would it take for the plasma concentration to reach this
   state?

PROBLEM #2

A 55-year-old man weighing 100 kg presents to the ER after experiencing
severe chest pain. Drug X is an anticoagulant that has recently been
approved for use in the management of acute myocardial infarction. The
following pharmacokinetic data are available for drug X:

Oral availability = 50%
Clearance = 10 mL/min*kg
Volume of distribution (V_d) = 1.0 L/kg
Therapeutic concentration (conc) = 5 $\mu g/mL$

1. As an attending in the ER, your goal is to administer an intravenous bolus
   (loading dose) of drug X so that the therapeutic concentration is reached
   rapidly. What is the loading dose of drug X?
2. After some time, the patient's condition is stabilized, but further
   management using drug X is necessary. Calculate the infusion rate

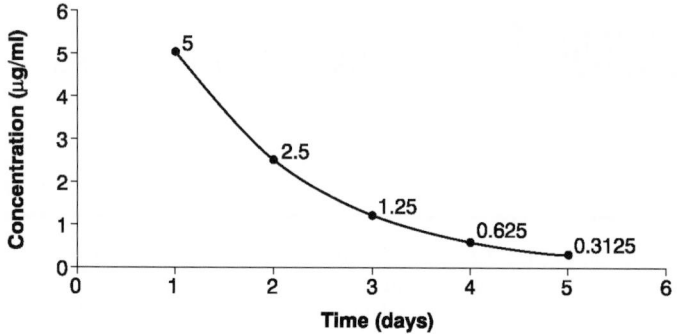

Figure A. Plasma concentration vs. time for Drug Y (see Problem #1).

(maintenance dose) to keep the average plasma concentration of drug X at 5 µg/mL.
3. If drug X's toxic dose is 20 µg/mL, what is its therapeutic index?

ANSWERS AND EXPLANATIONS

PROBLEM #1

1. $t_{1/2} = 1$ **day.** From inspection of the graph, you can see that it takes exactly 1 day for the concentration of drug Y to be reduced by half.
2. $V_D = 3$ **L.** To determine the volume of distribution, you must extrapolate the data to "time 0" to find C_0, the initial plasma concentration of drug Y. The plasma concentration on day 1 was 5 µg/mL. Since the half-life is 1 day, the initial concentration of drug Y (C_0) = 10 µg/mL. Since the route of administration was intravenous, 100% of the drug will reach the systemic circulation ($F_0 = 1$). Use the initial concentration to determine the volume of distribution:

$$V_D = \text{drug dose (D)} \div \text{plasma concentration } (C_0) =$$
$$30 \text{ mg} \div 10 \text{ µg/mL} = 3 \text{ L}$$

3. **Cl = 1.44 mL/min.** Use the information in answers 1 and 2 to find the clearance:

$$Cl = (0.693 \times V_D) \div t_{1/2} = (0.693 \times 3000 \text{ mL}) \div$$
$$1440 \text{ min} = 1.44 \text{ mL/min}$$

4. **Cav = 2 mg/mL. It would take at least 4 days to reach this value.** Again, since this is an intravenous delivery, 100% of the drug will reach the systemic circulation ($F_0 = 1$). If the infusion rate (dose over time, or D/T) is set to 2.88 mg/min and the clearance was determined to be 1.44 mL/min, the average plasma concentration at steady state would be

maintained at **2 mg/mL.** This can be explained using the following equation:

$$C_{av} = D/T \div Cl = 2.88 \text{ mg/min} \div 1.44 \text{ mg/min} = \textbf{2 mg}$$

It takes approximately **4 half-lives** to reach the steady-state plasma concentration on a continuous maintenance infusion. Since the $t_{1/2}$ was determined to be 1 day, it would take **4 days** to reach the average plasma concentration of 2 mg.

PROBLEM #2

1. **Loading dose = 500 mg.** The bolus depends on the V_d:

   Loading dose = conc $\times$ Vd = 5 μg/mL $\times$ 1000 mL/kg = 500 mg

2. **The infusion rate (maintenance dose) is 5 mg/min.** The maintenance dose (D/T) depends on the clearance (Cl):

   D/T = conc $\times$ Cl = 5 μg/mL $\times$ 10 mL/min*kg $\times$ 100 kg = 5 mg/min

3. **The therapeutic index is 4.** The therapeutic index equals the ratio of toxic dose to therapeutic dose:

   Therapeutic index = 20 μg/mL $\div$ 5 μg/mL = **4**

*Remember to match units while performing all the above calculations.

Appendix B

Recommended Antimicrobial Agents Against Selected Bacteria

Bacterial Species	Recommended Antimicrobial Agent*
Alcaligenes xylosoxidans (*Achromobacter xylosoxidans*)	IMP, AP Pen, ceftaz, MER
Acinetobacter calcoaceticus—baumannii complex	IMP or MER or [FQ + (amikacin or ceftaz)]
Actinomyces israeli	AMP or Pen G
Aeromonas hydrophila	FQ
Arcanobacterium (C.) haemolyticum	Erythromycin
Bacillus anthracis (anthrax)	CIP or doxycycline
Bacillus cereus, B. subtilis	Vancomycin, clindamycin
Bacteroides fragilis (ssp. *fragilis*), "DOT" group of *bacteroides*	Metronidazole
Bartonella (Rochalimaea) henselae, quintana	Azithromycin
Bordetella pertussis	Erythromycin
Borrelia burgdorferi, B. afzelli, B. garinii	Ceftriaxone, cefuroxime axetil, doxycycline, amoxicillin

Bacterial Species	Recommended Antimicrobial Agent*
Borrelia recurrentis	Doxycycline
Brucella **sp.**	Doxycycline + either gentamicin or streptomycin
Burkholderia (*Pseudomonas*) *cepacia*	TMP/SMX or IMP or CIP
Burkholderia (*Pseudomonas*) *pseudomallei*	Ceftaz (continuous IV) (*AAC 39: 2356, 1995*) or AM/CL
Campylobacter jejuni	Erythromycin
Campylobacter fetus	IMP
Capnocytophaga ochracea (**DF-1**)	Clindamycin
Campylobacter canimorsus (**DF-2**)	AM/CL
Chlamydia pneumoniae	Doxycycline
Chlamydia trachomatis	Doxycycline or azithromycin
Chryseobacterium (*Flavobacterium*) *meningosepticum*	Vancomycin
Citrobacter diversus (*koseri*), *C. freundii*	IMP or MER

(continued)

TMP/SMX: trimethoprim/sulfamethoxazole; *AP Pen:* antipseudomonal penicillin; *P Ceph:* parenteral cephalosporins; *PRSP:* penicillinase-resistant synthetic penicillins; *APAG:* antipseudomonal aminoglycosides; *FQ:* fluoroquinolones [ciprofloxacin, ofloxacin, lomefloxacin, enoxacin, pefloxacin, levofloxacin, trovafloxacin (not norfloxacin or sparfloxacin unless specifically indicated)]; *AMP:* ampicillin; *CIP:* ciprofloxacin; *IMP:* imipenem + cilastatin; *RIF:* rifampin; *AM/CL:* amoxicillin clavulanate; *TC/CL:* ticarcillin clavulanate; *AM/SB:* ampicillin sulbactam; *Ceftaz:* ceftazidime; *PIP/TZ:* piperacillin-tazobactam; *MER:* meropenem; *DOT group:* B. distasonis, B. ovatus, B. thetaiotaomicron; *NUS:* not available in the United States; *BL/BLI:* β-lactam/β-lactamase inhibitor (AM/CL, TC/CL, AM/SB, or PIP/TZ)
(Adapted with permission from Gilbert DN, Moellering RC Jr, Sande MA. *The Sanford Guide to Antimicrobial Therapy 2005*, 35th ed. Hyde Park, VT: Antimicrobial Therapy Inc., 2005.)

Bacterial Species	Recommended Antimicrobial Agent*
Clostridium difficile	Metronidazole (PO)
Clostridium perfringens	Pen G ± clindamycin
Clostridium tetani	Metronidazole or pen G
Corynebacterium jeikeium	Vancomycin
C. diphtheriae	Erythromycin
Coxiella burnetii (**Q fever**)	
Acute disease	Doxycycline
Chronic disease	CIP or doxycycline + RIF
Ehrlichia chaffeensis, *Ehrlichia phagocytophila*	Doxycycline
Eikenella corrodens	Penicillin G or AMP or AM/CL
Enterobacter spp. (*aerogenes, cloacae*)	IMP or MER or (AP Pen + APAG)
Enterococcus faecalis	Penicillin G (AMP). Add gentamicin for endocarditis or meningitis.
Erysipelothrix rhusiopathiae	Penicillin G or AMP
Escherichia coli	Sensitive to BL/BLI, cephalosporins, FQ, TMP/SMX, APAG, nitrofurantoin, IMP. Selection of drug depends on site of infection, i.e., UTI multiple PO agents; meningitis P Ceph 3 or MER.
Francisella tularensis (**tularemia**)	Streptomycin or gentamicin
Gardnerella vaginalis (**bacterial vaginosis**)	Metronidazole
Hafnia alvei	Same *Enterobacter* spp.

Bacterial Species	*Recommended Antimicrobial Agent**
Helicobacter pylori	Bismuth (B) + metronidazole (M) + tetracycline (T) + omeprazole (O) = 96% cure. BMT × 1 wk *or* BCT × 1 wk = 86%–90% cure.
Haemophilus aphrophilus	Penicillin or AMP ± gentamicin, or AM/SB ± gentamicin
Haemophilus ducreyi (chancroid)	Azithromycin or ceftriaxone
Haemophilus influenzae **Meningitis, epiglottitis and other life-threatening illness**	Cefotaxime, ceftriaxone
Non–life-threatening illness	AM/CL, O Ceph 2/3, TMP/SMX, AM/SB
Klebsiella pneumoniae, oxytoca	P Ceph 3, FQ
Klebsiella ozaenae (rhinoscleromatis)	FQ
***Lactobacillus* sp.**	Pen G or AMP ± gentamicin
***Legionella* sp. (36 species recognized)**	Erythromycin ± RIF; FQ; or azithromycin
Leptospira interrogans	Penicillin G or doxycycline

(continued)

TMP/SMX: trimethoprim/sulfamethoxazole; **AP Pen:** antipseudomonal penicillin; **P Ceph:** parenteral cephalosporins; **PRSP:** penicillinase-resistant synthetic penicillins; **APAG:** antipseudomonal aminoglycosides; **FQ:** fluoroquinolones [ciprofloxacin, ofloxacin, lomefloxacin, enoxacin, pefloxacin, levofloxacin, trovafloxacin (not norfloxacin or sparfloxacin unless specifically indicated)]; **AMP:** ampicillin; **CIP:** ciprofloxacin; **IMP:** imipenem + cilastatin; **RIF:** rifampin; **AM/CL:** amoxicillin clavulanate; **TC/CL:** ticarcillin clavulanate; **AM/SB:** ampicillin sulbactam; **Ceftaz:** ceftazidime; **PIP/TZ:** piperacillin-tazobactam; **MER:** meropenem; **DOT group:** B. *d*istasonis, B. *o*vatus, B. *t*hetaiotaomicron; **NUS:** not available in the United States; **BL/BLI:** β-lactam/β-lactamase inhibitor (AM/CL, TC/CL, AM/SB, or PIP/TZ)
(Adapted with permission from Gilbert DN, Moellering RC Jr, Sande MA. *The Sanford Guide to Antimicrobial Therapy 2005*, 35th ed. Hyde Park, VT: Antimicrobial Therapy Inc., 2005.)

Bacterial Species	Recommended Antimicrobial Agent*
Leuconostoc	Pen G or AMP
Listeria monocytogenes	AMP
Moraxella (Branhamella) catarrhalis	AM/CL or O Ceph 2/3, TMP/SMX
Morganella sp.	IMP or MER or P Ceph 3 or 4 or FQ
Mycoplasma pneumoniae	Erythromycin, azithromycin, clarithromycin, dirithromycin, or FQ
Neisseria gonorrhoeae (**gonococcus**)	Ceftriaxone, cefixime, cefpodoxime
Neisseria meningitidis (**meningococcus**)	Penicillin G
Nocardia asteroides	TMP/SMX, sulfonamides (high dose)
Nocardia brasiliensis	TMP/SMX, sulfonamides (high dose)
Pasteurella multocida	Penicillin G, AMP, amox
Plesiomonas shigelloides	CIP
Proteus mirabilis (**indole** −)	AMP
Proteus vulgaris (**indole** +)	P Ceph 3 or FQ
Providencia sp.	Amikacin or P Ceph 3 or FQ
Pseudomonas aeruginosa	AP Pen, P Ceph 3 AP, IMP, tobramycin
Rhodococcus (C. equi)	Imipenem + cilastatin, APAG, erythro, vanco
Rickettsiae species	Doxycycline
Salmonella typhi	FQ, ceftriaxone
Serratia marcescens	P Ceph 3, IMP, MER, FQ

Bacterial Species	Recommended Antimicrobial Agent*
Shigella sp.	FQ
Staph. aureus, **methicillin-susceptible**	Oxacillin/nafcillin
Staph. aureus, **methicillin-resistant**	Vancomycin
Staph. epidermidis	Vancomycin
Staph. saprophyticus (UTI)	Oral cephalosporin or amoxicillin/clavulanate
Stenotrophomonas (*Xanthomonas, Pseudomonas*) *maltophilia*	TMP/SMX
Streptobacillus moniliformis	Penicillin G or doxycycline
Streptococcus, anaerobic (**peptostreptococcus**)	Penicillin G
Streptococcus pneumoniae	
Penicillin-susceptible	Penicillin G
Penicillin-resistant (MIC ≥ 2.0)	Vancomycin
Streptococcus pyogenes (**Groups A, B, C, G, F**), *Strep. milleri* (*constellatus, intermedius, anginosus*)	Penicillin G or V (some add gentamicin for serious Group B strep infections) *(continued)*

TMP/SMX: trimethoprim/sulfamethoxazole; *AP Pen:* antipseudomonal penicillin; *P Ceph:* parenteral cephalosporins; *PRSP:* penicillinase-resistant synthetic penicillins; *APAG:* antipseudomonal aminoglycosides; *FQ:* fluoroquinolones [ciprofloxacin, ofloxacin, lomefloxacin, enoxacin, pefloxacin, levofloxacin, trovafloxacin (not norfloxacin or sparfloxacin unless specifically indicated)]; *AMP:* ampicillin; *CIP:* ciprofloxacin; *IMP:* imipenem + cilastatin; *RIF:* rifampin; *AM/CL:* amoxicillin clavulanate; *TC/CL:* ticarcillin clavulanate; *AM/SB:* ampicillin sulbactam; *Ceftaz:* ceftazidime; *PIP/TZ:* piperacillin-tazobactam; *MER:* meropenem; *DOT group:* B. distasonis, B. ovatus, B. thetaiotaomicron; *NUS:* not available in the United States; *BL/BLI:* β-lactam/β-lactamase inhibitor (AM/CL, TC/CL, AM/SB, or PIP/TZ)
(Adapted with permission from Gilbert DN, Moellering RC Jr, Sande MA. *The Sanford Guide to Antimicrobial Therapy 2005*, 35th ed. Hyde Park, VT: Antimicrobial Therapy Inc., 2005.)

Bacterial Species	Recommended Antimicrobial Agent*
Vibrio cholerae	Doxycycline, FQ
Vibrio parahaemolyticus	Antibiotic Rx does not ↓ course
Vibrio vulnificus, alginolyticus, damsela	Doxycycline ± ceftaz
Yersinia enterocolitica	TMP/SMX or FQ
Yersinia pestis (plague)	Streptomycin, gentamicin

TMP/SMX: trimethoprim/sulfamethoxazole; *AP Pen:* antipseudomonal penicillin; *P Ceph:* parenteral cephalosporins; *PRSP:* penicillinase-resistant synthetic penicillins; *APAG:* antipseudomonal aminoglycosides; *FQ:* fluoroquinolones [ciprofloxacin, ofloxacin, lomefloxacin, enoxacin, pefloxacin, levofloxacin, trovafloxacin (not norfloxacin or sparfloxacin unless specifically indicated)]; *AMP:* ampicillin; *CIP:* ciprofloxacin; *IMP:* imipenem + cilastatin; *RIF:* rifampin; *AM/CL:* amoxicillin clavulanate; *TC/CL:* ticarcillin clavulanate; *AM/SB:* ampicillin sulbactam; *Ceftaz:* ceftazidime; *PIP/TZ:* piperacillin-tazobactam; *MER:* meropenem; *DOT group:* B. distasonis, B. ovatus, B. thetaiotaomicron; *NUS:* not available in the United States; *BL/BLI:* β-lactam/β-lactamase inhibitor (AM/CL, TC/CL, AM/SB, or PIP/TZ)
(Adapted with permission from Gilbert DN, Moellering RC Jr, Sande MA. *The Sanford Guide to Antimicrobial Therapy 2005*, 35th ed. Hyde Park, VT: Antimicrobial Therapy Inc., 2005.)

INDEX

Page numbers set in italics denote figures; those followed by a t denote tables.